Dr. YOUNGSAM KIM'S 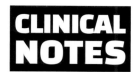 Easy Simple
Safe Efficient

MASTERING

Dr. Youngsam Kim's —————————

Mastering Dental Implants

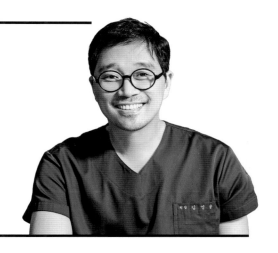

DENTAL IMPLANTS

Youngsam Kim

Young-hoon Pyun
Jisun Kim
Youngmin Park

The Essential Elements for Success in Dental Implants

KOONJA

Dr. Youngsam Kim's
Mastering Dental Implants

1st Print	2022-04-10
1st Publication	2022-05-15

Author	Youngsam Kim
Editor	Su-in Han
Designer	Jin-young Lim
Illustrator	Hak-yeoung Yu

Permissions may be sought at Koonja's rights department:
Tel: (82)-31-943-1888
Fax: (82)-31-955-9545
www.koonja.co.kr

Printed in South Korea
First Edition, © 2022 Koonja publishing, Inc.

ISBN 979-11-5955-859-7

USD 220.00

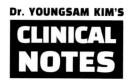

Dr. YOUNGSAM KIM'S
CLINICAL NOTES

Dr. Youngsam Kim's ————

Mastering Dental Implants

Easy Simple Safe Efficient

Authors

Youngsam Kim
DDS, MS, PhD

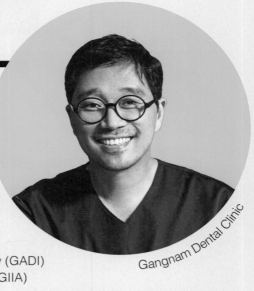

- Chonbuk National Univeristy School of Dentistry
  DDS, MS, PhD
- University of Toronto Faculty of Dentistry
  Periodontics-Implant CE
- UCLA school of Dentistry Periodontics
  Preceptorship
- UCLA School of Dentistry Oral Maxillofacial
  Surgery Preceptorship
- Faculty member of Ostem (Hiossen) Implant Korea
- Head director of Dentis Implant continuing education
- Director of Gangnam Academy of Dental Implantology (GADI)
- Director of Gangnam International Implant Academy (GIIA)

Gangnam Dental Clinic

 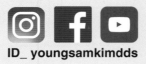

ID_ youngsamkimdds

Young-hoon Pyun

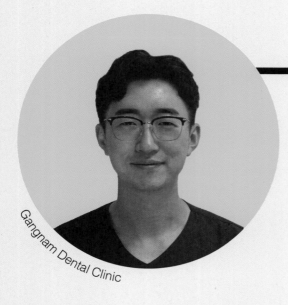

Gangnam Dental Clinic

- Chosun University School of Dentistry DDS
- Inha University School of Medicine MS
- Inha University Hospital Department of Oral
  Maxillofacial Surgery
- Faculty member of Gangnam Academy of
  Dental Implantology (GADI)
- Faculty member of Gangnam International
  Implant Academy (GIIA)

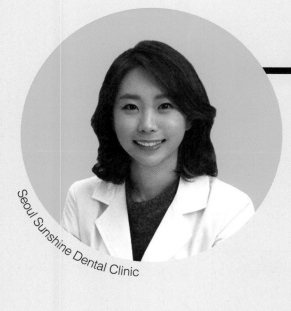

Jisun Kim

- Seoul National University School of Dentistry DDS, MS
- KEPCO Medical Center Department of Dentistry
- Seoul RED CROSS Hospital Department of Dentistry
- Faculty member of Gangnam Academy of Dental Implantology (GADI)
- Faculty member of Gangnam International Implant Academy (GIIA)

Seoul Sunshine Dental Clinic

Youngmin Park

- University of Pisa School of Dentistry DMD
- University of Pisa School of Dentistry MSc
- Seoul National University Department of Oral and Maxillofacial Surgery PhD Candidate
- Faculty member of Gangnam Academy of Dental Implantology (GADI)
- Faculty member of Gangnam International Implant Academy (GIIA)

Gangnam Dental Clinic

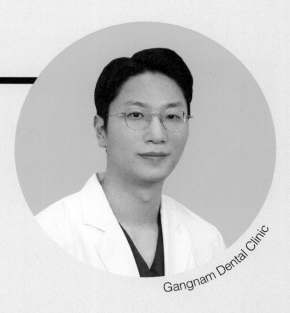

Translators

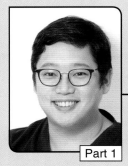

Part 1

Dr. Taehee Lee

University of Otago
Faculty of Dentistry

Melbourne, Australia

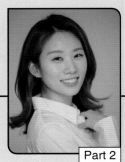

Part 2

Dr. Addie Y. Chang

Tufts University School
of Dental Medicine

Seattle, Washington, USA

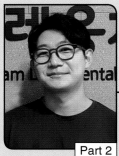

Part 2

Dr. Hector Shin

Griffith University
School of Dentistry

Brisbane, Australia

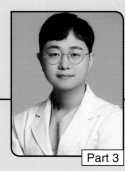

Part 3

Dr. GiTae Kwon

New York University College
of Dentistry

Connecticut, USA

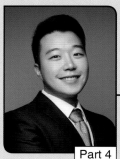

Part 4

Dr. Jong Wook Hur

Griffith University School of
Dentistry

New South Wales, Australia

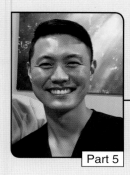

Dr. Joung Lee

🇺🇸 Nova Southeastern
   University
🇺🇸 San Antonio, TX, USA

Part 5

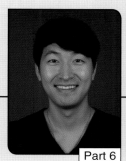

Dr. John Yun

🇨🇦 University of Toronto Faculty
   of Dentistry
🇨🇦 Ontario, Canada

Part 6

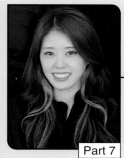

Dr. Chungmi Kim

🇺🇸 University of Texas
   Health San Antonio
   School of Dentistry
🇺🇸 Texas, USA

Part 7

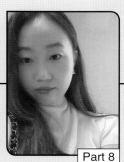

Dr. Shinyoung Park

🇨🇦 University of Toronto Faculty
   of Dentistry
🇨🇦 Toronto, ON, Canada

Part 8

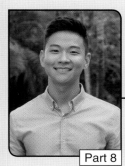

Dr. Byung Jun (Chris) Song

🇨🇦 University of Toronto Faculty of
   Dentistry
🇨🇦 Toronto, ON, Canada

Part 8

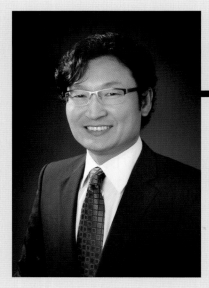

Eugene Kim
DDS

- Certificate in Advanced Prosthodontics, UCLA School of Dentistry
- DDS UCLA School of Dentistry
- BS in Biological Science, University of California, Irvine

Present
- Member, American College of Prosthodontists
- Member, Academy of Osseointegration
- Member, American Dental Association
- Member, California Dental Association
- Member, Orange County Dental Society
- President, Pacific Implant Academy, LLC
- Director, Advanced live implant surgery training in Baja California, Mexico
- Dental Board of California, Continuing Education Registered Provider
- Implant study club director, Pacific Implant Academy
- Course director, AIC Implant Mini Residency

✉ eugenekimdds1125@gmail.com
🌐 www.PerfectSmileOnline.com

One of dentistry's most respected clinicians and educators, Dr. Kim is the founder and director of Pacific Implant Academy. His lectures, seminars and live implant surgery courses have made a huge impact on countless number of dentists.

Dr. Kim was a clinical instructor of the department of removal prosthodontics at University of California at Los Angeles, School of Dentistry. He maintains a private practice in Buena Park limited to implant surgery and prosthodontics.

Dr. Kim earned his dental degree in 1996, and a specialty certificate in advanced prosthodontics in 2004, both from the University of California at Los Angeles, School of Dentistry.

After completing my first implant book⋯

Some say that if modern dentists did not have implants, all dentists would have become poor. I think that the catastrophe that doubled the number of dental schools in Korea in 1979 was a foresight with the popularization of implants in mind. I just managed to graduate from Chonbuk National University College of Dentistry, one of the dental schools that opened at that time. I am not that intelligent and lack the ability to hold a lot of knowledge in my head, but others say that I am very creative.

Although I have written many books before, my life has changed since my first clinical book 'wisdom tooth extraction', became a hit. As this book was published in English, it became an opportunity to make my name known worldwide, and this year, it will be translated and published in Spanish, Italian, and Japanese.

Wisdom tooth extraction is not a topic of great interest worldwide. This is also because, in developed countries, specialized treatment systems are in place for each department, and most wisdom tooth extractions are performed by oral surgeons.

However, unlike wisdom teeth, implants are a field of interest to most dentists around the world maybe except for some specialists like pediatric dentists and orthodontists. So, I plan to translate this book into English and other languages at the same time when it is published in Korean. There are so many books on implants on the market, but due to readers of my previous books all over the world, I am expecting that this book may be a bigger hit than 《Wisdom Tooth Extraction》. Yuna Kim, 2010 Vancouver Olympics gold medalist, once said, "Don't be afraid from the beginning. There are a lot of things in the world that are nothing when you actually get there." When I went abroad, I realized that Korea's implant technology was already the best in the world. So, in addition to my cases, this book introduces many implant masters in Korea that I respect, and provides an opportunity to share their cases as well. This is because, as my book becomes a bestseller around the world, not only me, but also my fellow dentists in Korea who I studied together can become a major pillar of the global implant education market.

This book feels like an autobiography, written to commemorate the 20th anniversary of my dental practice. This is because, unlike other treatments, implants contain the history of my practice. So, apart from the sales performance of this book, just writing this book seems to have fulfilled my dream, and I am already feeling very happy. But beyond this, if this book becomes widely known and becomes a global hit, I would like to give the credit to the entire dental industry in Korea who taught me, cared for me, and followed me. These days, they often add 'K' to Korean products and cultures popular abroad and now, I dare to say that the era of K-implant and K-dental has come and I want to enjoy that era with my Korean colleagues. I love you, all my fellow Korean dentists!

July 2021 in Gangnam

Acknowledgements

Thank you to so many people who have made this book possible.

Thank you for teaching me,

- Dr. Cho Yong-Seok, Director, 22nd Century Seoul Dental Hospital
- Professor Choi Young-jun, Department of Oral and Maxillofacial Surgery, Chung-Ang University Hospital
- Professor Dongseok Son, Daegu Catholic University Hospital
- Director Kim Ki-seong, Namsang Dental Clinic
- Professor Kyungwon Kim, Osstem Implant Education Research Institute
- Directors Ji-hye Kim, Jeong-ju Park, Eun-ju Kim, Choi Sang-jin, and Ji-eun Song, Human Love Dental Clinic
- Director, Yong Ahn, Jung Dental Clinic

My co-worker oral surgeons at Gangnam Leong Dental Clinic

- Dr. Lee Jae-wook, Dr. Kim Dong-seong, Dr. Lee Kyung-jin, Dr. Park Seul-ji, Dr. Pyeon Young-hoon
  I often scolded you guys, but I also learned a lot from you. Well done and thank you guys...

My co-worker prosthodontists and integrative care specialists who did my implant crown at Gangnam Leong Dental Clinic

- Dr. Jang Hyun-min, Dr. Kim Kyung-ae, Dr. Yang Mi-ra, Dr. Kim Min-ji Kim, Dr. Kyung Kyu-young Kyung, Dr. Park Young-min.
  Thank you for trying to restore those poorly placed, and for guiding me to place implants properly by making restorative treatment plan when I was struggling... Thank you all...

My sincere gratitude to the faculty members Dr. Lim Jong-hwan, Dr. Seo Min-kyo, Dr. Lee Jae-wook, Dr. Kim Dae-yong, Dr. Choi Geun-rak, Dr. Kim Hyeon-seop, Dr. Pyun Young-hoon, Dr. Kim Min-jae, Dr. Lee Ji-hye, Dr. Hong Jeong-pyo, Dr. Baek Su-hyeon, dr. Noh Hee-jeong, Dr. Park Young-min, and Dr. Kim Ji-sun, who have helped with live surgery seminars in Korea for nearly 10 years.

Thanks to my colleagues around the world Dr. Eugene Kim in the United States who opened my eyes to dental implants. Dr. Jin Kim, Dr. Jae-eun Jeong, and Dr. Ki-duk Park, who taught me. And those sharing knowledge with me from US, Canada and Australia, Dr. Jung-woo Lee, Dr. Chan-wook Ahn, Dr. Ki-tae Kwon, Dr. Jae-woo Cho, Dr. Hye-jin Jeon, Dr. Jong-ho Yoon, Dr. Yu-jeong Jang, Dr. Tae-eun Yoo, Dr. Jong-un Kim, Dr. Ga-mi Huh, Dr. Yong-kwon Kim, Dr. Shin-young Park, Dr.

Byung-jun Song, Dr. Tae Hee Lee, Dr. Oh-cheol Shin, Dr. Jong-wook Huh, Dr. Jeong-ho Lee, Dr. Yong-kwon Kim and Dr. Shin-young Park.

And to all my hygienists, especially Woo Soo-jin, Kim Jung-min and Kim Hee-jeong who I love most and from 2009, when I started preparing for lectures, worked hard to take and organize photos of patients.

Lastly, Su-in Han, team leader of Koonja Publishing Inc., who oversaw the production of this book; Director Hak-yeoung Yu who continued to take charge of the illustrations following the first clinical book, "Wisdom tooth extraction", editor Gyung-min Ku and designer Jin-young Lim for editing this book beautifully, and I would also like to thank Director Ju-yeun Chang, who regularly pays me book royalties. 😛

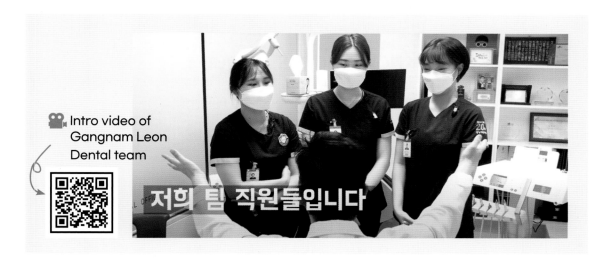

🎥 Intro video of Gangnam Leon Dental team

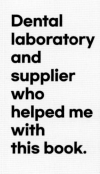

Dental laboratory and supplier who helped me with this book.

Dental supplier

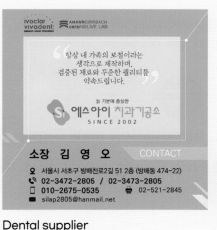

Dental laboratory

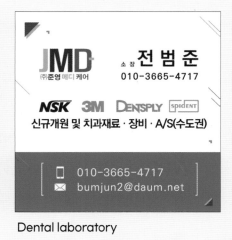

* The photos used in this book have been used as they are without any color changes or corrections. Only the symmetry and sizing are modified as needed for accurate content delivery.

Contents

Introduction

There is no future for dentists
who have forgotten history

1-1 History and Latest Trends in Implants _ 21
1-2 Korean Occlusion _ 44

Implant Basic Fundamentals

Knowledge is power

2-1 Dental Implant Materials and Surface Treatments _ 60
2-2 Implant Shape and Thread _ 85
2-3 Classification and Understanding of Abutments _ 116

Choosing Implant Fixture

Your choice will last a lifetime

3-1 Choosing Implants Length _ 166
3-2 Choosing Implant Diameter _ 211

4

Ideal Fixture Position, Angulation and Depth (PAD)

What's wrong with having a high standard?

4-1 The Pickaxe _ 248
4-2 Fixture Position & Angulation _ 265
4-3 The Depth _ 284

Implants and Soft Tissue

Soft tissue can deform hard tissue

5-1 Attached Gingiva and Vestibule _ 328

Bone Grafting in Implant Dentistry

No free lunch

6-1 Membrane _ 364
6-2 Bone Graft Material _ 394

Abutment Selection and Crown

You are stuck with me!

7-1 Abutment and Crown Shape _ 428
7-2 Why Screwmentable? _ 459

Implant Failures

Implant failure is
not the mother of success

8-1 Peri-implantitis _ 472
8-2 Fracture of Fixtures and Abutments _ 507

Dr. YOUNGSAM KIM'S

CLINICAL NOTES

EASY SIMPLE SAFE EFFICIENT

MASTERING DENTAL IMPLANTS

The Essential Elements for Success in Dental Implants

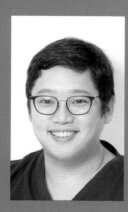

Dr. Taehee Lee

University of Otago, New Zealand BDS graduate
CEO and Principal Dental Surgeon
Bass Coast Dental Group
Melbourne, Australia

Introduction

There is no future for dentists who have forgotten history

1-1 History and Latest Trends in Implants

1-2 Korean Occlusion

•Introduction

There is no future for dentists who have forgotten history

My Implant Journey

In November 2001, I decided to jointly open a clinic with my senior colleague and treated my first paitent on February 18, 2002. It was a small 128 square meter, 3 chair clinic on the 5th floor of the building where my current clinic Gangnam Leong Dental is. My first implant patient was high school friend of mine, who also happened to be an employee of the dental company which supplied dental chairs to our clinic. He came to me in May of that year with missing tooth 46. I registered for an implant seminar in a hurry and that is how my implant journey started.

That first implant seminar I attended was 3 day seminar from Friday the 10th May 2002 to Sunday the 12th May 2002 and costed me 3.7million won. It was relatively expensive seminar however at that time the average cost of implant procedure was 2.5 million won using Korean implants and 3.5 million won using imported implants, so I was able to take the seminar without much financial burden. Considering the circumstances I remember only charging 900,000 won to my first patient

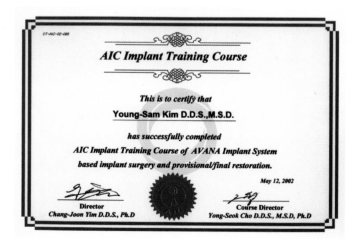

1.1 My first implant seminar certificate

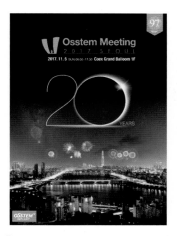

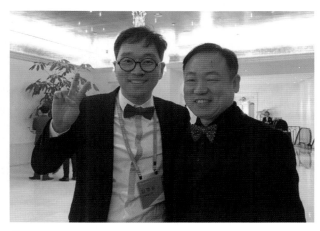

📷 1.2 Osstem 20 years anniversary world symposium poster

📷 1.3 **With Dr. Yongsuk Cho** at 2017 Osstem world symposium.

just to cover the cost of materials. That's how my implant journey started. The lecturer of the seminar was Dr. Yongsuk Cho who is still lecturing and in my opinion he is the best lecturer. Fast forward to 2017, I lectured at Osstem world symposium and Dr. Yongsuk Cho was there too as a lecturer. I was overwhelmed by the fact that I was standing on the same stage with the person who taught me 15 years ago. Moreover, it was a symposium commemorating the 20th anniversary of the implant that I first placed. It was an experience of great significance for someone like me who lives in memories all the time. I am sure that there is no disagreement that Dr. Yongsuk Cho is the best implant teacher (both in research and lectures) at present time in Korea. Under the motto, "once a teacher, a teacher forever", I attended Dr. Cho's seminars at various academic conferences.

Back in those days, when I placed the first implant, long implants were preferred. The first one I

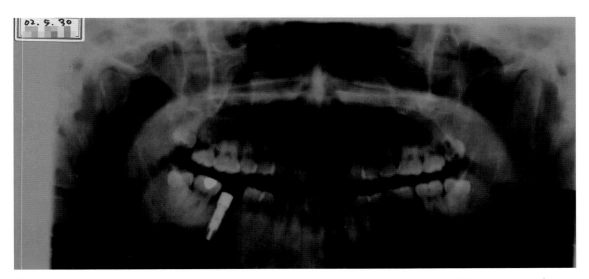

📷 1.4 Panoramic x-ray of my first implant case. x-rays taken back then were all film x-rays and most of them discoloured after statutory storage period of 5 years. However I scanned this one and kept it to commemorate my first implant.

placed was 4.8 mm * 15 mm Avana (now Osstem) implant (📷 1.4).

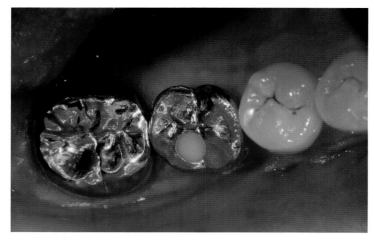

📷 1.5 Clinical photo 10 years after the placement

As always noticed on beginner's cases, you can see that the implant is placed slightly disto-buccally. It was restored with screw retained crown on extrenal hexa type gold UCLA abutment which was popular at that time. For some reason, probably due to lack of confidence in dental implant, it was common to see impant crown being slightly smaller than usual and you can see that the crown is slightly smaller bucco-lingually.

My friend (my first implant patient) has worked for 10 years before leaving the company and is now working as a dental material dealer. Because of my inclination to not change things, or because of my friend's great service, he still supplies dental materials to my clinic. So naturally, I get to review the case every year and over last 19 years I have had little trouble (📷 1.6). The external hexa type implants are known to cause marginal bone loss due to the micro gap formation and the movement at the abutment-fixture junction however I have not observed the marginal bone loss in this case. It is probably due to gold UCLA abutment's ductility which creates margin sealing effect. Prior to the

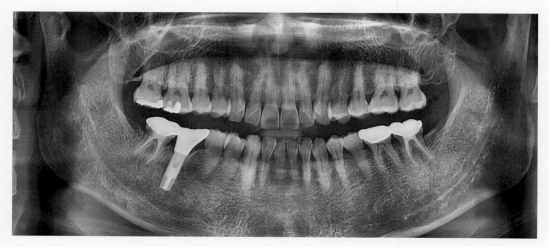

📷 1.6 The most recent panoramic x-ray taken on May 4, 2021. There are no more missing teeth because of good care for 19 years. Only two crowns were added.

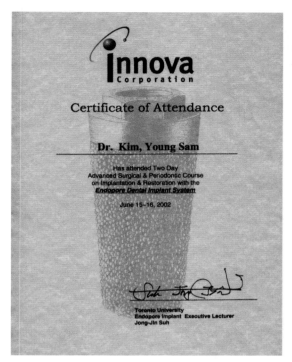

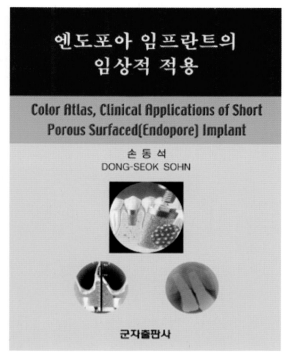

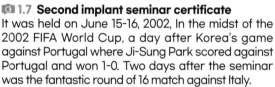

1.7 Second implant seminar certificate
It was held on June 15-16, 2002, In the midst of the 2002 FIFA World Cup, a day after Korea's game against Portugal where Ji-Sung Park scored against Portugal and won 1-0. Two days after the seminar was the fantastic round of 16 match against Italy.

1.8 Professor Dong-Seok Sohn's endopore implant book I studied.

surge of gold price in 2006, it was common to make both abutments and crowns using gold and surprisingly I rarely observed bone loss with these cases.

In June 2002, the dental material supplier who was selling "Endopore" implant from Canada explained me the advantages of the implant and suggested me to attend their seminar. It was a two day seminar over the weekend and costed me about 1.2 million won (1.7). I, for some reason, thought that this seminar was only one day long. The practical part of the seminar was so simple and Sunday afternoon was spent doing nothing. Maybe that is why I thought that the seminar was only a day long.

I have learned the basics from the endopore seminar, but in actual clinical practice I learned more from Professor Dong-Seok Sohn's books and lectures (1.8). The Endopore implant system and what I learned from the second implant seminar are still strongly remembered. At that time, endopore implants were placed by using a mallet and due to the fear of damaging patient's mandible or TMJ I did not use them on mandible. I mainly used Avana (Now Osstem) implants for mandible and endopore for maxillar.

Back then the fees charged for Korean implants and imported implants were different and I had to persuade any patients wanting imported implants for mandible to use Avana implants instead. Due to relatively higher price of implants, most patients were persuaded.

Panoramic x-rays of early endopore cases have become unrecognizable, but intra-oral x-rays were digital and well preserved (📷 1.9-1.12).

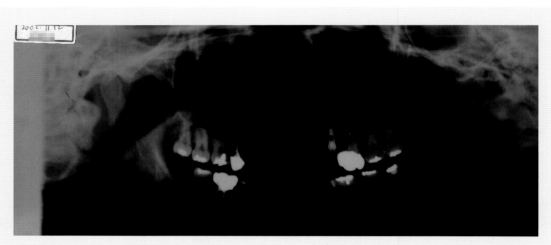

📷 1.9 **Early endopore cases from 2002.** I remember this patient as she was my comedian friend's ex-girl friend. She moved overseas few years after the procedure and review was not done.

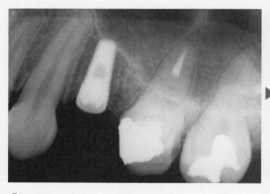

📷 1.10 Immediately after the placement of endopore implant

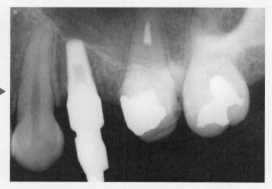

📷 1.11 Impression coping placement

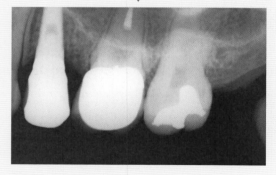

📷 1.12 2 years after the crown placement

In December 2002, about six months after my implant journey began, a senior colleague who trained in periodontology in Michigan, USA joined my practice. He purchased internal hexa type implants from Zimmer in the US for the mandible, and I started to place them as well as I had accumulated some skills by this point (📷 1.13). If I had known that I would become famous I would have collected a lot of old data, but it's a pity that I lost them due to computer issues.

Anyway, I started implants in this way, and since 2003, I mainly implanted Osstem's tissue level implant SS2 in the molars to minimize the need of second surgery (📷 1.14).

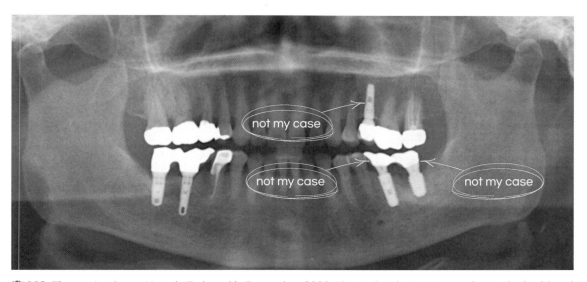

📷 **1.13** Zimmer Implants 46 and 47 placed in December 2002. The patient is my aunt, and now she is old and find it difficult to come to Seoul, so she sees my junior colleague nearby. The above panoramic photo was sent to me in 2016

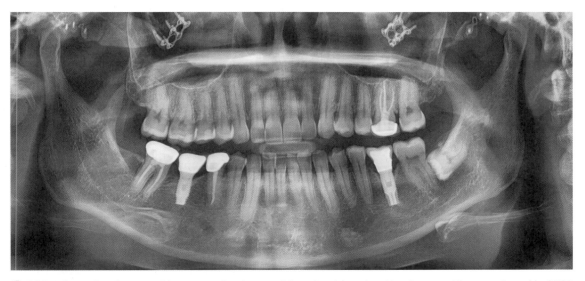

📷 **1.14** A bone-level external hexa type implant on 36 and a tissue level implant on 46 were placed in 2003 to a female patient in her early 20s. This panoramic x-ray was taken before the lecture at the symposium commemorating the 20th anniversary of Osstem in 2017. A typical 1.5 mm crestal bone loss is observed around the 36 external hexa type implant.

Afterwards, I went to the Department of Periodontology at Toronto Dental University from september to december 2005. At that time endopore implants were not as popular but still around.

During my time in Toronto, I learned a lot about cultural differences between countries and also spent time reading journals and learning theoretical aspects of implantology with Korean colleagues who were there. It was also a time that satisfied my intellectual needs to the point where I read and organized a lot of implant-related papers at the university library. I seem to have read so many articles that there are no more papers to read.

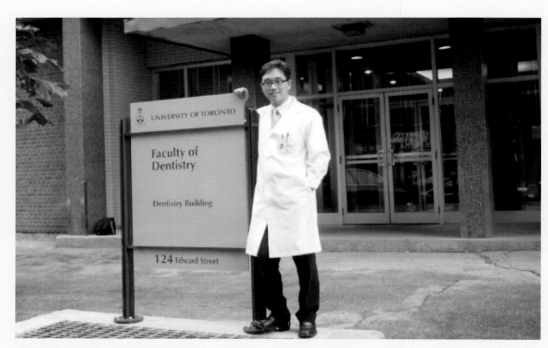

📷 1.15 September 2005, at the Toronto university dental school

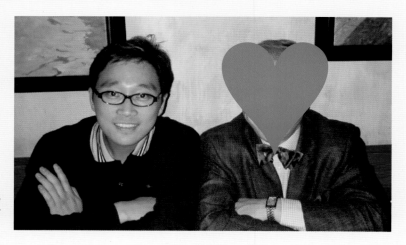

📷 1.16 December 2005, with professor at the peri-odontlogy department

*please understand that photos are mosaiced unless prior permissions were given.

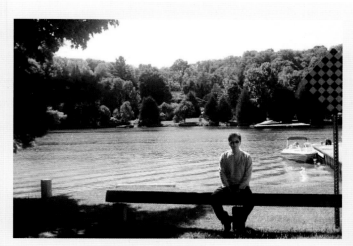

📷 1.17 Autumn in Canada East coast

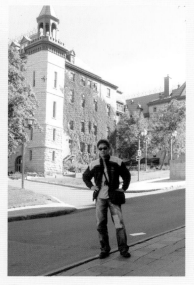

📷 1.18 In Quebec

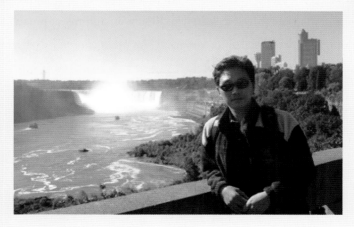

📷 1.19 Niagara Falls

I was having good time studying on weekdays and traveling around Eastern Canada on weekends.

At night, I went to the pool to swim, read a book in the library, and went out for 10 minutes every hour exercising. Maybe that's why I was the healthiest, slimmest and strongest back then. When I returned back to Korea, I was told that I had a structural problem with my spine and had operation. I am still suffering from the aftereffects of the operation and probably that's why I miss my time in Toronto so much.

And after returning to Korea in 2006, I started to place bone-level implants (Implantium) for the first time. At that time, only relatively larger practices were placing implants and I was able to place more implants than many other dentists.

I always had a busy social life and never worked alone. In 2004, I was lucky enough to have a great prosthodontist joining my team. He was really smart and had good skills, and that allowed me to focus on surgery. For most large cases the prosthodontist planned the treatment and oral surgeons and periodontists performed procedures according to the prosthodontist's plan. I also had an oral surgeon who joined me in 2004 and he was very meticulous person doing textbook treatment. So we discussed and helped each other with surgery that required precision and difficulty. I don't know if it was because I thought I was not as good as the oral surgeon or I liked doing simple cases but I tried to find a simple and safe procedures rather than doing big and fancy cases. Whenever I had cases beyond my capabilities I referred to the oral surgeon colleague and coordinated with the prosthodontist in the same way.

The oral surgeon colleague had very good surgical skills but there were cases where he did not agree with the prosthetic treatment plan or the patient's consent was not easily obtained due to the high cost and complexity of the treatment. When that happened I often offered simpler treatment options. At that time, the sinus lateral approach alone was priced at around 2 million won, and most blockbone grafts and large surgical bone grafts were priced at least 1 million won and my approach to minimize the surgical procedures by doing simpler crestal sinus elevation was often chosen by patients as a second option.

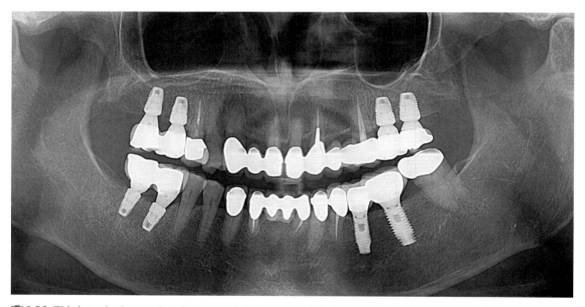

📷 1.20 This is typical case showing my style in the mid to late 2000s. External hexa type implants were rarely used, and bone level implants, dentium and SS2 of Osstem were used. Since 2009, I started to place Osstem's GS3 and TS3 implants and tissue-level implants were rarely used as well. Since then I only used bone level internal friction type implants.

Thanks to my business partners, I was able to leave the practice and study abroad in Canada. However, the time in Toronto was not enough to satisfy intellectual curiosity and I went to the US to do preceptorship for 1 year at UCLA periodontology department.

At first, it was not easy to be there but I became friends with a Japanese dentist named Reiji Suzuki and things got easier. In early 2008, a Spanish dentist named Xavi Costa came to the department for about 3 months. He was very sociable person and brought everyone (we had 2 Iranian, 2 Filipino, 1 Spanish and 1 Japanese colleauges) there together (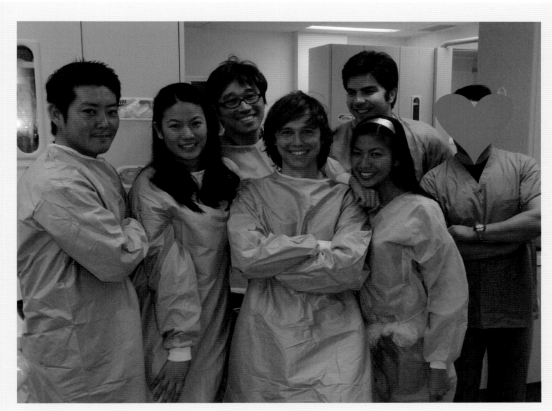 1.21). At that time, I was able to learn a lot about implant style and philosophy at UCLA Periodontology department. Unlike the Department of Periodontology at Toronto, UCLA did not have its own differentiated style and was similar to any other universities. It was a place that produced a world-famous professor named Carranza, but the building was not large and flashy, perhaps due to its limitations as a state university. I got the impression that it is a place where education and research are conducted according to the original purpose of a university hospital rather than focusing on clinical aspects. Nevertheless, it is clear that it was a valuable time to learn the differences between the American and Korean systems, and to learn the methods and culture of other countries from colleagues I met there.

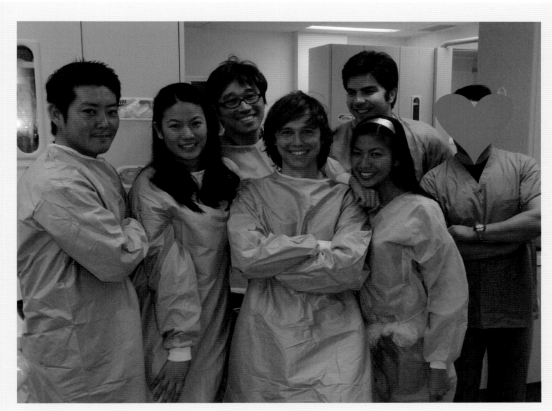

1.21 wth colleagues from other countries. March 2008

After returning to Korea in 2009, I expanded my clinic and hired more dentists and started to do more lectures. From 2013, I started live surgeries with dentists from other clinics at my office however it often caused issues with my co-workers who did not like the idea of it. I had to separate equipments for clinical use and seminar use and even had to purchase handpieces separately for my seminars. Then, after long persuasion, I managed to open a new clinic on a building next door (the building where my very first clinic was) in 2014 under the name of "Gangnam Leong Dental Clinic". My employees and patients followed. It was small but under my complete control. It was an opportunity to look back on my dentistry once again and to improve my skills. In fact, back then, I was mistaken to think that I do the best dentistry. But now thinking about it, I was a fool to think so. I still have long way to go. The reason I don't have as much confidence now is because I notice that my skills are still improving especially when I teach others. This is why I like doing seminars.

As I was seeing patients alone at the new Gangnam Leong Dental Clinic, I started to realize issues I am facing with prosthodontic aspect of the implant dentistry. I started to think how foolish I was and realized that I've practiced under the guidance of a great prosthodontist and just doing the surgery in the past. After that, I changed the way I do the implant dentistry. I made the treatment plan and performed the surgery and referred patients to the junior associated dentist for the prosthodontic aspect and it allowed me to at least slightly improve on diagnosis and treatment planning skills. Of course, even now, my skills in those areas are not that good, but at least, it allowed me to have a broader view on cases. And also seeing some cases done by other associate dentists which did not go very well, I have gained greater reassurance and confidence in the "ESSE, Easy, Simple, Safe and Efficient Surgery" method that I have been doing for a long time.

Also, my live surgery courses in Korea, which initially was a one off course, has been changed and now it goes for about 6 months with monthly meetings. It's the one I'm most nervous about but also my favorite. The course is usually full just by referrals from the previous participants and the advertisements are rarely done.

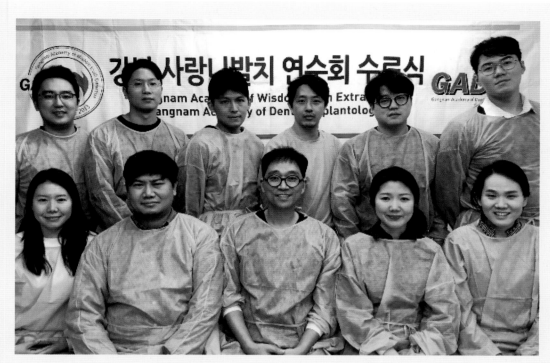

📷 **1.22** Completion ceremony for the 5th live surgery course in Korea in 2018

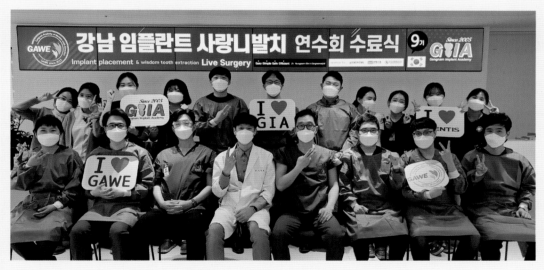

📷 **1.23** Completion ceremony for the 9th live surgery course in Korea. May 2021

In April 2018, 10 years after studying at UCLA, USA, I went back to UCLA Oral Surgery for a preceptorship. At that time, implants had already reached a certain level in Korea, so it was an opportunity to learn more about the cultural differences and methods of extracting wisdom teeth and others that are different from how they are done in Korea. Also at UCLA Oral Surgery, the dexterity of the trainees was so good that I was even thinking that they were selected based on their dexterity when they were interviewing for residency. Korean dentists with good dexterity often get frustrated by American dentists operating, however those residents doctors were very talented in implants and extraction, although they were little slower than us probably due to the cultural difference. Of course, it could be due to the long training period of 6 years, but all of those trainees were well equipped with the basics, and they had a great potential to become excellent oral surgeons in my opinion.

Even while I was in the US, I came to Korea once a month and spent a week each time for almost two years. As the covid-19 spread in March 2020, I returned to Korea a little earlier than planned.

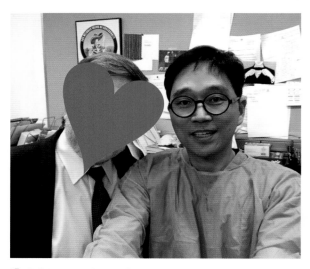

📷 **1.24** **Together with a professor at UCLA Oral Surgery department**
He is a man of great talent and character. Strangely, he does not shave his beard from Thanks Giving Day (4th week of November) until February of the following year. This has become established as the tradition of UCLA oral surgery, and residents also do so.

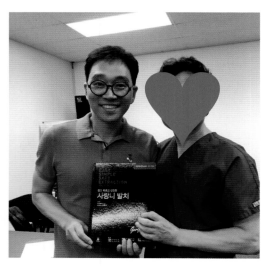

📷 **1.25** **In the summer of 2018, with the prosthodontist who place implants the fastest and the best.**
He invited me to do a wisdom teeth lecture at his Academy (PIA). This is a commemorative photo of the first time we met. I had no idea that I would learn so much from him about dental implants.

While in the United States, I met a prosthodontist who had very similar philosophy to mine and it allowed me to be convinced that my philosophy was right. Even considering the cultural differences and the different life paths we had, I can assure you that this prosthodontist are the **fastest and best implantologist** I have personally met. I think the implant path is the most important thing, and my standards are very strict and when I see this prosthodontist's cases, it is so well placed that I wonder if they are done by me. You may not like it but self bragging can be good for the mental health. Sometimes he sees my cases and jokes that he thought they were done by him. Our cases look so similar except the length of implants used. some surgical methods such as bone graft are very different though and it's more to do with differences in each countries. He emphasizes **"PAD (Position, Angulation, Depth)"** and these are what I also emphsize when I teach others. In fact, I called it **"LDH (Location, Direction, Height)"** in English but I am sure that his English terms are more appropriate than my Konglish (Korean English) expression. I have stopped using the term LDH and use his term PAD instead as a sign of respect to him.

Most American dentists perform live surgeries in Latin America or Mexico. Potential litigation issue is probably the biggest reason why they are performed there. This fastest and the best prosthodontist also runs a live surgery course in Tijuana, Mexico, which faces the border with the United States, and he generously helped me run the live surgery course there as well, so the students who like my lectures (who claim to be a part of Youngsam cult😅) come and participate my live surgery courses there.

So, until February 2020, about 100 American, Canadian, and Australian dentists participated over 8 courses and I discovered that my skills had improved significantly. I think the old saying is true that teaching is the best way to learn.

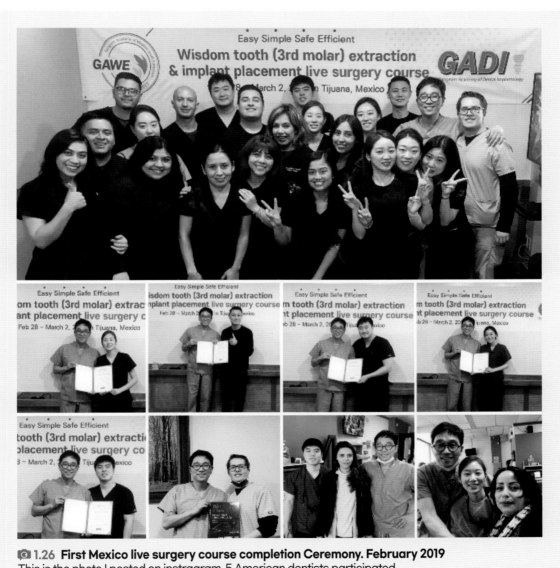

📷 1.26 **First Mexico live surgery course completion Ceremony. February 2019**
This is the photo I posted on instragram. 5 American dentists participated.

In particular, cases which were not experienced much in Korea due to cultural differences, such as immediate implants, were done in Mexico and it helped me a lot. The National Health Insurance scheme in Korea makes extraction very cheap (only few thousand won) while the implant costs around 100 times more than that and it is not easy to discuss both together. Also as a rule of thumb, **I never talk about money with patients**, so I leave it to the staff only. As a result, there weren't many patients who wanted to do both at the same time, and I was also reluctant to suggest patient to undergo expensive treatment while they are in pain. However, at Mexico live surgery, since there are many patients who want to get as much treatment as possible in the shortest possible time, there were many cases of immediate implants, and I naturally came across many of them.

As a result when I came back to Korea, I was able to offer many patients to do more implants immediately. During this time, my skills improved significantly. Looking at my skills that are still growing rapidly, I have thought a lot about the need to put aside the pride that I am always the best

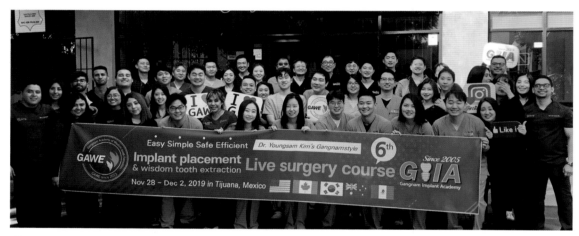

📷 1.27 **6th live surgery. December 2019**
8 dentists from US, 6 from Canada and 2 from Australia participated.

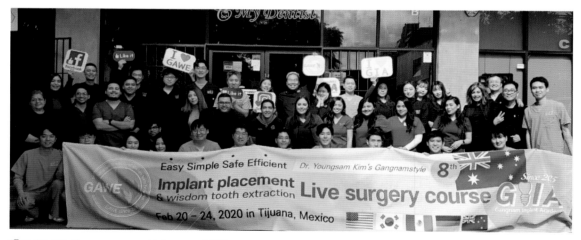

📷 1.28 **8th liver surgery. February 2020**
We had 14 dentists from Australia. You can see that the number of participants significantly increased.

and work harder in the future.

The UCLA School of Dentistry was also very good at implants. As mentioned earlier, I have very strict rules on placing implants, however residents there were not too bad with what I consider the most important, 'position, angulation and depth'. The use of PRF or bone grafting were not too excessive either. (although I am negative about those procedures).

They used Neo Biotech's SCA kit for sinus surgery and when lateral approach was performed, Dentium's DASK kit was used. When I see them being used, my pride as a Korean made me to brag about Korean implant systems. At that time another Korean implant company, Dentis, was sponsoring my seminars and they donated Dentis' crestal surgical kit to them and I took a commemorative photo. As the residents there liked Korean products, I have given them Korean Osstem Osteotome as gifts to final year residents. One of the residents returning to his hometown of

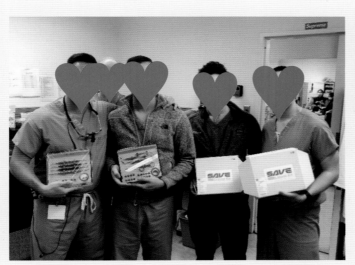

📷 **1.29 Commemorative photo after Dentis donation**
UCLA Oral Surgery had a really good atmosphere. They were respecting, caring and proud of each other. Everyone also had very good dexterity.

📷 **1.30 Chief Resident taking a commemorative photo with Osteotome, which I gave as a gift**
Although they have to compete with each other, they are very friendly and attractive people. Sometimes I think of these friends. They really liked Dentium's DASK kit and Neo's SCA kit made in Korea. They also liked Straumann implant's Korean surgical kit. If I ever have to go back there, I'd like to bring one and give it to them as a gift.

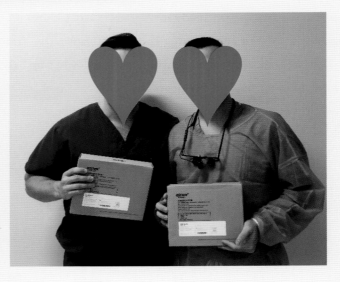

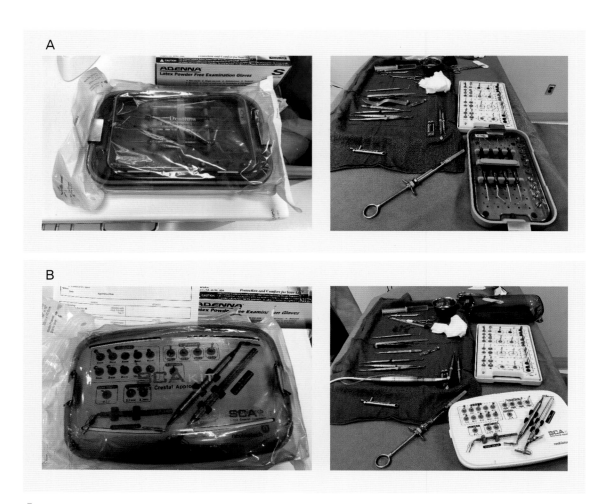

📷 **1.31 Implant Surgery Instruments at UCLA oral surgery department**
A is Dentium DASK kit used for lateral approach sinus cases. According to the reisdents, 80% of oral surgeons in US use DASK kit for their lateral cases. B is Neo-biotech's SCA kit used for crestal approach.

San Francisco was particularly interested in using Hiossen Osstem implants as the clinic he will be working there were already using Hiossen implants.

Now, let's talk about actual implants. The following are basically my lecture contents put in writing. I have **noted my implant experience and philosophy over last 20 years.** Since it is easy to become a banal book if it leans too far on the format, I will describe it while emphasizing the key contents in an easy and concise arrangement of my own style.

1-1

History and Latest Trends in Implants

Mastering dental implants

History and Latest Trends in Implants

Some of you may think 'here it goes again.' A book that is talking about the history from the first chapter. However, implants are different from other treatments. We always see 'the history' that has nothing to do with us remain intact in our patients' mouths, and we have to keep repairing and maintaining them. Also, like the famous saying in Korea, "There is no future for a nation that has forgotten history," I believe that **your implants have a future only when you know the history of implants.** As everyone already knows, I'm the type of person who explains things in a fun way, so trust me on this and follow me!

It was only in the 1990s, when I was at dental school, that implants started to be clinically recognized. Still, at that time, implants were not a very common treatment in Korea or around the world, so dentists who performed implants were recognized as pioneers. A professor who started implants relatively early in Korea once showed me a picture of the mandible of a Mayan with ground shells used as implants. I thought to myself, 'He must have died from that... '

In any case, studying the beginnings of modern implants going back to the 1960s and 1970s is meaningless. This is because most of the products used at that time have either already disappeared or have been completely transformed (📷 **1.32**). When I was at UCLA Oral Surgery department, we often did the removal of blade implants and subperiosteal implants, but I don't think the general practitioner needs to worry about it nowadays.

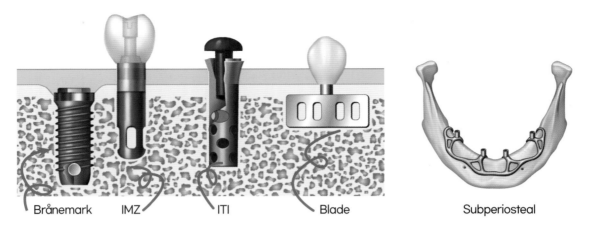

| Brånemark | IMZ | ITI | Blade | Subperiosteal |

📷 **1.32** I am sure you have seen this picture before showing old style implants

Therefore, if we consider the origin of the modern implants in terms of the shape and structure, 1980s is when the history starts. 📷 **1.33** is the figure I use when giving a lecture. The shape of the implant still being used are basically from one of these. Endopore is only included as I would like to discuss about its strengths and weaknesses in this book and the Bicon implant is included as they are still well used although their shape and implantation technique are unique. Nobel Biocare and Straumann (ITI) can be said to be the basis of modern implants that are still produced and sold today.

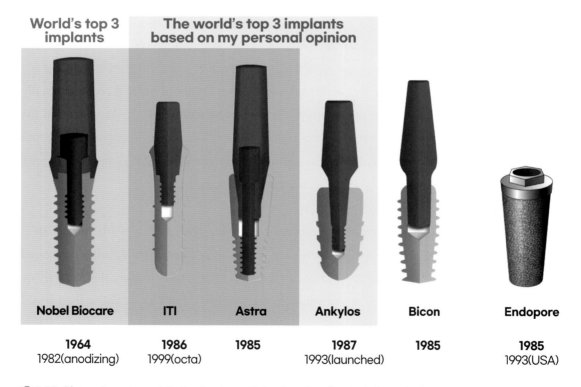

World's top 3 implants	The world's top 3 implants based on my personal opinion				
Nobel Biocare	**ITI**	**Astra**	**Ankylos**	**Bicon**	**Endopore**
1964 1982(anodizing)	**1986** 1999(octa)	**1985**	**1987** 1993(launched)	**1985**	**1985** 1993(USA)

📷 **1.33** Picture I use to explain the fundamentals of modern implants in my lectures.

Although they are still in use, it is true that the main products currently being sold by the two companies are completely different forms and different to modern implant concept. As a result, Nobel Biocare ,ITI and Astra with their original internal friction type implants are often considered top 3 implant systems (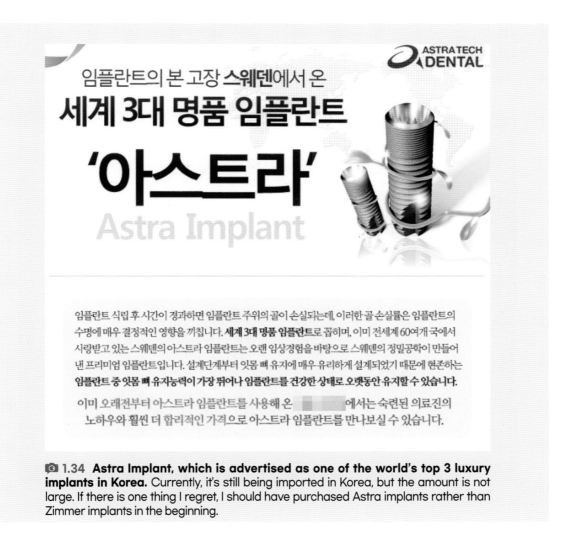 1.34).

However, I would say that Straumann (ITI), Astra and Ankylos implants are the world's top three implants instead. In my opinion, modern implants are made with the advantages of these three implants. These are 'Ankylos' fixture shape', 'Astra's fixture-abutment connection structure', and 'Straumann's surface treatment'. Most modern implants are made with the advantages of these three implants, and it is expected that there will be no significant change for a while. The details are covered in detail in **Part 2 Implant Basic Fundamentals**.

In 2002, the year I opened my own practice, Korean Havana (now Osstem) implants produced similar products to Nobel's external hexa type (US2) and Straumann's tissue-level implants (SS2), and the Korean domestic implant market began to become active. And around at same time, Dentium

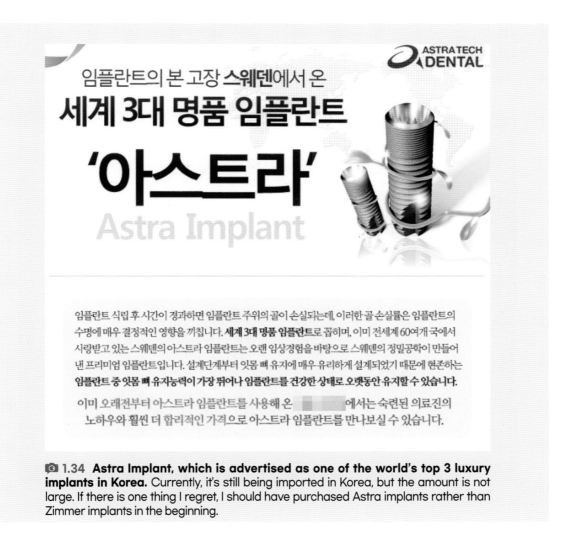

📷 1.34 **Astra Implant, which is advertised as one of the world's top 3 luxury implants in Korea.** Currently, it's still being imported in Korea, but the amount is not large. If there is one thing I regret, I should have purchased Astra implants rather than Zimmer implants in the beginning.

produced the implantium implants, copy of Astra, and the market share of imported implants gradually reduced in Korea. Later Dentium produced Superline system by removing micro thread and Osstem started to produce TS3 system and they are used as main products in Korea.

In the mid-2000s, when Korean implants started to gain more market share, one imported implants brand suddenly introduced, "Swiss Plus Implant" (📷 1.35). The name is Swiss Plus, but it is actually tissue-level implant from Zimmer in the US. Although it was from Zimmer, the Korean distributor was different and there was a big difference in price and their initial sales strategy worked well. The Zimmer implants imported by the company called Paragon was sold for 340,000 won for a fixture and over 100,000 won for an abutment. However, a company called Denix Co., Ltd., which imported and sold Swiss Plus implants were selling their implants for 270,000 won and even advertised that the mount can be used as a permanent abutment. As a result, as advertised, the cost was reduced by around 50% and it was possible to offer imported implants to patients at reduced cost. At that time the implant treatment cost was on a downward trend, and the imported implant treatment cost fell by about 1 million won to 2.5 million won, so it seems to fit well with the trend at that time. I also purchased them in a package of 40 to begin with and later purchased more. However, problems started to arise from the mount when used as a permanent abutment.

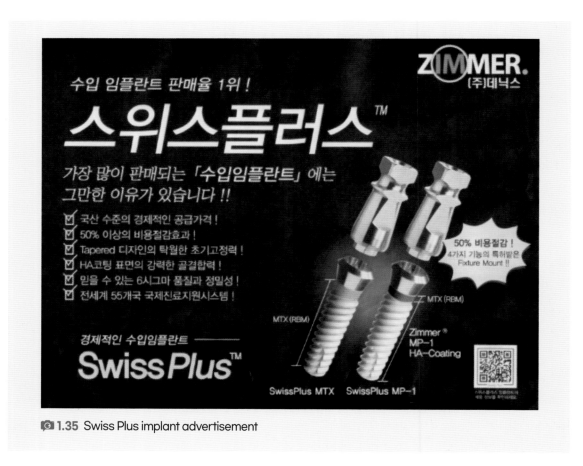

📷 1.35 Swiss Plus implant advertisement

Dr. YOUNGSAM KIM

What characteristics shuld mounts have? Let's think about which mount is a good mount. The mount is like a handle that the surgeon holds until the implant is placed in the jawbone. Without a screw, an external hexa type implant that has no holding force or a tissue level implant that does not have an octa structure cannot be implanted by a surgeon holding the implant. Therefore, the mount was absolutely necessary for implant placement. So, which mount is a good mount? Two things can be made clear. First, it must be weaker in strength than implants. This is because if the strength is stronger than the implant, the implant may be damaged during the placement process. Inevitably, even if excessive force is used during the placement process, it is better to damage the mount than to damage the implant. The second important factor is that the mount should be easy to remove once it has been placed. In particular, if the bone quality is poor, everyone must have experienced the case of the implant falling out while removing the mount. If these two are the characteristics of the mount, even a well-made mount would not be suitable for use in a permanent abutment.

Many dentists have started experiencing abutments loosening from fixtures and when the complaint was made to the distributor, their response was to use the original permanent abutment. This, not only caused the inconvenience to patients, but also meant that the crowns had to be remade and new abutments which costed over 100,000 won had to be purchased. As a result, the use of this implant system substantially reduced. In addition, Korean implants gained more popularity and the drop in implant costs due to excessive competition meant that imported implants lost their popularities and I also stopped purchasing them. Swiss Plus implants had a body design borrowed from Straumann tissue level and a slightly tapered form. Personally, I liked the tapered body. However, the tapered shape had a fatal weakness that it is not easy to adjust the height. Still, the implant product itself was satisfactory.

Foreign implant manufacturers do not easily apply the characteristics of other companies to their products, but dynamic Korean implant companies have developed products that borrowed the good points of various companies. As a result, we see that most Korean implants systems are almost identical in terms of forms and methods of placing them.

Anyway, if you ask me, "Which implant is the best implant?", I can answer, **"The verified Korean implant is the best implant in the world,"** as it is manufactured by combining the strengths of numerous companies for the convenience of customers only. The reason I use the expression "verified" is because I have many memories of being disappointed because the product was released too quickly that the long-term verification process was omitted and problems arose later. The problem mainly occurred in the surface treatment, and in the past, many dentists were troubled by the thread or shape issues of some company's products. Also, there is a recent issue of the one particular company's poor surface treatment, which was confirmed to have occurred during the manufacturing process and because of these reasons, when a new product with new surface treatment comes out, I often wait for at least 1-2 years to decide whether to use it or not. Surface treatment will be dealt with in more depth in **Chapter 2-1**.

I have one patient who carries a history of implants in Korea with her. She is the older sister of a close high school friend of mine, who had a Straumann tissue level implant placed at my alma mater hospital in 1996 (📷 **1.36**). As the patient had to travel long distance from Jeonju to Seoul, she was not able to find the right timing for treatment, so there are some regrets about the treatment, but she is still receiving treatment well. Let's take a look at this patient's treatment process.

In 2005, 17 was restored with an endopore implant (📷 **1.37**). Tooth 16's root anlge was not ideal and

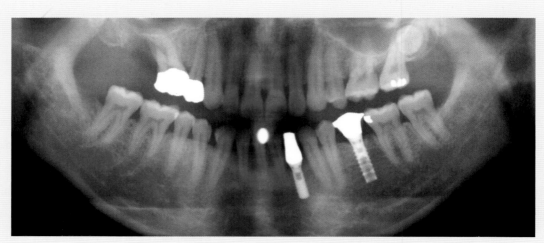

📷 1.36 A Straumann implant placed in 1996(the x-ray was taken at my clinic in 2005 when she first visited me)

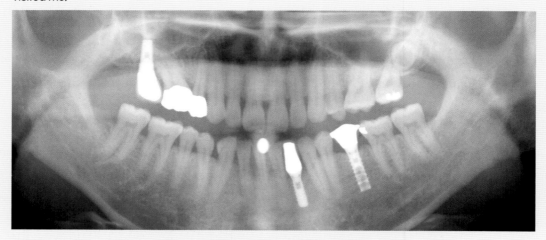

📷 1.37 Endopore implant placed to replace 17 in 2005

it was difficult to get the right path for the implant, but I thought that the treatment went well. The patient did not come back for a while due to the distance from her home, but in 2015, after 10 years,

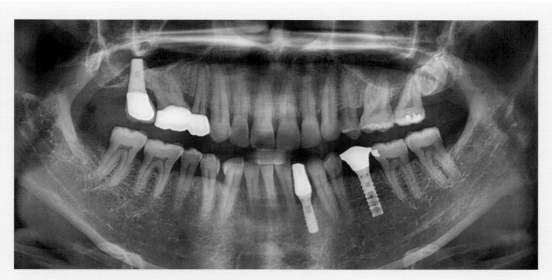

📷 **1.38** 10 year follow up x-ray taken in March 2015

she came back as one of the anterior veneers treated with the implant broke. 📷 **1.38** is a panoramic x-ray taken at that time and fortunately I could confirm that the implant was being used well.

Then, two years later, in 2017, she came back to me after visiting her local dentist in Jeonju because of gum pain. She was told by the dentist that the tooth 27 had to be extracted and wanted

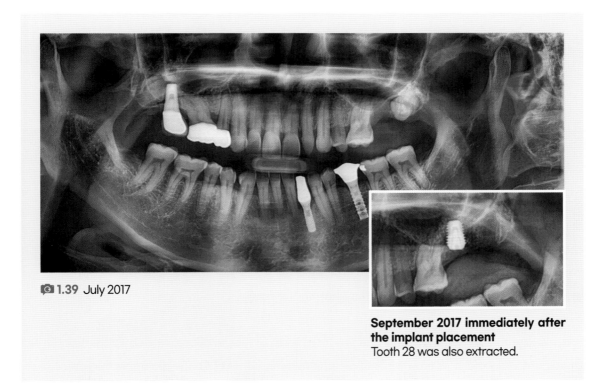

📷 **1.39** July 2017

September 2017 immediately after the implant placement
Tooth 28 was also extracted.

to get another implant done by me (📷 **1.39**). However, since it was immediately after the extraction, the implant was not possible. In principle, I usually place implants about a month and a half after tooth extraction. Although the bone heaing is acceptable, the soft tissue takes at least a month and a half (6 weeks) to become thick enough to handle. Although there was almost no alveolar bone, I was confident to some extent with crestal approach sinus elevation and placed the implant. But the primary stability was not very good and I had to use 6 mm diameter wide implant. I rarely use implants larger than 5 mm in diameter and wide implants are only used when the primary stability is not achievable with narrower implants (refer to **Chapter 3-2**). Due to the fact that the patient had to travel long distance, the restoration was placed 6 months later in April 2018 (📷 **1.40**).

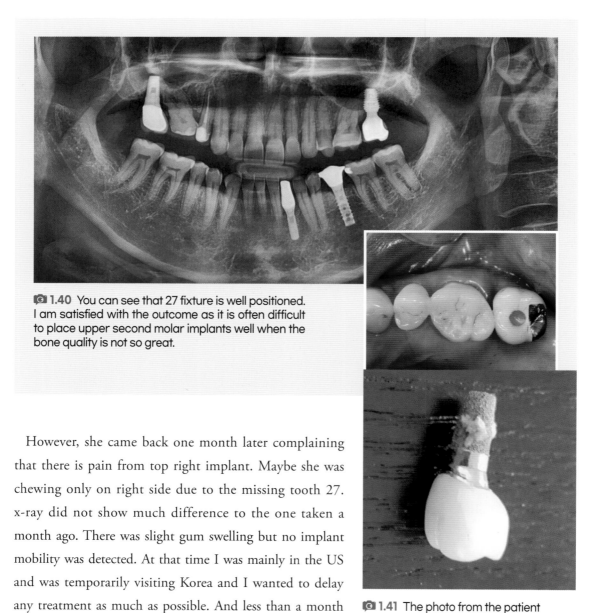

📷 **1.40** You can see that 27 fixture is well positioned. I am satisfied with the outcome as it is often difficult to place upper second molar implants well when the bone quality is not so great.

📷 **1.41** The photo from the patient

However, she came back one month later complaining that there is pain from top right implant. Maybe she was chewing only on right side due to the missing tooth 27. x-ray did not show much difference to the one taken a month ago. There was slight gum swelling but no implant mobility was detected. At that time I was mainly in the US and was temporarily visiting Korea and I wanted to delay any treatment as much as possible. And less than a month later when I was in the US she sent me a photo showing that the entire implant came out (📷 1.41). You may wonder how the implant which did not show any mobility less than a month ago could come out like that. The big disadvantage of the endopore implant is that when it gets inflamed it progresses so fast and the advantage is that it comes out so easily and minimizes the clinical effort required to remove the implant. Anyway, the patient replaced the implant on 17 in Seoul. Osstem's TS4 implant was used and I reviewed and took the x-ray of the implant recently 1 year after the placement (📷 1.42, 1.43). You can also see that the implant crown on 35 is re-manufactured as well as she was complaining that it was moving (📷 1.44). Information on this re-manufacturing process and tissue-level implants is discussed in **Chapter 2-3** and I will explain the crown method of tissue-level implants and points to be aware of.

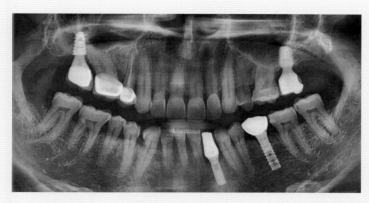

📷 **1.42** X-ray taken in July 2020.

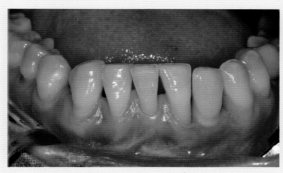
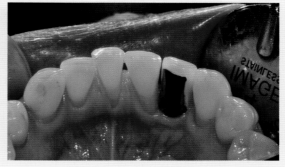

📷 **1.43** Photo of lower anteriors taken in July 2020. You can see that the condition of the crown is good even after 24 years of placement.

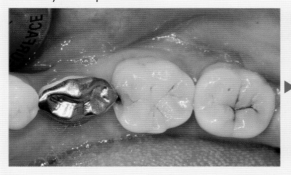
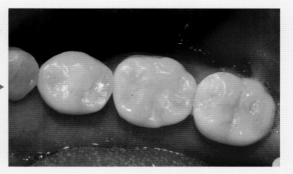

📷 **1.44** Caries developed adjacent to the implant crown on 35 which caused the mobility of the crown. A new Zirconia implant crown was placed after treating caries.

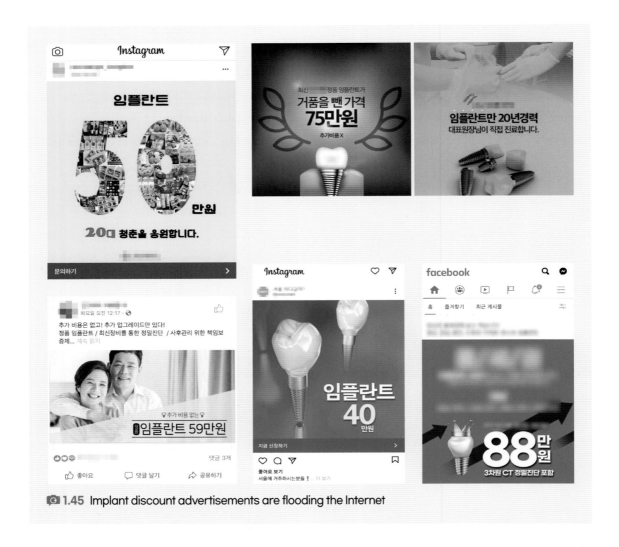

1.45 Implant discount advertisements are flooding the Internet

As the government insurance started to cover dental implants from July 2014 and the eligible age was reduced to the age of 65 as of July 2018, the co-payment was reduced to 30% just like other dental treatments in Korea. There are some dentists who complain that the cost is too low, but most seem to be somewhat satisfied with it as they know that **the trend of implant cost reduction is inevitable.** Compared to 2002, when I first started dentistry, the cost of dental implants are decreasing. We are even seeing the advertisement where the implant is advertised cheaper than what the insurance is covering. On the street of Seoul, tissue wipes with "Implant 500,000 won" advertisement are handed out for free to people and social media like Facebook and Instagram are full of advertisement for low cost implant (📷 **1.45**). Of course, I know that only few people actually end up getting implants at such low price, but due to the popularization of the implant procedure and the

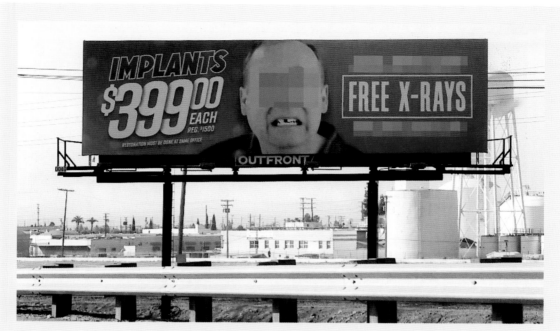

📷 **1.46** An implant advertisement sign on the Highway 5 in Los Angeles where I drive through often.

drop in implant material cost, it is unlikely that anyone can stop this trend (📷 **1.45**). Is this decline in implant treatment costs only an issue in Korea? This is already happening all over the world. In the case of the United States as well, this dumping of implant treatment costs initially started with immigrants from underdeveloped countries in large cities, but later it has spread to the main stream white society as well (📷 **1.46**). Of course, due to the hierarchical social structure of the United States, expensive implants and inexpensive implants coexist but in Korea, the cost of implant is low in all places except for a few university hospital clinics. Australia and Canada are still relatively immune to this change, but I think it is only a matter of speed of change and the trend will be same. In case of Europe, even considering their socialistic medical system, I think it is inevitable that the price of implant treatment will drop as implant treatment is not usually covered under the insurance scheme.

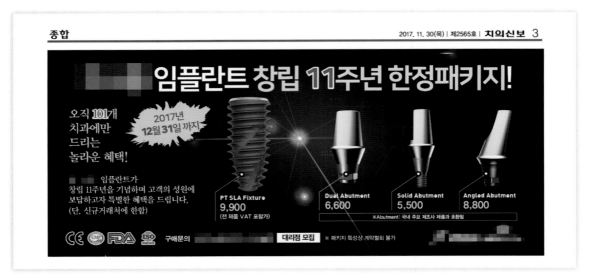

📷 **1.47** Advertisement of cheap implant fixtures that cost less than 10,000 won per fixture.

The one of the probable cause of the decline is the price drop of implant fixture itself (📷 **1.47**). Implant treatment became mainstream service provided by most dentists and the use of stock abutment increased. I hear that not many dentists these days take impression at the fixture level (less than 5% according to laboratory technicians) as it is so much cheaper just to make a crown on top of the stock abutment due to the reduced laboratory cost in recent years. So, in a way, we should not say that the price drop in implant is necessarily wrong or bad.

So, is cheap always good? In the end, the quality of implant treatment rather than the price is what matters. And even if we take price into consideration, the focus should be the the cost-effectiveness rather than just the price. I believe that if you follow my **"Easy Simple Safe Efficient" philosophy, you can improve your cost-effectiveness as a implant provider and set you free from future failures.** After reading this book to the end you will know what the important points are, and I guarantee that it will help increase the cost-effectiveness of your service.

The biggest trend of modern implants is "digitization" including computer-guided implants. Since 3-4 years ago, most implant seminars were focusing on digital implants. Most of the large-scale symposiums and seminars organized by companies were also focusing on digital implants. Dental newspapers and magazines also show advertisements for digital seminars and guide systems from various companies.

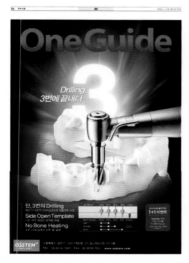 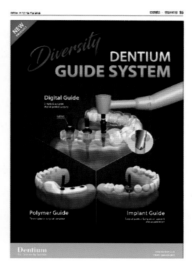 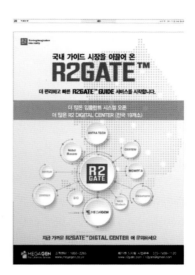

📷 **1.48** Digital implant advertisements from various companies

A few years ago, I went to the Implant World Symposium on the topic of digital implants. It was a timely seminar for me because I had just arrived from the US and I was also thinking a lot about whether to adopt digital or not. At the time, I had emphasized the importance of placing implants in the correct position, and I did not feel the need for guide implants because I thought I was doing pretty well.

On that day, live surgery was being broadcasted from early on. The surgery was performed by a pioneer and the best in the field of implant development in Korea. I watched the live surgery with the thought that 'this company is not behind in the guide field either'. In a completely edentulous maxillary patient, 8 implants were placed flapless with a digital guide and immediately loaded using a temporary crown. It appeared to be going well, and suddenly the surgeon started to open the flap. When the flap was opened, the implants were completely away from the alveolar bone and placed in the wrong position. Perhaps the operator also felt this way during the operation and raised the flap. As someone who does a lot of live surgery as well, I watched with a heart of sympathy. How frustrating, trembling, and embarrassing it must be right now. The 2,000 dentists sitting there must have been watching with concern rather than blaming the doctor. In the end, the operation was carried out with free hand drilling and grafting, and due to time constraints, the next lecture had to be continued. Later they showed the post operative photos, however, only 5 implants were placed and they were in completely different positions from the original plan.

There will be no one who will deny that the operating doctor is one of the finest surgeon. Not only that due to the nature of the live surgery, they would have selected an easy case, and there would have been thorough preparation. The company also would have wanted to promote its advanced digital technology in front of 2,000 dentists from all around the world. But the result was not satisfactory. The point of this story is that even the finest surgeon who thoroughly prepare for the procedure can have such outcome. I often say this at the lectures. **"Master the analog first, then digital can be done."** Those who have not mastered the analog implant will not be able to experience the true taste and beauty of digital technology. In the end, the fact that the surgery could finish reasonably well was ultimately due to the surgeon's analog surgery skills.

One professor who was the chairperson of a recent digital seminar said these words after all presentations were finished. "No matter how good a car you drive, even if the car is Maybach, if driven by a novice driver, it means nothing" It was the comment that particularly touched the audience as the seminars were about digital equipment.

Among the people I met in America, there was a doctor who was a great inspiration to me. I call her 'Guide Goddess'. She graduated from dental school at relatively later stage of her life after moving to America. Although her dentist career is short, she has been a tremendous inspiration to me in the digital field. I heard it later, but she even tried to come to my lecture in Dallas all the way from LA back in 2017. She eventually could not make it as there were no more space and I first met her in my first LA wisdom teeth extraction seminar in July 2018. And thankfully, she also brought many of her colleagues and friends with her.

I visited her clinic for an observation and saw a guided implant surgery which was impressive (📷 **1.49)**. When it comes to the implant path, I thought I was more confident than anyone else and it is not usually easy to please my high standard. However, her implant path was amazingly good especially considering her short career as a dentist. And her surgery was really fast as well probably because she's already placed around 2,000 implants with Dionavi system. At that time I was not very happy with my associate dentists' implant cases in Korea. When I was in Korea, I would have replaced any of their implants I was not happy with but since I was far away, I couldn't check every single one. So I have made a decision to introduce digital guide system and started to use Dentis simpleguide

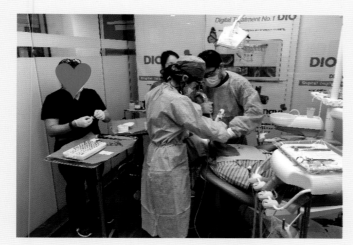

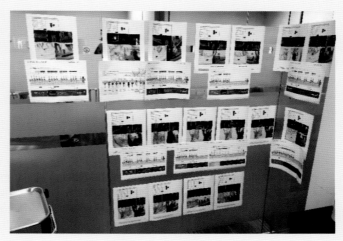

1.49 Surgery being done by the guide goddess

1.50 A wall full of digital guide information for the patient to be operated on that day.

system. The digital technology was the answer as I could not check and control all the implant cases at my clinic. All our implant dentists were specialist oral surgeons and therefore the surgical skills were not a concern. However I was not satisfied with their implant paths and I made a policy to use digital guides for all implant cases at my clinic. It was also a decision I made so I can learn the guide system as well. Anyway, this was the reason why I gave her the nickname 'Guide Goddess,' and, in every lecture, I mention this story to everyone.

And not long after, I was doing an implant seminar as a presenter. When she was asked to come, she was bit hesitant to participate. She wasn't too sure if she needs to attend my implant seminar as she already placed over 2,000 implants. As I didn't have many participant, I asked her to just come and help me out and the seminar finished well.

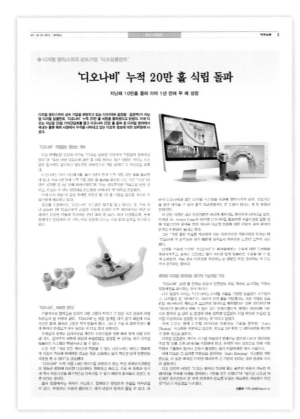

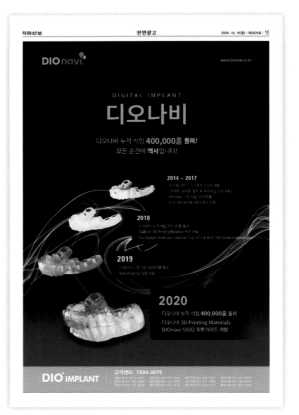

📷 1.51 Dio Implant advertisement in November 2018 celebrating 200,000 DioNavi cases. DioNavi contributed greatly to popularize the guide implants.

📷 1.52 **Advertisement celebrating DioNavi's 400,000 cases**

In less than two years, there was another advertisement saying that it had surpassed 400,000 cases. 'Guide Goddess' doctor had already completed 4,000 cases a year before this article was published. So she did more than 1% of the world's DioNavi system.

After my seminar, the guide goddess was impressed with it and started showing her failed cases to me. This allowed me to analyze the cause of failures in a traditional analogue way, while she taught me her digital know-hows and we could learn from each other. The doctor is currently participating as a faculty in the Mexican live surgery that I am conducting, and teaches the guided surgery. Also she is learning analog surgery skills which she was lacking. She was also changing her system from DinoNavi to Osstem's oneguide system and I am sure that she could learn alot from the live surgery course.

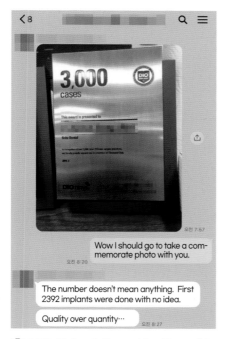

On June 19, 2019, I received a KakaoTalk (text) message. It was a photo of a plaque stating that she did 3,000 guided cases (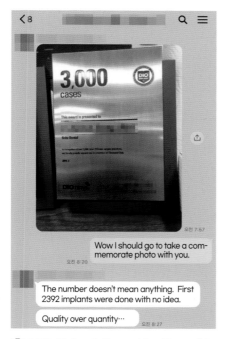1.53). Since she took 2,000 authentication photo with me, I told her that I should go and see her to get another photo to celebrate 3000 cases. She replied me back saying that the 2392 she implanted before taking my lecture should not be counted as she did not know the real stuff. That's probably the best compliment for me. Perhaps she knew that I will capture her message and use it on my lectures and made that number up.

📷 **1.53 Kakaotalk sent by the guide goddess.** I know that she said this to make me feel good but I took it to mean that even a digital expert should know about analog implants.

After the LA implant two-day course in 2018, a few 'evangelists' like the guide goddess appeared, and favorable reviews for the lecture spread among Korean American dentists. That's how I started my implant lectures in Seattle and New York, and I got a cult of Dr. Youngsam followers. Especially in Seattle, there were a few doctors who were friends with the guide goddess, and they still treat me like an idol. I have the most Korean fans in New York, but there are many people who like me enough to say that Seattle has the highest number of quality fans.

After that, the guide goddess also took an interest in the traditional free hand implant seminars and participated them. It was quite an impressive day for me. 📷 **1.55** is a commemorative photo taken

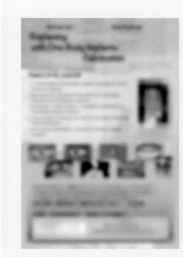

📷 1.54 Analogue God's implant seminar poster

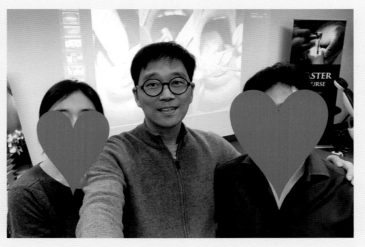

📷 **1.55 Photo with guide goddess and analogue god after his lecture**
Guide goddess realized the importance of free hand surgery and started to participate in these seminars with me.

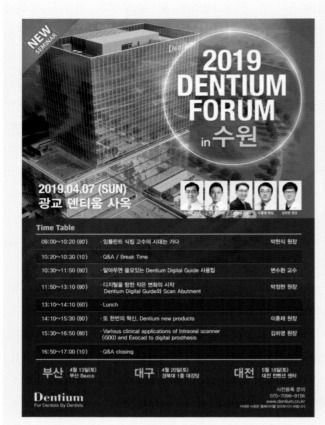

Dentium implant forum poster in 2019

with the guide goddess and another doctor I call analog god. Both of them like and support me, so I'm even more grateful and like them.

Although I was not able to participate as I was in the United States, the Dentium Symposium held in 2019 was also a digital-related topic. If you look at the title of the first lecture, it is <The era of implant placement experts is gone>. Now, as digital guide implants become popular, implant cases that are well planted can be seen commonly on Instagram and Facebook. To be honest, as someone was was quite proud of my implant path without using guides, I am also bit sad to see this digital age coming.

There is one good case as an example of how digital guide implantation worked really well for me. In March 2019, I had an implant seminar scheduled in Boston and was scheduled to catch an overnight flight to New York. However, my employee called an hour before I should leave for the airport and asked to do the surgery. Even though it was all prepared with the guide, there were too many implants to be inserted.

The patient was one of my associated dentist's uncle. He had a heart valve surgery and had other systemic diseases, so he was worried about the implant surgery. So, after consulting with the associate dentist, I decided to perform the guided surgery. the timing was also good as Osstem started to produce guides for edentulous arches but I didn't expect to do this one hour before I scheduled to leave for the airport. Not too sure what my staff were thinking... Did they think that New York is just a stone's throw away from the clinic or I can just catch next flight if I miss it? However, **the advantage of guided surgery is in the shortening the procedure time.** It was the first ever edentulous guide and we had to do sinus elevation. I also took all the clinical photos, but I was able to finish it within an hour. After the procedure I packed my bags in a hurry and took a taxi without even checking the panorama x-ray. On the way to the airport, I asked my staff to send a photos to me so I can post them on my instagram. I checked in at the airport and tried to post them on Instagram in the lounge, but while I was enlarging and checking the photo... Oh, no, what is this? I could see the perforated left sinus

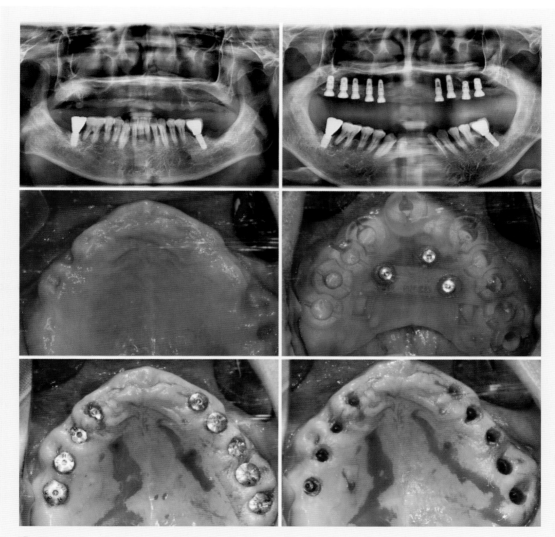

📷 1.57 This is the case I prepared to post on instagram but ended up not doing so due to sinus perofration.

with bone particles in it. Since I rarely experienced tear during sinus elevation in the past, I placed the implant after bone graft as usual. However this time this happened and I believe that it is the biggest drawback of guided surgery (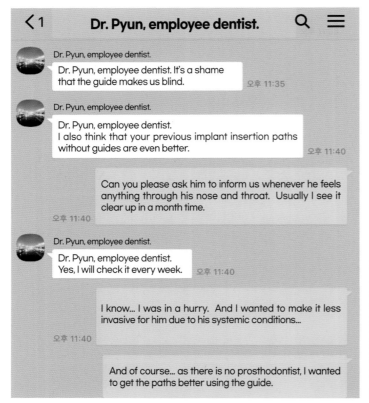 **1.57**). Later Osstem developed the sinus elevation kit for the guided surgery, but at that time there were no such systems and I did it just using osteotome. However, with the guide installed, it was different from what I expected. It was a case that usually worked well with almost no failure, so I didn't worry and followed the usual rules, but it seemed that when the drilling was done through the guide, it already perforated the sinus membrane. It would have been better if I had calculated the distance manually as I usually do, but it seemed that I was overdoing it by just trusting the guide. In the end, I could not post the case on instagram and sent a message to my colleague asking for help and got on the plane (**1.58**).

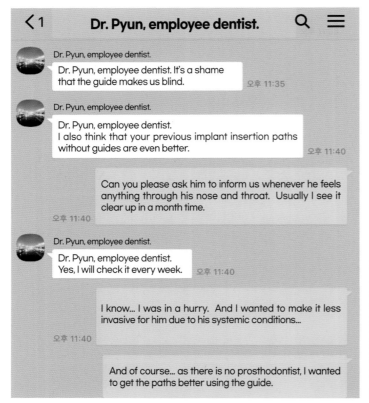

1.58 Text messages with the my colleague who helped me with the case. He is also one of co-authors of this book
He was my employee at that time but now he is my partner and co-director. He is such a nice person who said that it would have been better to implant them free hand with my skills to make me feel better.

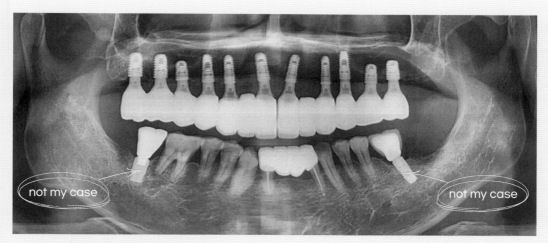

📷 **1.59 Final panoramic radiograph**
Two more implants at location of 11 and 21 were added after a few months for a better support.

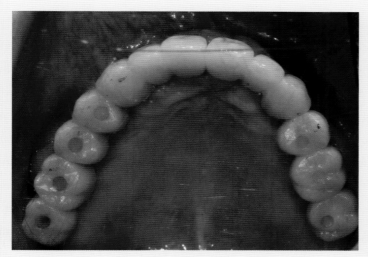

📷 **1.60 Photo after setting the final prosthesis**
I understand that it was done after watching for a long time with a temporary prosthesis. Because I was in the US, a new prosthodontist did the prosthesis, but there were many things I didn't like about it. It's also the reason why I can't even show the picture from the front. I feel that it would have been better if the final impression was taken after reshaping the gingiva more with the temporary prosthesis. Considering only the cosmetic aspect, it would have been better to place only one of the two implants.

After returning to Korea, two more implants were placed in the anterior region to finish. The two anterior teeth were considered from the initial planning stage, but decided not to do so initially. I did not like the posterior implant, so I decided to place an additional implant to separate the posterior and anterior bridge, and I proceeded with the analog placement. My associate dentist suggested that we add 27 and 37 implants, but I politely refused. If you look at the final occlusal clinical picture, you can see that the hole location is not as ideal despite the fact that the entire surgical process from drilling to final implant placement was done guided (📷 **1.60**).

Let's anticipate the future trend of digital guide implantation. I participated in the Osstem Faculty Seminar in December 2017. At this time, I had no interest in digital guides at all and it was a place to listen to the experiences of pioneers. The lecturer listed the issues he had experienced while doing the guided implant, and wrote the expression "Moments of deep frustration" as the title. From the title, I could feel the agony. However, now that I am interested in digital guides and look back at the slides, most of the problems have been solved or improved. That's a lot of progress in such a short period of time.

In a recent digital-related seminar, there was a slide showing how short it took to develop from 1G → 2G → 3G → 4G → 5G. It must have been to show that the pace of change in the future will be faster than the path we have taken so far. No one knows how and how much digital dentistry will develop, but even if you do not immediately switch to digital dentistry, you should always turn on the antenna and watch the degree of change. Of course, **if analog skills are still insufficient, increasing analog implant skills should be given priority.**

Lastly, I want to show you the advertisement from Dr. Young-Goo Huh, director of Neo-Biotech, who is known as the Edison of the dental world. He created a guide in less than 30 minutes using the system he developed and placed implant in his jaw himself (📷 **1.61**). I'm still a beginner in the digital field, and I'm not particularly interested in Neo products, so I have not studied the system yet but if you are already a Neo-Biotech user or interested in the digital technology, you should try this system. It seems that the companies that were at the forefront of the digital field are now being a little neglected in the market. I think the reason is because the focus was on making and selling guides. I think the era of companies making guides and selling them to dentists for a fee is over. Rather, I wonder if such implant companies would have been able to remain as a world-famous guide company if they opened their software early and focused more on program sales and advanced technology promotion than guide sales.

Gone are the days of the expert in implant placement. Now you can easily create a guide so that you can place the implant straight up right away. **The key is, "Which implant is the best placed implant?"** Now is the time to raise your bar with me. The era has come that allows you to place implants as you want by making guides and **now it is rather more important to know which implant design is a good design.** To do that, you must now understand the implant itself.

(주)네오바이오텍 임상 네오바이오텍이 지난 10월 13일 '2019 월드심포지엄'을 개최했다. 이날 허영구 대표가 환자가 돼 진행된 라이브 서저리 증례를 소개한다.

"네오, 바로가이드로 임플란트 자가 식립!"

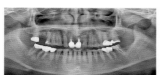

환자(허영구 원장)는 16번 치아가 Missing 된 상태였고, 잔존골이 9mm, 클래스 3로 Sinus Lifting 과정을 진행하기로 했다.

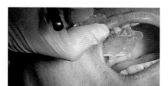

우선, 구강에 알맞은 Pre-Guide를 사용하기 위해 Trial-Tray로 Bite를 측정한다.

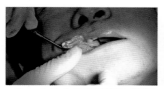

Composite Resine이 충전되어 있는 PGS13을 식립할 위치에 알맞게 위치시킨 후 수직으로 지긋이 누른다.

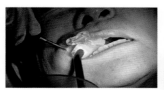

Buccal과 Occlusion, 교합면에 20초 정도 Curing을 한다. 중간중간 차가운 물에 담궈 Cooling을 시킨다.

Pre-Guide를 수직으로 분리한 후 치아가 닿은 부분도 20초 정도 Curing을 한다. Curing을 마친 Pre-Guide를 구강 내에 다시 장착하여 움직임이 있는지 확인한다. 움직임이 없는 것을 확인한 후, Pre-Guide를 문 상태로 CT를 촬영한다. 촬영한 CT 데이터는 바로가이드 소프트웨어로 전송되며 대략 2분 정도의 시간이 걸린다.

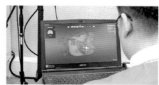

CT 데이터를 DICOM 파일 형태로 전용 소프트웨어에 옮긴다.

VARO Plan S/W는 CT 데이터 하나로 Surgical Guide를 제작 할 수 있기 때문에 구강 스캔 또는 모델 스캔 과정이 필요 없다.

Radiopaque Marker 5개 중 3개의 점을 골라 CT 데이터와 PGS13 트레이와의 데이터를 정확히 정합시킨다.

미리 치아를 디자인 하여 이를 토대로 자동으로 임플란트가 위치되며, 사이즈나 각도를 자유롭게 움직여 원하는 곳에 식립 계획을 세운다.

환자(허영구 원장)에게는 직경 5mm의 임플란트를 식립하기로 하고 Planning 과정이 마무리됐다. Planning을 마치면 STL파일이 NC파일로 자동 변환된다. 이 데이터를 VARO Mill로 전송한다.

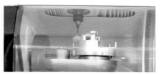

Tray를 알맞은 곳에 위치시키면 10분 안에 Milling이 완성된다. 환자(허영구 원장)는 스스로 뼈 상태는 Crestal D2, 중간부분 D3, Apical D2 상태로 진단했다. 수술은 직경 5mm, 길이 10mm Fixture를 식립할 예정이며, 상악동 거상 2mm와 뼈 이식을 계획했다.

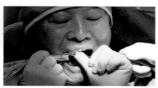

바로가이드를 Positioning 한 후 Initial Drilling 이 시작됐다. 무절개 시술을 위한 Tissue Punching 이 진행됐다. Bone Planner를 통해 뼈를 평평하게 했다. Pilot Drill 직경 2.2 직경, 길이 8.5로 드릴링이 시작되었다. 모든 과정은 환자(허영구 원자)가 직접 시술했다.

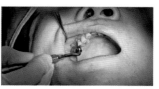

Sinus Imperial Cortical을 열기 위해 S-Leamer을 사용했다. 뼈이식은 DM Bone(합성골)을 수화시켜 뼈이식을 진행했다. 상악동 내부로 골이식이 진행됐다.

골이식을 끝낸 후 바로가이드를 다시 위치시켜 Final Drill이 진행됐다.

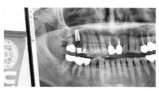

환자(허영구 원장)는 활성화 된 임플란트를 엔진 핸드피스에 연결하고 식립을 진행했다.

가이드 준비까지 걸리는 시간은 25분도 채 되지 않았다. 김종엽 원장이 토크 렌치를 사용해 마무리를 하고 초기 고정력을 확인한 결과 40Ncm로 좋은 수치가 나왔다.

허영구 원장은 "바로가이드를 직접 사용해 보니 고정이 잘 되어 가이드를 붙잡고 있지 않아도 되었다. 정확한 Impression으로 고정력이 우수했다"고 전했다.

또한 "30년간 임플란트 수술을 했지만 직접 식립하는 것은 처음이라 많이 긴장됐다. 환자, 술자, 경영자로서 큰 결단이 필요했다. 그러나 Self-Surgery를 진행하기로 결정한 것은 바로가이드에 관심을 갖고 계신 분들께 보여드리고 싶었다. 정확한 가이드가 있다면 가능하다고 생각했다"고 말했다.

네오바이오텍 관계자는 "Sinus Case에서 가이드를 활용한 Self 임플란트 식립 퍼포먼스는 전세계 최초다. 이번 라이브 서저리는 환자(허영구 원장)와 술자의 설명이 덧붙여졌고 Sinus까지 진행했으나 디지털 가이드 준비까지 30분도 채 걸리지 않았다. 신개념 디지털 가이드 '바로가이드'의 환자 상담 후 30분 만에 가이드 제작이라는 컨셉을 증명한 것"이라며 "본인이 개발한 제품에 대해 웬만한 자신감이 없었다면 시도조차 할 수 없는 일이었다. 허영구 원장님께 바로가이드의 정확성과 안전성을 전세계에 알렸다"고 전했다.

📷 **1.61 Neo-Biotech's Guide System**
Dr. Young-koo Huh, the Edison of dentistry became a patient himself by making a guide and self-implanteded using it.

https://youtu.be/1fpyB_VwBns

1-2

Korean Occlusion

Mastering dental implants

Korean Occlusion

While in the US, I met a lot of good people, and one of them is this handsome Periodontist (📷 2.1). He graduated from the Department of Periodontology at UCLA and conducted many international seminars. He is already well known in Korea. Since he majored in periodontology, he also lectured a lot on esthetic implants in the anterior region. He is also a great Marathoner.

When I visited him I saw a promotional poster hanging on the wall. It was a picture of an anterior esthetic implant case.

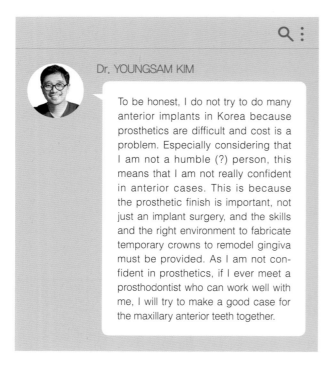

Dr. YOUNGSAM KIM

To be honest, I do not try to do many anterior implants in Korea because prosthetics are difficult and cost is a problem. Especially considering that I am not a humble (?) person, this means that I am not really confident in anterior cases. This is because the prosthetic finish is important, not just an implant surgery, and the skills and the right environment to fabricate temporary crowns to remodel gingiva must be provided. As I am not con-fident in prosthetics, if I ever meet a prosthodontist who can work well with me, I will try to make a good case for the maxillary anterior teeth together.

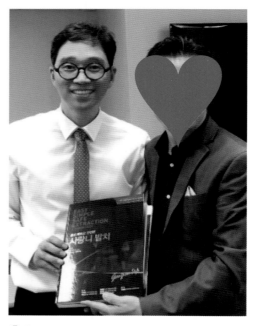

📷 2.1 Photo taken after wisdom tooth extraction seminar in LA

At that time, he was performing surgery on the maxillary anterior teeth and he took all the photos and even made temporary crown himself. Seeing a master like him doing them all by himself made me think, 'Have I not lived my life too easily?'

Anyway, going to the main topic, I noticed that ANKYLOS® was used in the implants placed in the maxillary anterior teeth in his seminar poster. Ankylos implant is the one I mention the most in my implant lectures. It is German-made implant system developed by Professor Georg-H Nentwig of Goethe university.

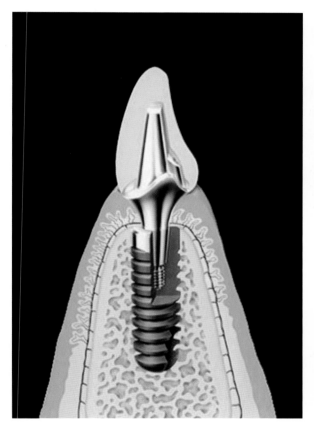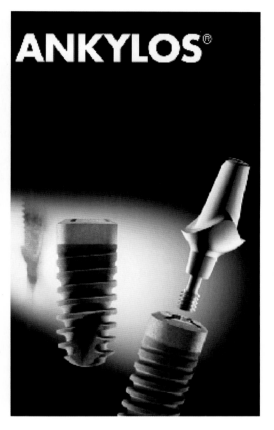

2.2 German ANKYLOS® Implant Poster

As I briefly mentioned earlier, modern implants use Astra's abutment connection structure, Straumann's surface treatment and the body shape of Ankylos. Looking at it now, there is nothing I find it strange, but in the past, I thought it was a very unusual and strange implant. As the fixture shape of other implants start to resemble that of ankylos, it doesn't feel strange anymore. The thread becomes deeper toward the apex and is almost non-existent towards the coronal making it like the cylinder shape. The body itself is straight, but the coronal part when drilling is enlarged almost to the size of the implant while the lower part with deep thread is drilled small in order to achieve better primary stability at the apex where the bone quality is not optimal. It is fair to say that all modern implant placement styles are from Ankylos.

Ankylos is probably not that famous for its name, but it has been around while maintaining its form and is a traditional brand name implant. In this chapter, I am going to talk about its thin and elongated abutment rather than the fixture shape of Ankylos (which is trending these days). The fixture shape of Ankyos system will be discussed in a later chapter.

Let's have a look the fixture shape of the world's top three implants system Nobel, Straumann, and

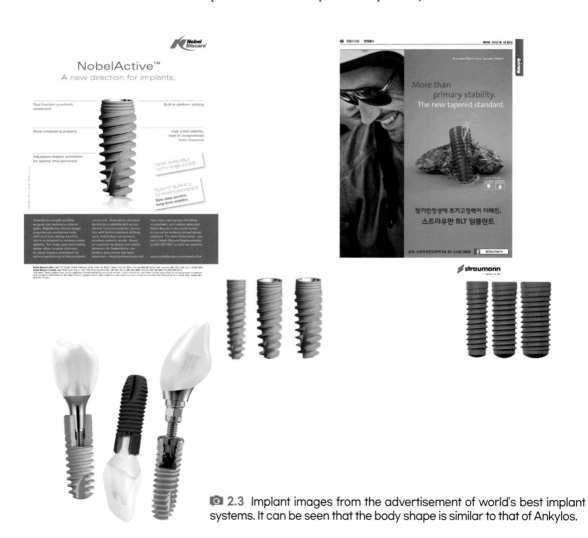

📷 2.3 Implant images from the advertisement of world's best implant systems. It can be seen that the body shape is similar to that of Ankylos.

Astra implant. It can be seen that most of them have a body shape similar to that of Ankylos.

Why did the handsome doctor do the anterior esthetic implant with Ankylos? It's probably because of Ankylos' thin and straight abutment. Ankylos is an internal friction type and its angle is "5.74°". so there is almost no gap and it achieves cold welding (there are many different opinions but it can be understood that it is attached almost like one body without gaps, and I call it clinical cold welding) and thanks to the long and thin abutment, it promotes thick and healthy periodontal tissues.

More importantly, the Ankylos is one of less common system which is still made from CP Titanium Grade 2.

Although the material of the abutment is not described in detail, some say that it is the same Grade 2, and others say that it changed to Grade 4 in last 1-2 years. (I recently asked a salesperson at Sidex and according to him there are no changes)

Anyway, Ankylos is an implant that has a long, thin abutment and it is its greatest strength. And another characteristic of Ankylos is that the diameter of the abutment does not increase even if the diameter of the implant increases. If you compare it to the typical Astra-type implant, it's like abutment used for a mini-size implant with a diameter of 3.5 is also used for 4.0, 4.5, 5.0, and etc (📷 2.4).

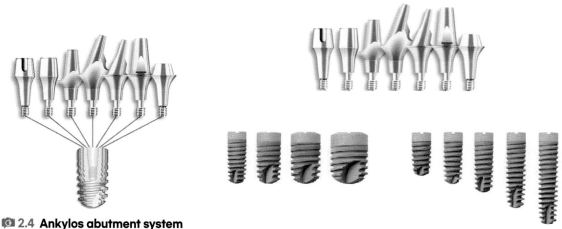

📷 2.4 Ankylos abutment system
Ankylos use the same abutment whether the diameter increases or the length increases.

In August 2017, I attended the Osstem Faculty Seminar and listened to a lecture from a dentist from Brazil, which was very interesting (📷 2.5). He graduated from São Paulo University, studied implants there, opened his own practice in Brazil and worked there for more than 10 years. In 2015, he obtained a Korean dentist's license and moved to Korea.

He said that 70% of his patients in Brazil were Asians and about half of them were Koreans, so about one-third of his patients were Koreans. He said he used a lot of German-made Ankylos implants. At the beginning of the lecture he listed advantages of Ankylos system and, as mentioned above, he cited healthy periodontal tissues as the greatest strength.

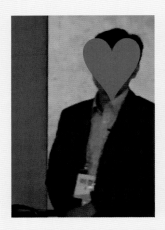
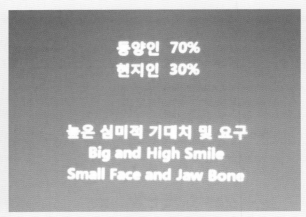

2.5 Osstem faculty lecture by the dentist from Brazil and his slide

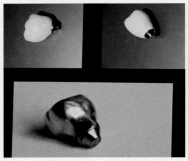
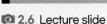

2.6 Lecture slide

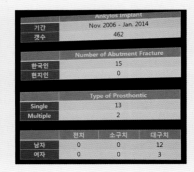

Ankylos Implant		
기간	Nov. 2006 - Jan. 2014	
갯수	462	
Number of Abutment Fracture		
한국인	15	
현지인	0	
Type of Prosthontic		
Single	13	
Multiple	2	

	전치	소구치	대구치
남자	0	0	12
여자	0	0	3

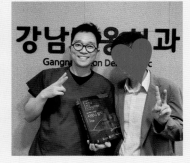

He is currently translating my wisdom teeth extraction book into Portoguese together with 3 other Brazillian and 1 Portuguese dentist.

However, as time passed, the abutment of Ankylos began to break. So he called the manufacturer however they said they couldn't figure out the cause as it was a product that sold well without any problems everywhere else. So he decided to analyze the cause himself and analyzed the fracture pattern. Of the total 462 he placed, 15 were broken, and as shown in 2.6, all 15 were from his Korean patients. Three of them were from female patients but most were from men and their molar replacements. 'Why only Koreans? After thinking for a long time, he came to his own conclusion that 'Koreans have large faces, strong masticatory muscles, and there is a big difference in food culture. Especially considering that they eat a lot of food like dried radish, dried squid, etc.

I also contacted a senior colleague who implanted a lot of Ankylos in Korea, He placed around 300 implants between 1998 and 2010 and had more than 10 fractures including 1 bridge failure and they were all from young male patients. So since 2010, he stopped placing them and around that time he was also asked by Ankylos sales person to help removing some broken cases that were placed at other clinics.

Then, suddenly, he remembered asking about this issue to a dentist who had a master's degree at Goethe University in Germany. The dentist asked this question to one of Ankylos advisor specialists and his answer was that it's probably due to the fact that Koreans eat foods like dried squid. The reason behind why a world class name brand like Ankylos was unusually failing in Korea was due to the Koreans' extremely strong occlusion force. I also remember hearing about many occlusal filling materials failing in Korea while there are no issues in other countries.

As another example, consider the occlusal material of the posterior implant. Since gold got expenive, PFM was mainly used. In Korea, unless a Zirconia crown is used, most male patients get metal occlusal surface. Even for female patients, even when they demand tooth coloured material, I always insist that at least the disto-occlusal surface of lower second molars were done with metal. The reason is otherwise it is just a matter of time before the porcelain start to break from the distal. Most Korean dentists would understand, but surprisingly, foreign dentists ask if it is necessary to do so.

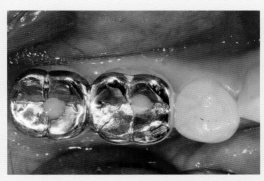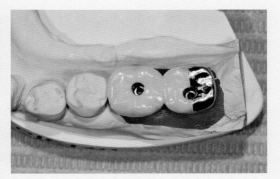

📷 **2.7 Common posterior implant crowns in Korea**
When a patient asks for tooth colored occlusal surface I insist on using metal for at least distal 1/3 of 7s.

This is probably why (along with many other reasons) inlays and onlays are more common instead of composite resins and after root canal treatment, crown is done most of times. Otherwise the strong occlusal force will easily wear and break materials.

As another example, let's talk about All On 4 which has been popular since around 15 years ago. All on 4 was not a huge hit in Korea. Why? This is because the prosthesis mostly fractured. No matter how strong 4 implants were the prosthesis fractures were very common and even when the prosthesis

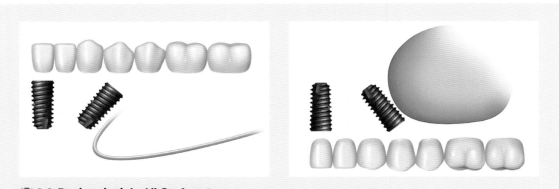

📷 **2.8 Basic principle All On 4 system**
The concept to avoid inferior alveolar nerve in mandible and sinus in maxilla. The apical of the implant is placed mesially and the coronal part is facing distal.

did not fracture, implants were overloaded sometimes. I personally don't like the concept but we still need to think about why the concept was not popular in Korea.

The basic principle of All On 4 is to allow the positioning of bridge teeth as far back as possible by tilting the implant distally while avoiding the maxillary sinus and mandibular canal when the maxillary sinus is too low or there is insufficient bone in the mandible (📷 **2.8**). However sometimes this concept of tilting the implant is used even when the bone is sufficient. The reason for this is that when the implants are placed straight the thread of the implant fixture receives the occlusal force, but when implanted at an angle of about 30°, the occlusal force is transmitted to the entire implant body, enabling immediate loading.

In fact, there is a study done on the ideal tilting angle required to allow the whole body to withstand the vertical loading well and the result was 30°. I don't quite agree with this part and I believe that if the bone is good, the immediate loading is possible without tilting the implants. And what is certain is that the more implant you place, the better. As a result, these all-on-four concept seminars were held by Nobel in Europe, where implant prices are expensive, and BioHorizon, a company that makes external hexa type of strong alloy in the United States.

These All On 4 concept was developed by the Portuguese Doctor named Paulo Malo. I held a lecture on wisdom tooth extraction in Italy in September 2019, and a dentist named Dr. Luis Beres from Portugal attended my lecture. As he traveled long distance for my lecture, we went to sightseeing together and got to know each other, and I had a chance to ask him about his opinion on All On 4. He joked that the Portugal is a relatively poor country in Europe (for reference, GDP per capita is around 20,000 USD), and people spend a lot of money on making them look better but not much for their oral health and it's hard for Portuguese dentists to make a living. He said that many patients even demand their front teeth to be fixed nicely for esthetic reason while they have mouthful of caries and this type of demand also created environment where concept like All On 4 can be introduced. (This is

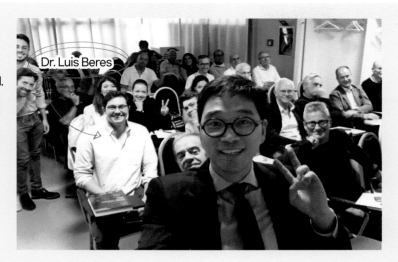

◎ 2.9 Photo of my first Italian wisdom tooth extraction class in September 2019
Dr. Luis Beres from Portugal. Currently, he is translating my wisdom teeth extraction book together with the Korean dentist from Brazil and three other Brazillian dentists.

Dr. Luis Beres

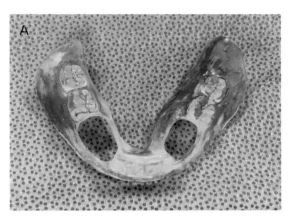

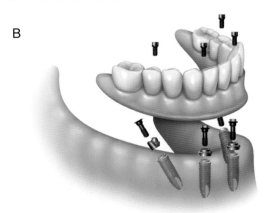

◎ 2.10 **A**: Stents manufactured for All On 4 surgery at UCLA School of Dentistry **B**: Basic All On 4 concept

purely his opinion and I do not know anything about dentistry in Portugal). Also when I was at UCLA Oral Surgery department, I often saw that four implants were placed with posterior implants tilted even when there was enough bone.

◎ 2.10 is the same case described. The prosthodontic deparment makes such guide and the distal implants are tilted as much as possible within that hole (which covers from canine to second premolar) so as you can see on the picture next the bridge is secured at the occlusal surface of the premolar. On the x-ray, the bone volume was good that even 16 implants could be placed without bone grafting. To me it seemed that they just wanted to do all on 4. I thought it could be done by just placing 6 implants straight.

If it was my case, I would have placed 8 or 10 implants and section the prosthesis for each area instead of placing just 4 implants especially considering that implant fixtures are not expensive. (of course, in the US they are expensive. Mostly these concepts are introduced by companies with expensive fixtures. I remember that BioHorizon external hexa was used in this case at UCLA.)

Case study

Let's have a look at one of my similar cases.

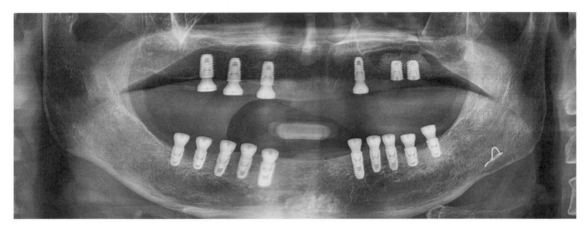

📷 2.11 A case where I placed more implants than what my prosthodontist planned. (I was told off by the prosthodontist for not following his plan)

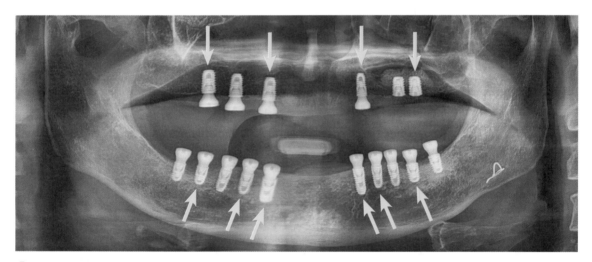

📷 2.12 The original plan by the prosthodontist in yellow arrow. (Fixed prosthesis on 6 implants on mandible and overdenture with 4 implants on maxilla was originally planned.)

In this case, the prosthodontic department asked me to only place where the yellow arrows are pointing, but the patient was the father-in-law of my comedian friend who was very close, so I placed a little more (📷 2.13) and it ended up being a fixed case for the lower and a temporary denture for the top (📷 2.13).

After the fixed lower was placed, the patient wanted to make the upper to be fixed as well. There are many patients who say that they feel like they are born again when a denture is replaced by a fixed prosthesis. So once they get lower fixed, many patients, especially male patients who don't care much

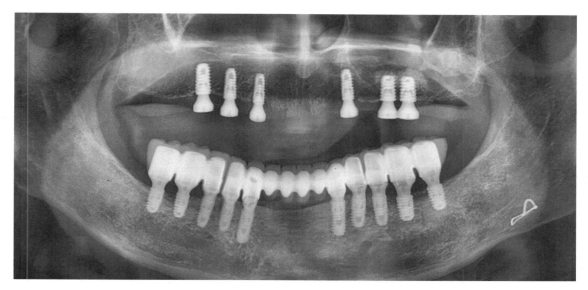

📷 **2.13** After the initial treatment

about aesthetics, often want a upper to be fixed as well. To us Koreans, being able to chew properly again is so important.

So, in the end, I placed additional implants and made fixed prosthesis for upper as well (📷 **2.14**).

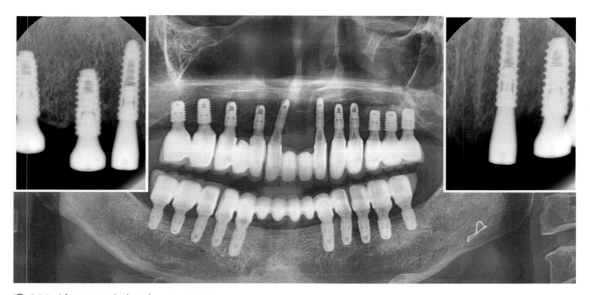

📷 **2.14** After completing the treatment

The panoramic x-ray on 📷 **2.14** shows that the implant placed on the position of 12 is angled. However this is due to the fact that it was placed palatally and two PA x-rays confirm that the angulation is not as much as it appears on the panoramic x-ray.

As shown in the case above, in Korea, distal cantilever is usually not done. Due to very poor prognosis caused by strong occlusal force in the posterior region, Korean dentists do not make prostheses with distal cantilever. However, I routinely see up to 2 distal cantilevers are done in other countries such as in the United States and Australia. Also many dentists there seem to think that second molars do not need to be replaced. Some even question me why I over-treat by placing implants to replace second molars when they see my cases on my lectures or instagram.

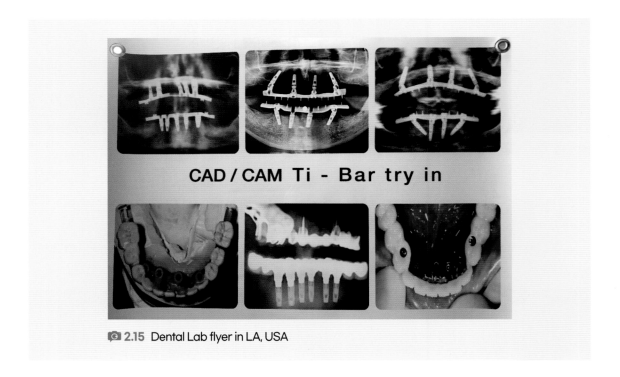

📷 2.15 Dental Lab flyer in LA, USA

When I went to an implant seminar of Korean dentists in LA there was a banner showing LA's Korean dental laboratory's work (📷 2.15). So I asked them, "I know that these types of prostheses are common in the United States, but do you do this to Korean patients as well?" and they said that this is for local Americans only and they do not suggest All On 4 or distal cantilever prostheses to Koreans. Koreans even break the world-class luxury implant like Ankylos. Distal cantilever of two teeth on implant bridge is almost impossible to Koreans. (Interestingly, the skills of the Korean dental technicians are also very good. Some even say that most famous American actors' aesthetic cases are done by Korean dental technicians...)

No surprise as Koreans are people who value their food and joy of chewing so much. So it does not make any sense to design prostheses with distal cantilever for people like this even when they have sufficient bone distally. I would rather place 6-8 cheaper implants than 4 expensive implants. And needless to say, in terms of maintenance, All On 4 or such a fixed cases are not very advantageous.

임플란트 만족도 최후방 치아 '최고'

후치부·전치부 순 저작·심리 기능 개선

임플란트 식립 후 환자들은 최후방치에 대한 만족도가 가장 높은 것으로 나타났다.

특히 임플란트 식립 후 삶의 질에서는 저작·사회·심리적 기능이 모두 증진되는 것으로 분석됐다.

박지영 씨(대구대 산업·행정대학원)가 석사논문인 '임플란트 매식 전·후의 구강건강관련 치료만족도에 관한 연구'에서 대구광역시 소재 6개 치과 내원 환자 145명의 자료를 분석한 결과에 따르면 임플란트 식립에 대한 치료만족도는 최후방치에서 96.6%로 가장 높았다. 이어 후치부가 85.9%, 전치부가 71.4%로 각각 조사됐다.

식립 후 재내원 의사에서는 최후방치(100%), 후치부(98%), 전치부(78.6%) 등 전 부위에서 전반적으로 높았으며, 임플란트 식립 후 추천 의사 역시 최후방치(96.9%), 후치부(93.9%), 전치부(71.4%) 등으로 높았다.

특히 이들 환자들의 경우 임플란트 식립 후에 삶의 질이 전반적으로 개선된 것으로 나타났다.

저작기능의 경우 2.67점에서 3.62점(5점 만점 리커드 척도), 사회적 기능은 2.67점에서 3.33점, 심리적 기능은 2.46점에서 3.75점으로 개선되는 등 저작·사회·심리적 기능에 대한 만족도가 높아진 것이다.

박 씨는 이번 논문과 관련 "임플란트 매식 전·후의 구강건강관련 삶의 질 변화와 치료 만족도를 측정해 분석함으로써 환자 관점에서 임플란트 매식의 효과에 대한 평가 자료를 축적하는 데 의미가 있다"고 밝혔다.

윤선영 기자 young@kda.or.kr

2.16 This is an excerpt from an article in the Korean Dental Newsletter dated June 10, 2013. Implant satisfaction was the highest for the most distal one. As expected...

Anyway, the reason why I talked about the occlusal power of Koreans in particular in this chapter is to tell you that **what works in Korea will work anywhere else.** When it comes to the length and the diameter of the implant, if it worked for Koreans you can assume that it will work in other countries too. Some people say that because westerners are usually bigger and stronger what works in Korea should not be applied to them but when it comes to occlusal forces I think it is a completely opposite. Koreans are not only at the top in the world with mobile phones, semiconductors, ship building and K-pop. They are at the top with the occlusal force. When Korean dentists say that it works, it will surely work anywhere in the world.

Dr. YOUNGSAM KIM'S

CLINICAL NOTES

EASY SIMPLE SAFE EFFICIENT

MASTERING DENTAL IMPLANTS

The Essential Elements for Success in Dental Implants

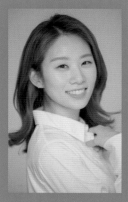

Dr. Addie Y. Chang

B.A. in Chemistry from Carnegie Mellon University D.M.D. from Tufts University School of Dental Medicine Private Practice in Tukwila, Washington, USA

It was a great honor to be part of Dr. Kim's implant book. He is an inspiration to lot of doctors and I enjoy learning by working closely with him at the live implant surgery courses in Mexico. He wanted me to put here how charming he is in person. If you haven't already, I hope you find the time to meet Dr. Kim in person!

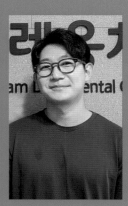

Dr. Hector Shin

I graduated from Griffith University in 2015 and am currently working in the Brisbane/Gold coast area for about 7 years. I started my implant journey about 2 years ago after attending Dr. Kim's Live surgery in Tijuana for about 2-3 times.

2

Implant Basic Fundamentals

Knowledge is power

2-1 Dental Implant Materials
and Surface Treatments

2-2 Implant Shape and Thread

2-3 Classification and Understanding
of Abutments

● Implant Basic Fundamentals

Knowledge is power

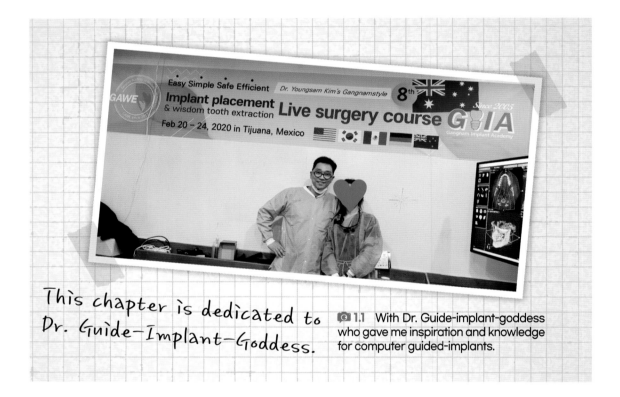

This chapter is dedicated to Dr. Guide-Implant-Goddess.

📷 **1.1** With Dr. Guide-implant-goddess who gave me inspiration and knowledge for computer guided-implants.

I talk to Dr. Guide-implant-goddess (I call her by this name because she did thousands of guided-implant surgeries.) We talk about implant quite often. One time I was talking to her about implant materials and alloy, and she asked me, "what is an alloy?" I was surprised when she asked me that question since she has already placed more than 2,000 implants in the last two years. I think it is critical to know the basics of implants because **sometimes you have to treatment plan for long term care for other doctors' implant surgeries.** I once had a lecture in Los Angeles for 1 hour about this topic, and a lot of doctors loved it so ended up being 2 hours instead. So this section about implant materials has always been part of my lecture ever since then.

Dr. YOUNGSAM KIM

I used to teach the most about the basic implant theory lecture in 2006. At the time, the basics were more important and taught more in lecutres than the clinical side of the implant surgery. In 2005, I read a lot of papers so I was able to teach in 2006 about the basics. After that, implant lectures have been more focused on the surgery itself, so I didn't lecture about the basics for over 10 years. I want people to know the basics about the implant materials, so please read it casually to understand the general idea.

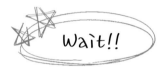

If you want to learn about placing implant first, please move on to **Part 3**. You can always come back to this chapter when you read this book again the second time. 😊

2-1 Dental Implant Materials and Surface Treatments

Mastering dental implants

Implant Materials

Everyone knows that implants are made of titanium. Unlike in the early days of implants, people are not very interested in the success rate of implants, so they do not seem to have much interest in the materials. However, you should know the basics to not be fooled when talking to implant company sales representatives. First of all, titanium is divided into pure titanium (commercially pure, CP) and titanium alloy (alloy). CP Titanium is classified based on the purity - Grade 1, being the purest, to Grade 4. As it goes to Grade 4, the mechanical properties improve. However, since casting becomes impossible, you can think that it can be machined only by cutting mechanically.

There are so many types of titanium alloy. Most of the things that are light and hard, from bicycles to airplanes, can be thought of as titanium alloys. Titanium alloy used in implants should be considered Ti-6Al-4V (Grade 5). These days, it is called the first-generation dental titanium alloy because it has been expanded a bit, but it is still the most important material. You can consider in 90% titanium, there is a mixture of 6% aluminum and 4% vanadium. The mechanical properties are twice stronger than that of CP Titanium. Recently, a material called Ti-6Al-4V ELI (Grade 23) has been used more widely in replacement of Grade 5 alloy for implants. You can consider Grade 5 as extremely low (Extra Low Interstitial Elements, ELI) contents of oxygen, nitrogen, hydrogen, and iron in Ti-6Al-4V alloy. I usually just call it titanium alloy (Grade 5) without distinguishing it.

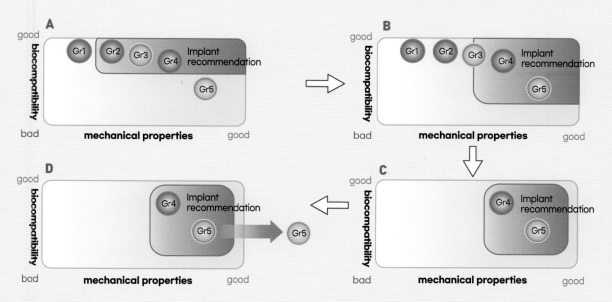

📷 **1.2** Changes in implant recommendation according to the type of titanium advertised by implant manufacturing companies

📷 **1.2A** is a figure from Osstem (Hiossen) implant company back when I was studying about the basics of implants. At the time, implant fixture was made in Grade 3, the abutment was made in Grade 2 since we don't want to damage it, and the screw was made in Grade 4 or alloy. Recently, it has changed to where the fixtures are made in Grade 4 and the rest of the abutment and screws are made in alloy, as you can see the change from 📷 **1.2A** to 📷 **1.2B, C**. If I want to make any changes to this illustration, I would move the grade 5 alloy to some where farther away (📷 **1.2D**).

Now you can safely assume that **the implant fixtures are made of CP Titanium Grade 4, and the screws and the abutments are mostly made of alloy (Grade 5).**

Is Titanium Alloy safe?

I searched "Titanium Alloy" on Wikipedia.

> Grade 5 also known as Ti6Al4V, Ti-6Al-4V or Ti 6-4 is the most commonly used alloy.
> It has a chemical composition of 6% aluminum, 4% vanadium, 0.25% (maximum) iron, 0.2% (maximum) oxygen, and the remainder titanium. It is significantly stronger than commercially pure titanium while having the same stiffness and thermal properties (excluding thermal conductivity, which is about 60% lower in Grade 5 Ti than in CP Ti). Among its many advantages, it is heat treatable. This Grade is an excellent combination of strength, corrosion resistance, weld and fabricability.
>
> Source: Wikipedia

So is titanium alloy really harmful? When I was studying about implants in 2005, I read a lot of research papers. It was difficult to find all the papers that I read so I will state briefly here from what I remember.

First of all, there were some rumors where aluminum causes alzheimers and banadium causes cancer but there is not enough evidence for them. Also based on papers, lectures and my experiences, I have not noticed any difference. Since the Endopore implant is also made of alloy, I was able to learn a lot about related research from researchers at Endopore.

15 years later, I can only remember this one phrase - "only minimally toxic." No one has stated that titanium alloy is perfect. There are many controversies and quarrels, and we need more research about the toxicity, it is still "only minimally toxic". **Remember that although alloy is different from CP titanium, it is "only minimally toxic."** The more important thing is the allergic reaction to various metals. When we are talking about amalgam, mercury is the main concern, but some have different allergic reaction to different metals in the amalgam. Therefore, in the case of implants using alloys, I think that unpredictable failure may occur with extremely low probability due to an allergic reaction to aluminum, vanadium, or trace metals used. In addition to the aforementioned amalgam and titanium alloy, this can happen with all the metals used in dentistry. Even after considering all the other reasons of failure, maybe you could consider failure due to allergic reaction to some metals.

📷 **1.3** shows the materials used for different implant companies. You can consider most of them as Grade 4. However, it is said that the Ankylos, which is brittle, is made of Grade 2, and the abutment is also made of the same material which is why it is even more brittle. It is said that attempts

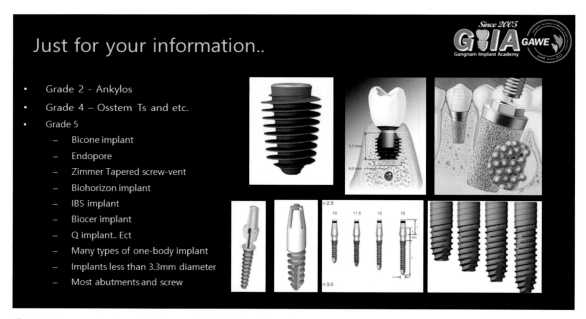

📷 1.3 From my lecture slide to explain Titanium Grade

📑 1.1 Titanium Grade Strength Comparison

Material	Modulus (GPa)	Ultimate Tensile Strength (MPa)	Yield Strength (MPa)	Elongation (%)	Density (g/cc)	Type of Alloy
Cp Ti grade I	102	240	170	24	4.5	α
Cp Ti grade II	102	345	275	20	4.5	α
Cp Ti grade III	102	450	380	18	4.5	α
Cp Ti grade IV	104	550	483	15	4.5	α
Ti–6Al–4V– ELI	113	860	795	10	4.4	α+β
Ti–6Al–4V	113	930	860	10	4.4	α+β
Ti–A1–7Nb	114	900–1050	880–950	8–15	4.4	α+β
Ti–5Al–2.5Fe	112	1020	895	15	4.4	α+β
Ti–15Zr–4Nb–2Ta–0.2Pd	94–99	715–919	693–806	18–28	4.4	α+β
Ti–29Nb–13Ta–4.6Zr	80	911	864	13.2	4.4	β

Source: Adopted from Lemons, 1990 [5]; Craig, 1993 [6]; Wataha, 1996 [4]; McCracken, 1999 [15].

📑 1.1 Compares the titanium grade strength. I also graduated dental school a long time ago so I forgot all of it too. But let's not focus too hard on this topic. We let the implant companies and researchers to do all the work, and we can pick the ones that we like and do the implant surgery well.

have been made to increase the strength of the ankylos in the molar area for the past 1-2 years by increasing the thickness or increasing the grade. I am not too certain, but I have not verified it to provide accurate information.

Here, it is necessary to take a look at the types of implants made of alloy. The examples, as shown in the next page, are the Bicon and Endopore implants, two of the most popular short implants. Both are unique in shape and since the implant is placed by hitting it with a mallet, it is thought that strength is more important. And other examples include Zimmer and BioHorizon implants.

I know that there are still many implants that are made of alloy. In Korea, IBS implant company is one of them. They make threads thin and large, probably because the core (implant diameter excluding the thread) becomes thinner and thus weaker strength. Except for these small diameter implants, most of the implants of 3.3 mm or less which are designed to be thin are alloys, and 2.5 mm one-body implants can be considered as all alloys. The only alloy implant I'm using is Osstem's one-body implant, MS.

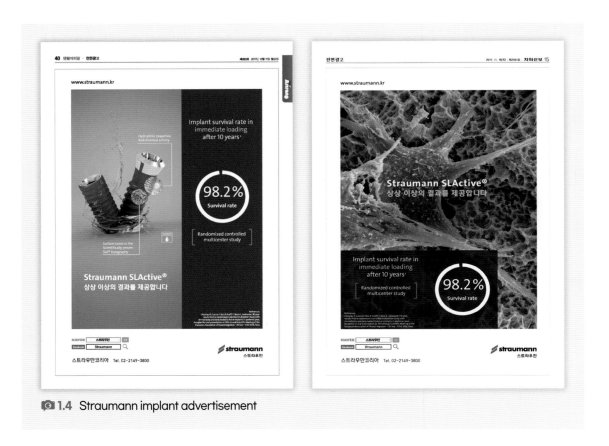

📷 **1.4** Straumann implant advertisement

The next thing to look at is Straumann's Roxolid, which is an alloy made of a mixture of 15% zirconium and 85% titanium (📷 **1.4**). Some people see this as a grade 4, but you can just consider as zirconia alloy Roxolid. I think it is named as Roxolid since is it hard as a rock. I consider this to be the most successful implant material, and whether it is because of patents or technology, the other companies are unable to produce similar products. According to Straumann's press release, Roxolid exhibits 70-80% higher tensile strength than Grade 4. You can consider this as slightly less than Grade 5.

Recently, the use of zirconia in implants has been increasing (📷 **1.6**). Zirconia usage started out as a crown, and then just as a titanium base on the upper part of the abutment, and now they are being made as the abutment itself and even the implant. It is still not common to see zirconia implants in Korea, but I have seen some cases abroad. I have seen a case of zirconia implant being placed where the patient asked the doctor to use the most expensive material out there.

You can see zirconia implants in the most recent catalog from Straumann implant, the leader of implant companies (📷 **1.7**).

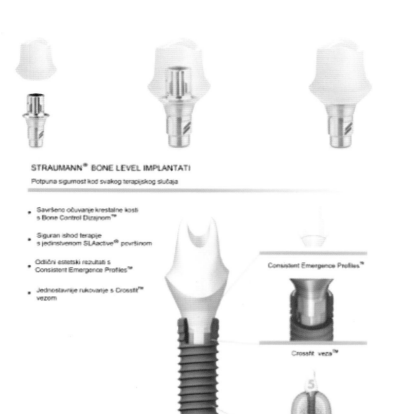

STRAUMANN® BONE LEVEL IMPLANTATI

Potpuna sigurnost kod svakog terapijskog slučaja

- Savršeno očuvanje krestalne kosti
  s Bone Control Dizajnom™

- Siguran ishod terapije
  s jedinstvenom SLAactive® površinom

- Odlični estetski rezultati s
  Consistent Emergence Profiles™

- Jednostavnije rukovanje s Crossfit™
  vezom

Consistent Emergence Profiles™

Crossfit veza™

Bone Control Design™

📷 1.5 Straumann Zirconia abutments

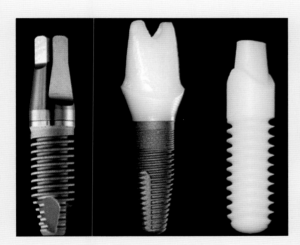

📷 1.6 Zirconia implant advertisement

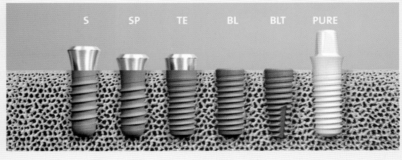

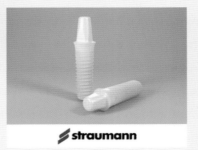

✦ straumann

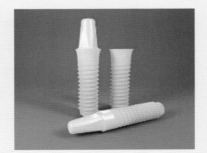

📷 1.7 Struamann zirconia implants

1.2 Tensile strength, compressive strength, modulus of elasticity comparison between titanium and zirconia

Features	Bone	Commercial pure titanium	Titanium alloy	Zirconia
Tensile strength (MPA)	104~121	662	993	1000
Compressive strength (MPA)	170	328	970	2000
Modulus of Elasticity (GPA)	10~15	103	113.8	200

Source: Paulo Leme. "Zirconia Implants-an overview". ISMI.

ISMI | INT. SOCIETY OF METAL FREE IMPLANTOLOGY

As you can see from the 1.2, zirconia has the highest tensile strength and compressive strength.

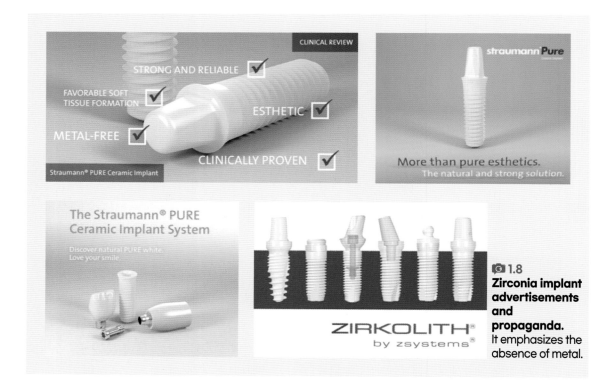

1.8
Zirconia implant advertisements and propaganda.
It emphasizes the absence of metal.

However, if you look at the zirconia abutments on the market, most of them have a one-piece fixture abutment. There seems to be a problem with the fit or the strength of the connection part. Even if it comes as a separate type, it is almost looks like a tissue-level implant or the connection part is made very thick. It is only recently that we can see zirconia abutments that are not too thick at the connection part, but considering that there are no threads in the coronal part, it seems that the problem of fit or strength in the connection part has not been resolved. Some doctors may utilize the zirconia implants already but I personally want to wait on it and use the safe-proven implants for now. Successful implant surgery cases are dependent more on the doctor's skills and ability more than the type of implant they use.

I would like to briefly mention the implant surface treatment as I do not want to waste the time on this topic. In fact, I think the **technology of the company is more important than the surface treatment method**. If it is on the market and has been verified for several years, you can trust it and use it.

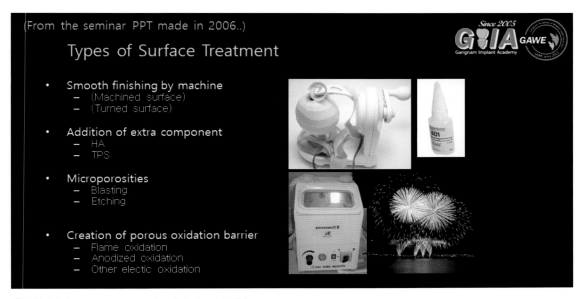

📷 1.9 My lecture power point slide from 2006

Different methods of surface treatments can be classified as follows.

- Grinding and machining to create smooth surface (machined surface)
- Methods to form a rough surface by additionally coating the machined titanium surface (HA coating, TPS coating, titanium sphere; sintering coating method)
- Methods of forming rough surfaces through acid corrosion or blasting (blasting, etching, SLA, RBM)
- A method of making the surface rough by forming a thick titanium oxide layer by an electrochemical method (flame oxidation, anodized oxidation, other electric oxidation)

For a while, hybrid surface treatment methods using a mixture of the above surface treatment methods were popular. The hybrid form can be thought of as implants that have been surface-treated in a complex way, such as treating the implant with two or more methods or treating the upper and lower parts differently.

Now let's look at each of the surface treatment methods.

A smooth surface treatment method that is formed only by cutting with a machine
• Machined surface

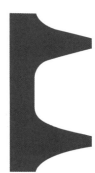

The surface of the implant is a smooth, machine-cut surface. I used to think that the materials for implant should be pure and the surface should be smooth to adhere well to the bone. But over time, I've learned that bones like rough surfaces. So I often say this: "the bone likes rough surfaces, and gingiva likes smooth surfaces." In other words, it can be said that bones stick better to rough surfaces, and gums do not like rough surfaces.

Methods of forming a rough surface by applying additional coatings to machined titanium surfaces
(HA coating, TPS coating, titanium sphere; sinter coating method)
• TPS & HA coating

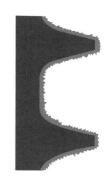

This method can be thought of as an adhesive (but not sticky) so that it sticks to the bone just like we use a glue to attach something to it. TPS is an abbreviation of titanium plasma spray, and titanium powder is sprayed on the implant surface. When TPS coating was used, it definitely adhered well to the implant, probably because of the wider surface. The problem, however, was that the powder sprinkled over time fell off the implant. Also, as mentioned above, since the surface is too rough, once exposed to inflammation, it progresses rapidly, causing peri-implantitis. HA followed the same process as TPS. However, HA is better to think that it is more effective than TPS and has less side effects. Some companies are still using this method, but because of the fast infection progress, its use has gradually decreased.

International Journal of Oral Maxillofacial Implants 2005;20:124~130

Human Histologic and Histomorphometric Analyses of Hydroxyapatite-Coated Implants After 10 Years of Function: A Case report

Method

Reporting of biopsy of a 73-year-old patient, who had cylindrical implant with HA coating placed 10 years ago.

Result

Satisfactory with BIC 78%

Loss of HA coating by 27%, yet osseointegration was satisfactory in such area.

No reporting of inflammation of soft tissue

Conclusion

It is deemed that HA coating was well maintatined for over 10 years in patients with adequate prosthetic treatment and good plaque control.

International Journal of Oral Maxillofacial Implants 2005;20:238~244

Marginal Bone Loss (MBL) Pattern Around Hydroxyapatite-coated Versus Commercially Pure Titanium Implants After up to 12 Years of Follow-up

Method

Masurement of MBL of normal CP titanium implant vs HA=coated implant, for the past 12 years

Result

With respect to MBL value, HA is better than CP initially, but starts to get worse after 2 years, then much worse after 4 years.

CP is stable with respect to MBL after 2 years

Long-term success rate (over 12 years) was higher for HA (93.2%) than CP Titanium (89%).

Conclusion

The fact that HA-coated implant has higher survival rate over 12 years (despite higher MBL after 4 years) disprove minimal failure, if any, of the surgical procedure.

Failure rate (12/156 Vs 26/232)

A brief and concise summary of the above two papers is as follows. The first is that "As a result of dissecting a person who died after having an HA implant 10 years ago, there was sufficient amount of

HA coating remaining."

The second paper is saying that "HA is susceptible to peri-implantitis, so inflammation progresses quickly, but compared to the comparison group, the initial success rate was quite high, so even after 12 years, the HA was higher." The problem here is that the comparison group was the machined surface implants. I think this conclusion is not too significant because any surface treatment these days are better than the machined surfaces. I've been searching for papers recently, but there aren't many research results because HA surface treatment is rarely used anymore. Rather, I identified some papers with negative research results as follows.

Influence of surface treatment on osseointegration of dental implants: histological, histomorphometric and radiological analysis in vivo
Clinical Oral Investigations 2014 DOI: 10.1007/s00784-014-1241-2

We conclude that even if there seems to be a tendency to obtain better BIC results with surface A (blasted-etched and covered with hydroxyapatite (HA), no statistical differences were obtained in this study. The study shows the influence of different implant surfaces in increasing osseointegation for immediate loading implants.

HA is rarely used alone and is often used in combination with other surface treatments. Since we are talking about something added onto the surface, we should talk about endopore implant as an example which has small beads added on the surface.

The porous surface is achieved by sintering Ti alloy spherical particles (📷 1.10).

The spheres attached to implants are very smooth, but when we look at the implant surface, since we don't look at implants microscopically,

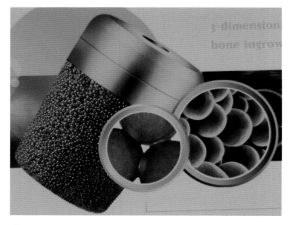

📷 1.10 Endopore implant advertisement

it can be seen clinically as the roughest surface. Therefore, even a short implant has been advertised as sufficiently functional. But why did it fail? That's because the surface was too rough. The endopore implant uses an external hexa type abutment, so it can assumed that due to marginal gap and movement, there is a bone loss of 1.5 mm as the default. However, there are two types of machined surfaces, 1 mm and 2 mm. Of course, 2 mm is also insecure, but for a 1 mm machined surface, the inflammation progresses out of control when the implant is incorrectly placed or if the implant and the abutment are slightly out of alignment. When I met the developer in 2005, he told me to place only 2 mm, not 1 mm, but it was already too late. Also at that time, the professor recommended to use the gold UCLA abutment rather than the company's titanium abutment. Why? Eventually, the micro-gap and movement create bone resorption, and the best material to stop that was the gold. Even now, among the external hexa type implants that I placed in my early days, there are many that do not have bone resorption at all. I think one of the reasons is that most of the abutments were gold. I think it's because it has no bad chemical effect on the human body and by having a good fit, it not only seals securely, but also blocks micro-gap and movement with excellent ductility. After all, because the bone likes a rough surface, dentists make other attempts to roughen the implant surface.

Methods of forming rough surfaces through acid corrosion or blasting (blasting, etching, SLA, RBM)

• Etching

When we put resin on our teeth, we etch it, probably because it is the easiest way to increase the surface area. In addition, since etching also has a strong cleaning action of impurities, the cleaning effect is obtained as an added bonus. Such etching has a fatal drawback. As with resin filling, if you etch on a smooth cervical area caused by abfraction, the resin will come off quickly. This is because the surface becomes wider, but the physical strength is too weak due to small surface roughness. And the reason why we tell you not to rub the etched surface hard when using resin is because the surface gets crushed. Even the etched surface of the implant is crushed when the implant is placed in the bone. So we need a bigger and stronger roughness.

• Blasting

If you look at the crown from the laboratory, you can see that the inner and outer surfaces are completely different even with the same material. This is because the inner surface is blasted to make it rough so that the adhesive adheres well. Blasting is a good way to create increased roughness. However, the biggest problem with blasting was that the blasted material was embedded in the implant surface and did not come off or the surface became dirty. When the surface is dirty, we know the best way to clean it. What is it? It's etching. So usually after blasting, it is etched - this is the most commonly used in implants these days and the example of it is Straumann's SLA surface. Osstem calls it SA. In fact, each company gave different names, such as S&E, SBE, and SMA, but they are all basically SLA.

• SLA (Sand blasted with Large grit and Acid etched)

As mentioned earlier in blasting, it was blasted with large grit and then cleaned by etching. It is the most popular surface treatment method in modern times because it can produce both large and small roughness. Most implants sold in Korea these days are SLA-based. It is said that the most important technology is to thoroughly clean the acid at the end of the processing stage. There is a rumor about a recent incident in Korea with one of the companies where the problem with the surface treatment of the implant was due to the poor cleaning of the acid.

• RBM (Resorbable Blasting Media)

Let's talk about RBM now. I mentioned the problem of the rough surface of HA earlier, and 'what if HA is attached only at the initial stage of implantation and then disappears gradually?' From this idea, RBM surface treatment came. In other words, the blasting material is an absorbent material that can induce osseointegration. In Osstem, the surface treatment of the implants I used in the early days was also RBM, but most of them changed to a more effective SLA. However, there are still products that insist on RBM. These are titanium grade 5 alloys. I mentioned earlier that you only have to know one thing: "Only minimally toxic." However, it is true that there is some burden on the surface being too wide. How wide will the surface be when even the acid etching is done? (I do not know in details, but it is also said that it is technically also not easy.) They say there may be ions that may be harmful to the human body. If it is lightly covered, it is possible to prevent excessive surface exposure while maintaining the unique mechanical strength of alloy. Therefore, most of the alloy products adopt the RBM method. The thin and large-thread IBS implants mentioned above are, of course, RBMs. Now you can see why Megagen's Anyridge was made of Grade 4 instead of alloy. This is probably due to the SLA surface treatment. It may have been difficult to SLA the alloy, and it is better to do it on the already roughened SLA if you want to have more effect on the implant surface.

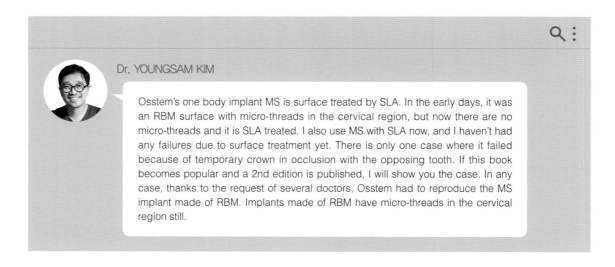

Dr. YOUNGSAM KIM

Osstem's one body implant MS is surface treated by SLA. In the early days, it was an RBM surface with micro-threads in the cervical region, but now there are no micro-threads and it is SLA treated. I also use MS with SLA now, and I haven't had any failures due to surface treatment yet. There is only one case where it failed because of temporary crown in occlusion with the opposing tooth. If this book becomes popular and a 2nd edition is published, I will show you the case. In any case, thanks to the request of several doctors, Osstem had to reproduce the MS implant made of RBM. Implants made of RBM have micro-threads in the cervical region still.

A method of making the surface rough by forming a thick titanium oxide layer by an electrochemical method (flame oxidation, anodized oxidation, other electric oxidation)

The typical method used in the current market is Nobel Biocare's anodizing

• Anodizing

It started in 1982 from Nobel Biocare but other companies could not do anodizing due to lacking technical skills. So it can be said that anodizing is Nobel Biocare implant's unique characteristic.

I know a few companies have tried in Korea too, but most of them have failed.

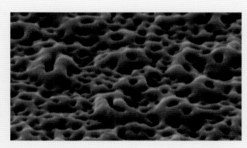

📷 1.11 Unlike the other surface treatments, instead of outer layer having protrusion, it has holes inside. Nobel calls this "cell nest."

I summarized some research papers here but things may have changed now. Let's look at a paper about surface treatment.

International Journal of Oral Maxillofacial Implants 2005; 20:425-431
Early wound healing around endosseous implants A review of the literature

Research method
Systemic review of 1095 literature related to wound healing of endosseous implants from 1997 to 2004.

Conclusion
Despite various types of machined surface with increased roughness, there's no conclusive evidence to which type is the best as of yet.

In this paper, it concluded that machined surface treatment is not the best, but not sure which one is better. I personally think that they were not able to say what was better (even though they knew already), due to connections with the implant companies and other issues.

Now let's take a look at the surface treatment advancement. For a while, hybrids were popular like hybrid cars these days. Hybrid form is when the implant surface is treated in complex way such as treated in two or more ways, or different treatment on upper and lower portion of the implant. Recently other methods were introduced that improved the existing coating method using biocompatible materials rather than the surface coating method that appeared before. Now let's take a look at these methods.

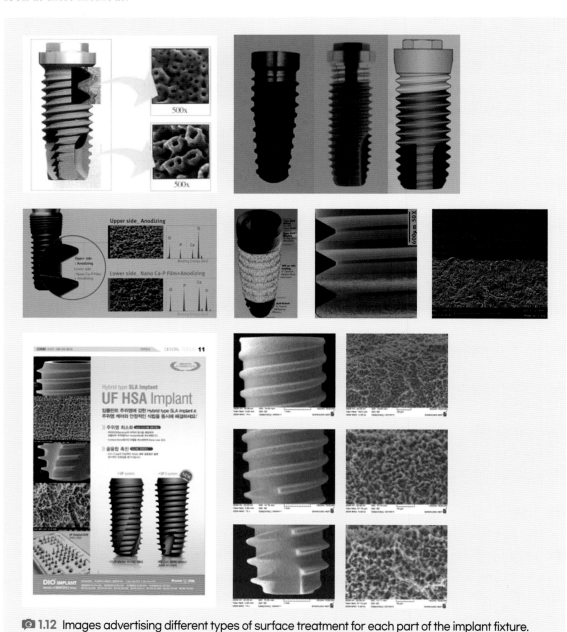

📷 1.12 Images advertising different types of surface treatment for each part of the implant fixture.

Looking at 📷 **1.12**, the lower part of the implant is made of surface treatment that are good for osseointegration, and the upper part is treated to be more favorable for periodontal disease management. For the external hexa type or internal type, which has a high tendency for bone resorption on the crestal side, was treated with machined surface under the premise that the there is bone loss of least 1.5 mm. On the other hand, for internal friction type which does not have a bone resorption in the crestal region, the most common method is to treat the upper area with relatively small roughness and the lower area with large roughness, or add HA.

Zimmer implant surface treatment

Among all the implants, there is one alligator-like implant. That's the Zimmer® implant. Why did I call it an alligator? This is because it has existed for a long time and has survived and sold without much change. Zimmer® implants are made of alloy, and since the abutment connection structure is an internal fit type, cervical bone resorption can occur frequently. As a result, the cervical part is machined or slightly rough, and the fixture body is coated with HA. I've used Zimmer implants a lot, but I've never used a surface treatment like this before. For reference, I used the Zimmer implant without any complaints and was satisfied with it. It was just expensive.

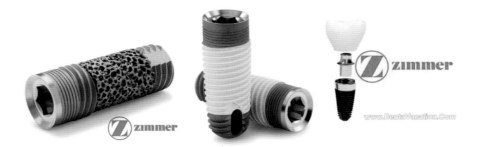

📷 **1.13 Zimmer® implants**
Zimmer® implants are available with two surface texture options, a hydroxylapatite (HA) particle blasted and acid washed surface (MTX™) or a dual HA coated (MP-1®), MTX™ surface. The acid wash of the MTX™ surface roughening process is designed to remove embedded HA particle and does not etch the titanium surface. Zimmer's MP-1® HA coating procedure increases the HA crystal density to around 90 percent on the surface of the implant.

In Zimmer® implant surface treatments, there is one called MTX - in the Zimmer implant catalog, there is a part that emphasizes that they did not wash with acid but with distilled water (micro textured surface where only HA particles were removed with weak acid after HA blasting). After all, there is no need to etch the alloy with acid to make a large surface. Occasionally I am concerned about the SLA surface of Osstem MS made of alloy. But I try to think that if the Osstem implant is defective, it will be a problem for many of us dentists and I trust that Osstem would have verified it well.

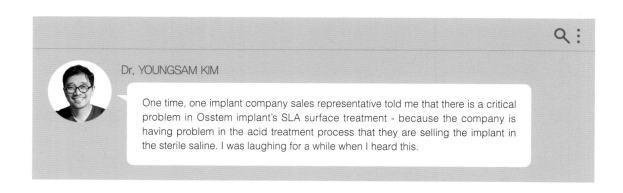

오스템 임플란트 표면

CA(Calcium SA)
CA이온 도입 및 **SA 대비 표면오염을 차단시킨 초친수성** 표면

치료기간			식립가능범위			
1개월	2개월	3개월	강한뼈	보통뼈	약한뼈	부위별 뼈의 강도
4~6주						
12주						

*골량이나 치아건강상태에 따라 기간 차이는 있음

📷 1.14 Osstem's CA surface treatment advertisement

Osstem CA surface is a product with improved hydrophilicity and blood affinity by storing it in an aqueous calcium solution after SA surface treatment.

Osstem's CA is the most frequently used implant surface treatment I used until last month, which the implant is immersed in a saline solution. The implant has a hydrophobic surface. As a result, to test the hydrophilicity of the implant, we often do a test in which only the tip is immersed in saline. I guess they didn't want us do these tests so they sell it in a saline solution. 😊 I have been using it satisfactorily without much concern except that the surgical cloth is wetted with saline and becomes messy. It's said that it sticks well because it contains CA ions, but that's a phrase they're trying to advertise to the general public... I probably wouldn't have told the dentists to believe it.

Dr. YOUNGSAM KIM

One time, one implant company sales representative told me that there is a critical problem in Osstem implant's SLA surface treatment - because the company is having problem in the acid treatment process that they are selling the implant in the sterile saline. I was laughing for a while when I heard this.

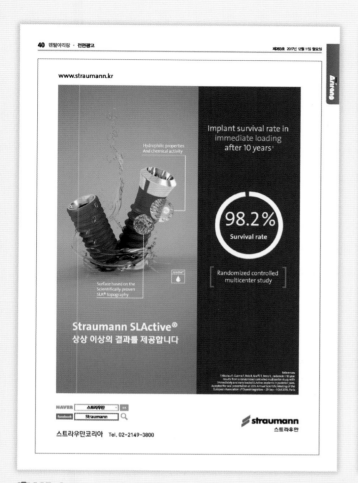
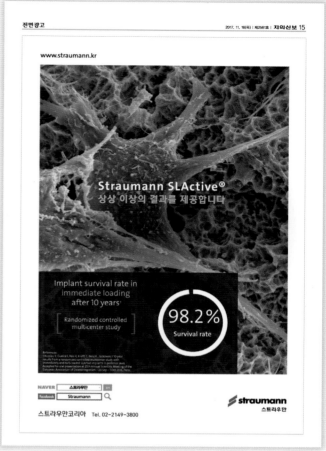

📷 **1.15** Struamann SLAactive implant (first implant to be contained in isotonic saline)

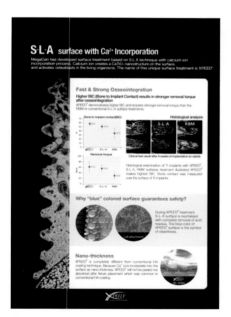
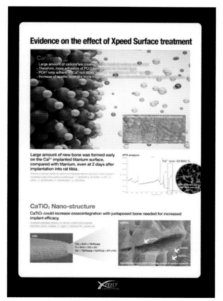
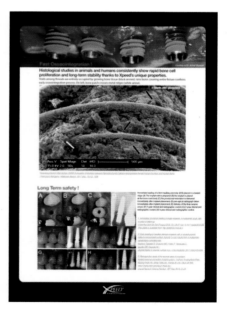

📷 **1.16** MegaGen Xpeed implant surface treatment

Let's look at MegaGen (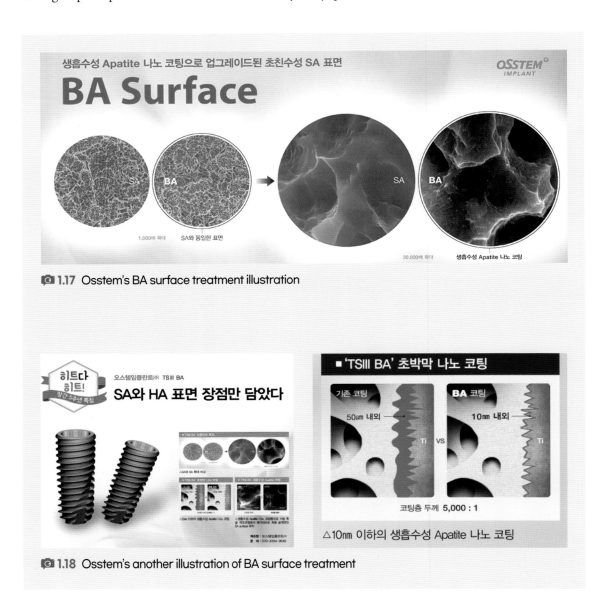1.16). I often see MegaGen advertising that their implants are blue, which I don't know why implant should be blue. It is advertised that Ca ions are attached to the SLA surface. Osstem uses a method of attaching nano-sized particles to a point that does not damage the surface treatment, and Megagen is also added a CaTiO3 nano-structure. It's called Xpeed, but I haven't tried it yet. I would like to try maybe after 2 years to see how they are.

If you look at Osstem's BA flyer, after SA surface treatment, apatite with properties that can be absorbed in the body is reduced to 10 nm or less.

It is said that it contains only the advantages of SA and HA as a product coated with nano thickness. An Osstem official explained that "Because in BA, an ultra-thin coating is applied with a thickness of 10 nm, there is no need to worry about the coating layer peeling off due to friction during implant placement unlike conventional hydroxyapatite."

📷 1.17 Osstem's BA surface treatment illustration

📷 1.18 Osstem's another illustration of BA surface treatment

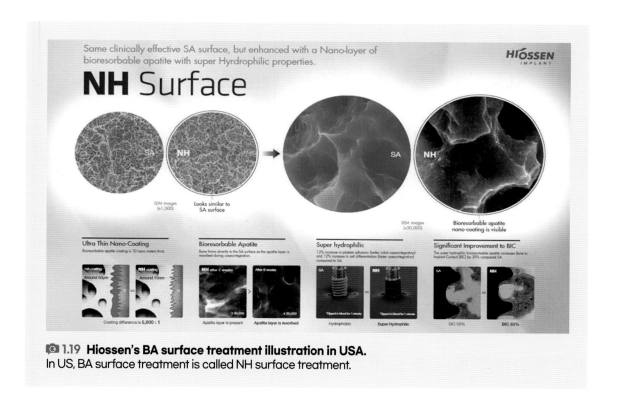

1.19 Hiossen's BA surface treatment illustration in USA.
In US, BA surface treatment is called NH surface treatment.

To put it simply, it is said that, like Megagen, a biocompatible absorbent material was attached to an implant that has already been properly surface-treated with SLA in a nano size. From my point of view, it seems that the advantages of RBM are also combined, rather than just the combination of the advantages of SA and HA, by exaggerating a little. As soon as it came out, I tried to use it, but I always like to wait 2 years before I try new things so I have been using it recently. Now it sells more than SA in Korea (in the US, this product was mainly sold). In the US, it is called Nano Hydrophilic. Note that Osstem no longer produces HA implants.

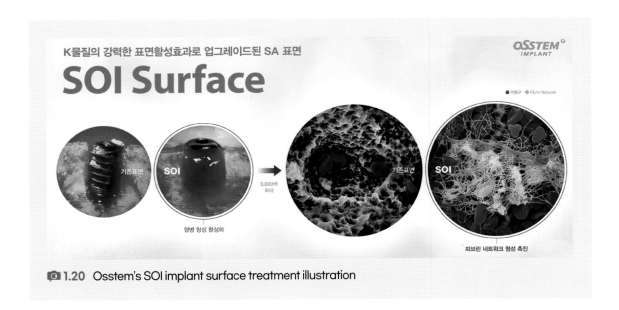

📷 1.20 Osstem's SOI implant surface treatment illustration

Osstem seems to have applied something different to the surface of SLA this time, unlike BA. They called it substance "K." I only saw the advertisement so I just came across the name. What does SOI stand for? It was abbreviation for Super Osseo-Integration.

Later, when I saw the advertisement for the BA surface, I don't know if I've seen it before, but the material they applied here is substance "A." Maybe they changed it from K to A to differentiate, but as of July 2021, this is the implant surface treatment that I used most commonly.

Ultraviolet Photofunctionalization of Titanium Implants

UV rays are a hot topic in dental implant surface treatment these days. Let's take a look at this video. Believe it or not, it looks pretty good.

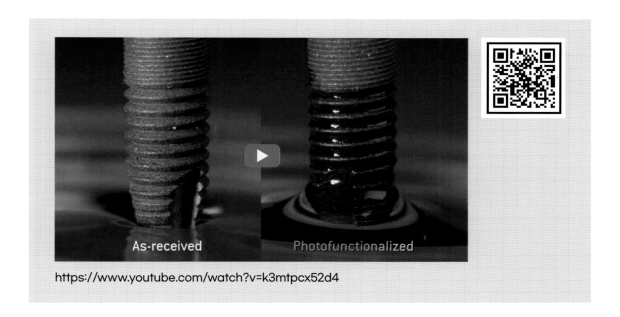

Recently, Pointnics, Dio, and Dentis etc. are making a lot of UV implants. In particular, advertisements targeting patients such as "implants also age" seem to work. That's why Osstem started talking about UV rays. In the lecture of the Osstem Institute Director, I remember him saying "The expression 'aging of implants' is wrong. The word 'stabilization' is more appropriate."

In any case, the implant surface is originally to be disinfected with ultraviolet rays (a lot of medical devices do that). Then the surface becomes hydrophilic and the performance is much better, but aging starts immediately and the effect of UV disappears after a few hours.

For this reason, UV implants sold these days use their own UV machine to treat the implant surface with UV right before placing implant. I don't think it's a bad thing to say. If it's really good, I thought that Osstem, my main dealer, would make it and sell it. I also noticed that Dentis made UV implant machine so I am wondering if I should buy one. It seemed like a good product that made up for the shortcomings of other products so far.

Recently, however, Osstem has mentioned the UV again. It was mentioned at the Denol TV opening seminar and recently at the faculty seminar. Osstem also said that they would continue to promote it in the future.

Here's Osstem's summary:

"I am not here to talk about ultraviolet rays. Originally, Osstem had been interested in UV light for 10 years. And in fact, Osstem is also doing UV treatment. However, since the effect disappears quickly, after surface treatment with ultraviolet rays on the implant, we attached a material that prevents aging and maintains the ultraviolet treatment effect. Those are the aforementioned substances K and A."

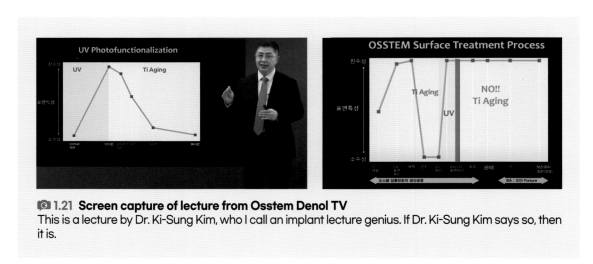

📷 **1.21 Screen capture of lecture from Osstem Denol TV**
This is a lecture by Dr. Ki-Sung Kim, who I call an implant lecture genius. If Dr. Ki-Sung Kim says so, then it is.

I am pretty gullible, and I have a lot of trust in Dr. Ki-Sung Kim, who conducted the lecture, so I decided to try SOI after listening to these lectures. And this is the product I use the most as of July 2021.

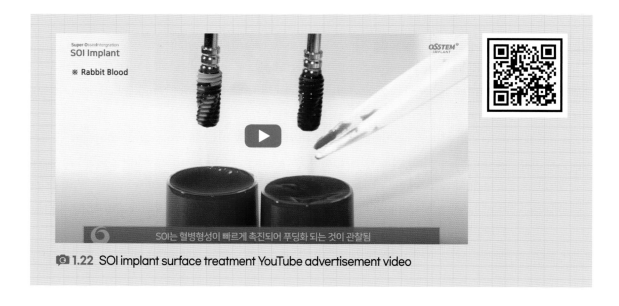

📷 **1.22 SOI implant surface treatment YouTube advertisement video**

Let's take a look at the video in 📷 **1.22**. This video is about a year older than the time I was writing the book. It's been over 2 years since the BA came out, so I decided to try and start using this.

Once again, it can be said that the case of surface treatment has already been concluded. Basically, **in the case of Grade 4, the SLA surface treatment method is recommended, and in the case of Grade 5, the RBM method is recommended.** All of the new hybrid methods have different pros and cons, but I think it can be trusted and used if it has been verified. As mentioned earlier, I believe that the company's technology is more important than the surface treatment method. As long as it is on the market and has been proven for several years, you can trust it and use it.

Recently, as I finished the renewal of this surface treatment part, I searched for some papers on it, but there were not many. Now, I think that it would be appropriate to view implants as an industry rather than a science. Let's take a brief look at two of them that are interesting.

Early osseointegration driven by the surface chemistry and wettability of dental implants
Journal of applied oral science : revista FOB 2015, DOI:10.1590/1678-775720140483

Conclusion The surface chemistry and wettability implants accelerate osseointegration and increase the area of the bone-to-implant interface when compared to those of other group.

As you can see, basically the paper is saying that it is better to soak implant in saline. I think this research is related to Straumann's product, who sells implants soaked in saline. Let's look at one more paper.

Dental implant surfaces after insertion in bone: an in vitro study in four commercial implant systems Clinical Oral Investigations 2017

Primary healing of dental implants is influenced by their surface morphology.
However, little is known about any alterations in morphology during their insertion.
Therefore, the aim of this study was to evaluate the surface morphology of four different implant systems···
Six new implants of four systems (Ankylos® 4.5×14 mm, Frialit Synchro® 4.5×15 mm, NobelReplace® Tapered Groovy RP 4.3 × 13 mm, Straumann SLA® Bone Level 3.3×14 mm) were inserted ··· Revealed that differences between the four systems were highly significant in the apical region of implants. ··· The insertion process had an impact on the surface of all four implant systems.
Anodized implant surface modification seems to result in more alterations compared with subtractive surface modifications.
Therefore, surgical planning should take into consideration the choice of surface treatment because the characteristics of the implants may be modified during the installation process. The given information is of value for daily implantation practice and the course of osseointegration.

Roughly speaking, it is saying that it is meaningless to analyze the surface before placing. This is because the surface is crushed after the implant is placed anyway. However, there is one that has only a small change in the surface before and after placing implant, that is, anodizing. Just by looking at it, it can be said that this is a research related to the Nobel Biocare implant company that uses anodizing surface treatment. This is not to say that this paper is wrong, but in fact, I would have reached another conclusion a little differently.

I would have added another saying, "don't place the implant too hard." If you place it too hard, the surface treatment will be crushed and there will be no significant difference, and the outer layer substances will come off. In addition, the internal hex structure can be damaged so **the implant should never be placed with a lot of force.** In fact, if the torque comes out too much than I expected, I remove the implant, drill again, and then put a new implant in. This is because I think that implants that have already been rubbed excessively once are of less value. I just think that I used the tap drill once for free and throw it away without any regrets. Korean implants are replaced free of charge, so there is no reason not to. This is because if you become proficient even a little, the rate of returning implant gets very low.

2-2

Implant Shape and Thread

Mastering dental implants

Implant Body Shape

There are so many different types of implants (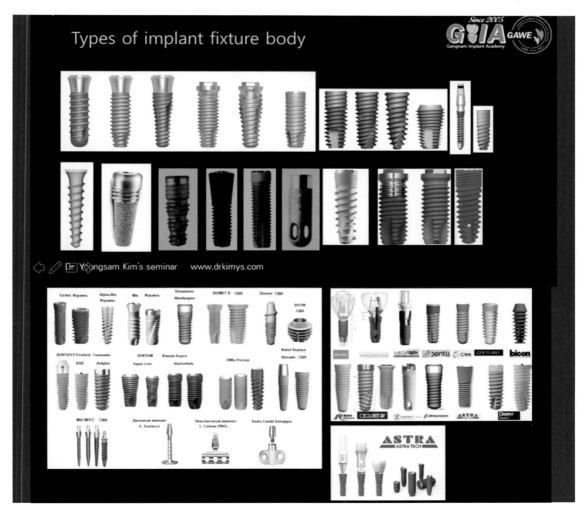 2.1).

2.1 My PPT slide that I use when teaching about implant shapes

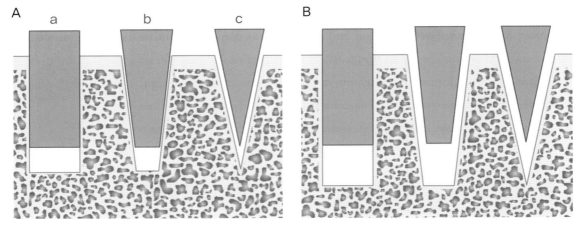

📷 **2.2** Comparison of space size around implant according to implant drilling cross section and implantation depth

📷 **2.2** shows a schematic diagram of implant placement according to body shape while ignoring threads. 📷 **2.2A** shows the drilled sites the same size as the implant. At first glance, the tapered shape looks advantageous for initial fixation.

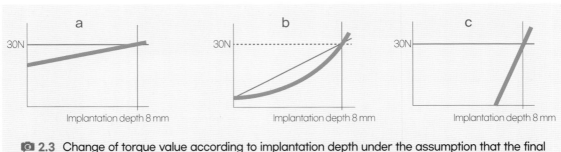

📷 **2.3** Change of torque value according to implantation depth under the assumption that the final implantation torque is obtained with 30N when placing 8 mm implants of a, b, and c in 📷 **2.2** above.

📷 **2.3** is a graph that roughly plots the change in torque value according to body shape. A parallel implant will maintain a relatively constant torque value from the beginning until the placement is complete. Depending on the degree of tapered shape like 📷 **2.3b** and 📷 **2.3c**, there will be no torque or weak torque when the apex of the implant passes through the coronal side, and the torque value will increase abruptly as the implant depth approaches.

The first reason that the initial fixation of parallel implants is inferior to that of tapered implants is that the initial fixation of parallel implants is mostly dictated by the screw thread, because the screw thread of the implant passes through the same spot several times. And the second reason is probably because the depth of the implant thread is limited at the same diameter.

What would happen if you drilled a little deeper to place the implant deeper in the same condition as in 📷 **2.2B**? In a straight form, the torque value according to the depth does not change much until the implant touches the drilled apex. Even if you take it out a little at the thought of 'Did you drill too deep?' there is no difference. As a result, in terms of depth adjustment, it will be easily adjusted without a large change in the torque value. However, it can be predicted that as the tapered shape increases, the torque value will be very low until the implant touches the apex. The torque value will increase abruptly as the implant approaches the apex. Thinking that the implant is placed too deep and you try to remove a little, the initial fixation is not good at all.

What are the advantages of tapered implants other than initial fixation? First, anatomically, it is less likely to damage the lingual plate, the inferior alveolar nerve, and even the adjacent teeth. The diameter is reduced at the apex. In addition, there are many places where the apex part is concave in the buccal of the maxillary anterior or premolar region, but the probability of coming out of the buccal bone here is very low. Because the occlusal force is not transmitted much, it does not need to be thick and strong. Therefore, in many ways, there is no need to dislike the fact that the implant gets smaller as the apex becomes smaller. Conversely, if the cervical diameter is maintained according to the diameter of the apex, problems such as implant fracture may occur. Most companies are trying to make implants with a thick cervical region and a thin apical end.

As in 📷 2.4, efforts were made to make the cervical region as thick as possible and the apex as thin as possible. Since the tapered part is advantageous for initial fixation and the straight part is advantageous for depth adjustment, it has both forms. On the other hand, if you have both forms, two disadvantages

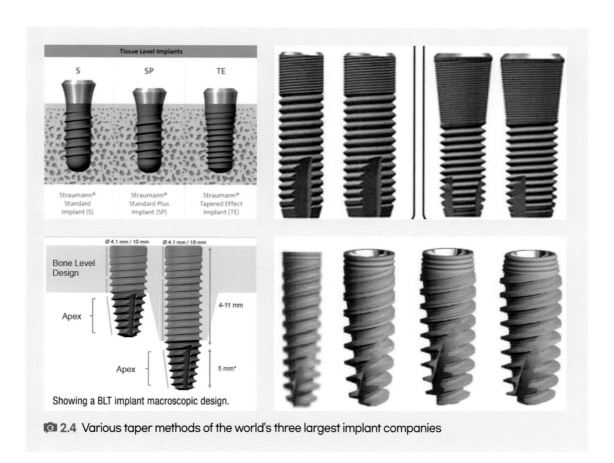

📷 2.4 Various taper methods of the world's three largest implant companies

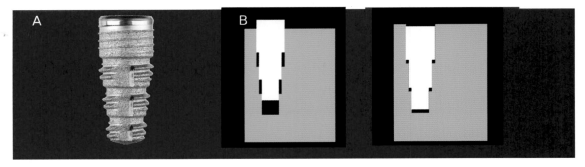

📷 **2.5 Stepped tapered implant (PPT material I use when teaching)**
A: FRIALIT Implant (Germany), **B**: Schematic diagram of the placement process of stepped taper implants

may occur. It is difficult to adjust the depth because of the tapered part, and the initial fixation may be difficult because of the parallel part. Anyway, if you have both straight and tapered shapes, drilling can be a bit complicated because you have to form both shapes. Thus, the stepped taper form emerged.

📷 **2.5** is a historical implant that once was popular with an implant called "Frialit". This design is what I call a "stepped taper," and consists of steps of 2-3 mm in parallel planes. If we consider that we adjust the implant height in 1-2 mm, tapered shape and straight shape has all the advantages. Although the overall shape of the implant is tapered, it is easy to adjust the depth because it consists of parallel surfaces. Based on this concept, it can be said that several companies developed the implant. These days, implants are made to take advantage of both the parallel and tapered surfaces by well considering the size and shape of the thread to this body shape. 📷 **2.6A** is a pictorial representation of the stage of change of the implant. You can see it gradually tapering in steps. However, as short implants have become popular recently, the number of steps has been reduced to about one or two. In particular, considering the structural stability of the implant, it is also because the diameter of the upper part cannot be reduced. As in 📷 **2.6B**, as short implants have become a recent trend, their characteristics are less evident, but the basic concept is a stepped taper shape.

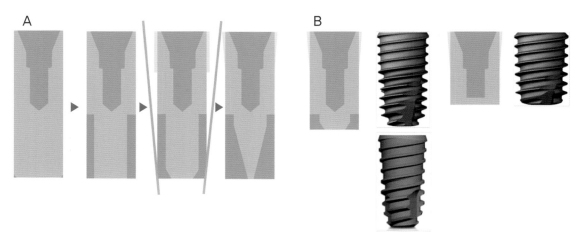

📷 **2.6 A**: Steps of applying various taper shapes to implants of 12 mm or more, **B**: Taper shapes applied to implants of 8 mm or less and short implants of 6 mm or less

In 2005, my interest in the structural contents of implants grew, and I read many papers. At that time, I thought about 'What if we could gather all the good things in the world and make an implant?' Then I saw something called "Oneplant."

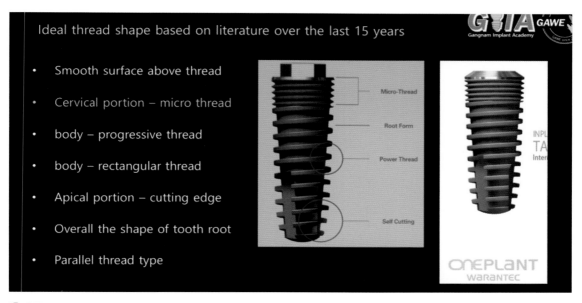

📷 2.7 Contents of slides I show in lectures

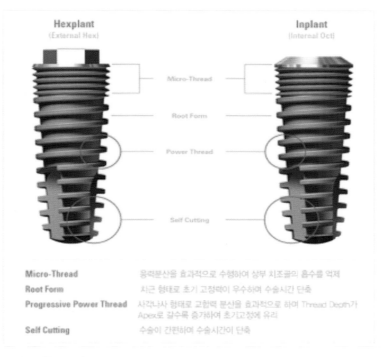

📷 2.8 Oneplant implant illustration

It seems that all the good characteristics of the implant thread have been put together. If you don't do a lot of implant surgery and make an ideal implant only based on theory, you can think that this is the best implant. In particular, I would like to say that the implant in the form of internal friction on the right side of 📷 2.8 is the best in theory.

So, what is the problem with this implant? As mentioned earlier, surgery is not easy. After implantation, it can be a very good implant, but it is not easy to place. **"Initial fixation" is the first factor in implant success,** and it is not easy to obtain initial fixation with these implants. To be more precise, it should be expressed that it is not easy to obtain initial fixation at the correct position and height. Now let's learn about threads one by one.

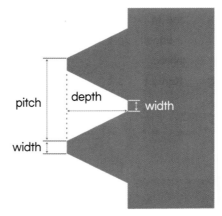

📷 2.9 Basic terms for the screw

📷 2.9 is a term commonly used to describe screws, and pitch and depth are one of the most important factors. Personally, I think it is better when the outer width is narrow and the inner width is wide, and when the pitch is relatively large and the depth is deeper. But the more you do, the more problems arise, so let's study about the the size and shape of the thread.

Take a look at the thread of the historic early implants in 📷 2.10. Early Branemark implants really have the same thread shape as when metal and metal are combined, and seem to arrange an equilateral triangle with a pitch of 0.6 mm. The depth of the thread is 0.3 mm as if the edge of the thread was slightly trimmed. The thread size of the Straumann implant is almost the same, but the distance between the thread and the thread is 1.2 mm, so it seems that the bone tissue, which has less strength than titanium, was intended to be contained between the thread and the thread thicker.

So, what about other companies that were created based on the design of these two companies? Most are initially made in medium size, with threads between 0.8 and 1.0 mm (📷 2.11). Recently, for the structural stability of implants, the cervical thread is small, but only for implants used in poor bone quality areas, you can see that the implant thread gets deeper and bigger as it goes toward the apex. It can be seen that it is composed to be well compatible with the implant body shape.

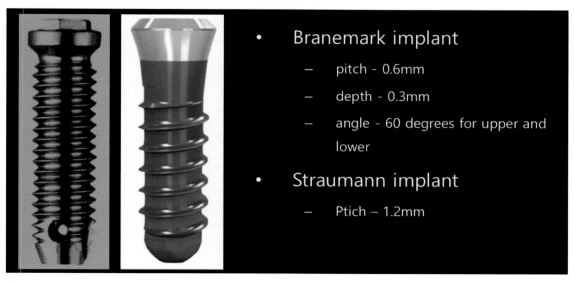

- **Branemark implant**
  - pitch - 0.6mm
  - depth - 0.3mm
  - angle - 60 degrees for upper and lower
- **Straumann implant**
  - Ptich – 1.2mm

📷 **2.10** Branemark implant (Nobel Biocare) and ITI (Straumann) implants

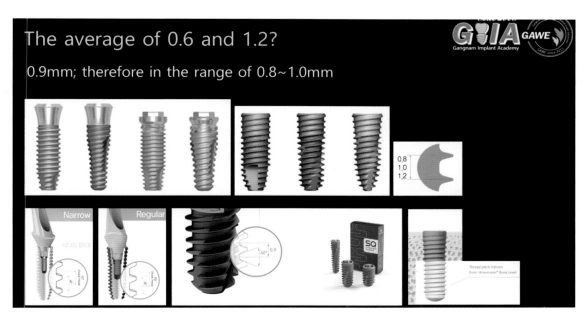

📷 **2.11** Implant thread shape

First, let's look at the shape of the thread. The sharper the end of the thread (the smaller the width), the better the self-cutting will be when placing the implant so the initial fixation will be good. However, in the distribution of occlusal force, it is said that a slightly larger width and an angled square parallel thread are advantageous. I don't know why, and I don't understand. ☺ Anyways, for this reason, the thread shape develops to a combination of the two (📷 **2.12**).

Shape of thread.

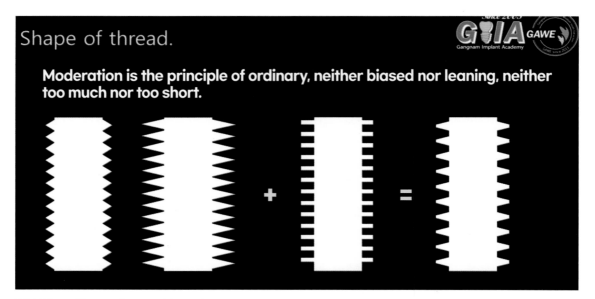

Moderation is the principle of ordinary, neither biased nor leaning, neither too much nor too short.

📷 **2.12A** Different shapes of thread

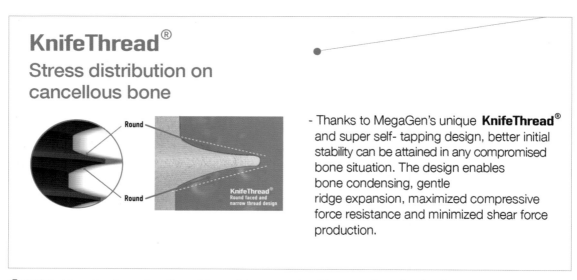

KnifeThread®
Stress distribution on cancellous bone

- Thanks to MegaGen's unique **KnifeThread®** and super self- tapping design, better initial stability can be attained in any compromised bone situation. The design enables bone condensing, gentle ridge expansion, maximized compressive force resistance and minimized shear force production.

📷 **2.12B** MegaGen's explanation of thread. It seems that Megagen is well reflecting the modern concept of implants. It was said that it was a round and sharp design unique to Megagen, but most implant threads seem to be changing like this these days. Because titanium is stronger than bone, it is better to think of it as a concave and thin design (rather than round) to contain as many bones as possible between the threads.

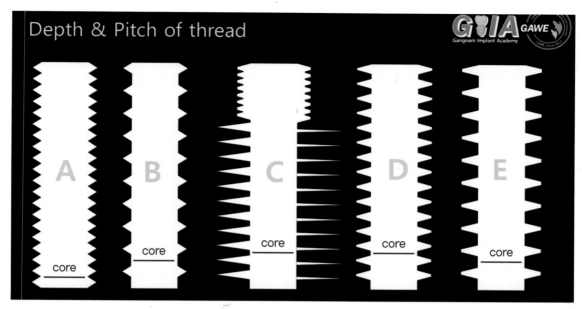

2.13 Implant core and thread shape and distance

Now let's look at the depth and distance of the thread. First, consider the core concept of Megagen Anyridge. In general, the size of the implant is said to be the size of the largest outer part, but the deeper and thinner the thread, the less the strength is proportional to the size of the outer size. So, the body part of the fixture, excluding the threads, is called the core in Megagen. We will refer to it as the core here as well.

First of all, comparing **2.13A** and **2.13B**, the thread size is the same, but the distance between the threads is increased. Although **2.13A** is stronger in terms of implant structure, since the strength of bone tissue is weaker than that of titanium, it can be seen that **2.13B** has greater stability in bone tissue after implantation.

As shown in **2.13C**, the size and shape of the implant thread can be made variously. All of them have their pros and cons. Considering that the shape of the implant thread has changed in general like **2.13D**, it seems that the thread has changed to a longer and farther way to contain a large amount of bone between the threads, as in **2.13E**.

So, what are the benefits of longer and larger threads?

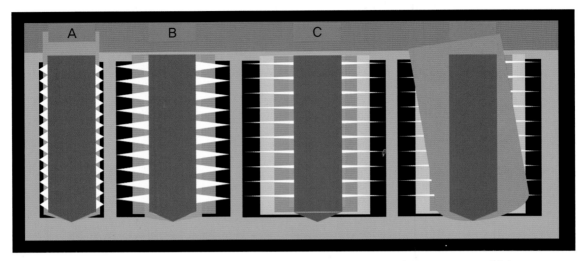

📷 2.14 Comparison according to drilled bone size and implant thread size (My lecture PPT slide)

Consider the 📷 2.14A, the most common Branemark-style implant. In general, the size of the implant refers to the outermost size, so the black size can be called the implant size. So how do you drill? If the bone quality is very poor, drill as much as red according to the size of the implant core, and generally drill as much as the size of pink. But, what happens if you drill a little bigger and closer to the black size because you think the bone is harder than expected? The implant will become loose, making it difficult to obtain an initial fixation, and even a little more or less drilling will interfere with the placement of the implant. Therefore, since bone quality and bone shape vary greatly for each patient and the area, correct initial fixation can be obtained by understanding them in advance and paying attention to them when placing implant.

Now let's look at 📷 2.14B. The size of the implant core remains the same, but the thread of the implant is increased. If only the thread of the implant increases like this, forgetting the core size and thinking only about the entire implant size and placing it in the posterior region carelessly can cause a big problem later. In any case, if you look here, you can see that the categories that can be drilled from pink to orange are forming a wide range. A little less or more, implants can be placed without significantly affecting the trend.

Let's look at 📷 2.14C, which is expressed in a more maximized way. Threads are a bit larger, but thinner. Whether the bone quality is good or bad, if it is moderately larger than the core, there will be no problem in placing implant. You can even place something completely different from what you drilled. That means there is a lot of space available. With proper drilling, the implant can be placed very easily and quickly. So, curious about how to solve this problem, I went to my colleague Dr. Jeon

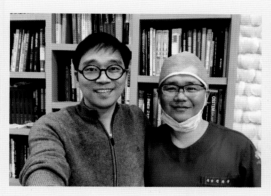

📷 **2.15** With Dr. Jeon Hee-kyung, the King of Anyridge implants

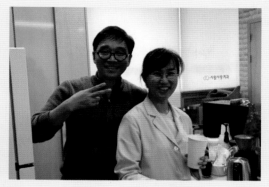

📷 **2.16** My colleague who works with me, Dr. Huh Mi-ja (a really nice person)

Hee-kyung, who placed the most Megagen Anyridge in the world. Director Jeon Hee-kyung, whom I call the Great Demon King of Anyridge, has trained in oral surgery and is even more special because he married our classmate. Because he is famous for being a great dentist, he has a lot of patients despite the high cost of treatment compared to other dentists. There are so many patients that he sees patients in order of visit time rather than appointment time. This does not mean that wisdom tooth extractions or other treatments are not available. As a result, he has to see the patient at an incredibly fast pace. Why is he using implants mainly with Anyridge? The reason for Megagen's Anyridge is that the thread is so thin and large that it can place implants quickly and reliably even with moderate drilling.

Obviously, thin and large threads are a big advantage. However, the problem is that, as mentioned earlier, it makes the implant core small and reduces structural stability.

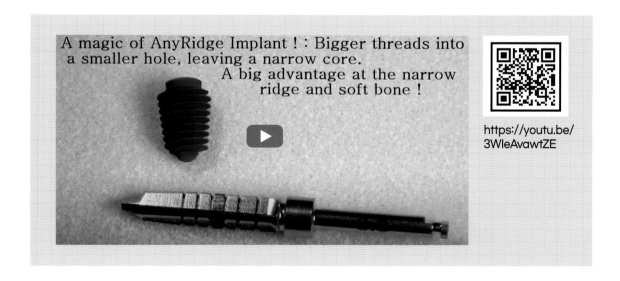

A magic of AnyRidge Implant ! : Bigger threads into a smaller hole, leaving a narrow core.
A big advantage at the narrow ridge and soft bone !

https://youtu.be/3WleAvawtZE

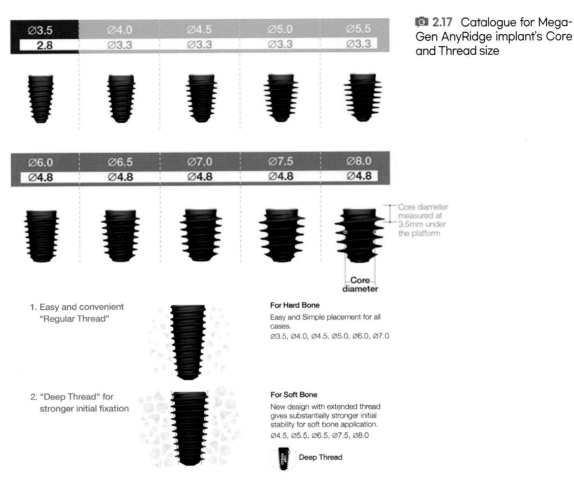

Ø3.5	Ø4.0	Ø4.5	Ø5.0	Ø5.5
2.8	Ø3.3	Ø3.3	Ø3.3	Ø3.3

Ø6.0	Ø6.5	Ø7.0	Ø7.5	Ø8.0
Ø4.8	Ø4.8	Ø4.8	Ø4.8	Ø4.8

Core diameter measured at 3.5mm under the platform

Core diameter

1. Easy and convenient "Regular Thread"

2. "Deep Thread" for stronger initial fixation

For Hard Bone
Easy and Simple placement for all cases.
Ø3.5, Ø4.0, Ø4.5, Ø5.0, Ø6.0, Ø7.0

For Soft Bone
New design with extended thread gives substantially stronger initial stability for soft bone application.
Ø4.5, Ø5.5, Ø6.5, Ø7.5, Ø8.0

Deep Thread

2.17 Catalogue for Mega-Gen AnyRidge implant's Core and Thread size

Let's watch this video. You can see how the thin thread makes the implant placement so easy. Not only you can get good initial fixation in poor bone density area, but also you can even take out the implant and place it again and still get good initial stability.

The **2.17** implant is very interesting. I haven't seen it myself, but I can feel the worries of the CEO of Megagen, who is well known for his love for implant surgery. I heard that Megagen's Anyone is an Astra type-like product, and Anyridge is an implant designed by Dr. Park Kwang-beom himself. Let's compare Osstem's 5.0-diameter wide implant and Anyridge's 5.0-diameter, which I use the most in the molar area in the early Anyridge product lineup (**2.17**). In Anyridge 5.0, the diameter of the core part minus the thread is marked as 3.3. This is about the same size as the core size of a 4.0 regular size implant on Osstem. Moreover, in Anyridge, the inner strength of the implant that holds the abutment is much weaker because there is not even a thread that holds the core in the crestal part. Even when the diameter is enlarged to 5.5 mm, the core size remains the same at 3.3 mm. Therefore, the implant placement of Anyridge 5.0 or 5.5 on the molars is considered to be weaker than the implant placement of Osstem regular size 4.0 without considering the abutment and fixture connection system.

If we review the implant material and surface treatment section in the previous chapter, it probably makes more sense to make this type of implant with alloy like an IBS implant. However, I think the reason why the implants that require such strength are made of Grade 4 instead of alloy is to base the basic surface treatment on SLA (only my opinion). In any case, despite its numerous strengths, Anyridge could not avoid the fracture issue. As a result, Anyridge created a product with an increased core size (in the case of 5.0 and 5.5 wide implants, 3.8 mm and 4.0 mm were added to one core size of 3.3). On the other hand, Anyone made a deep thread implant like Osstem's TS4 for the convenience of placement. Except for this abutment connection part, the fixture shapes gradually improve each other's shortcomings, so it can be said that they resemble each other.

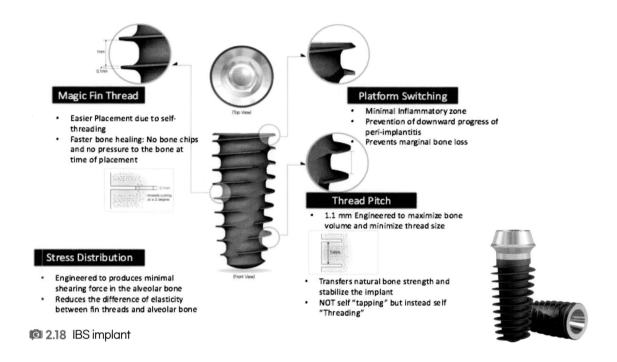

Magic Fin Thread

- Easier Placement due to self-threading
- Faster bone healing: No bone chips and no pressure to the bone at time of placement

Stress Distribution

- Engineered to produces minimal shearing force in the alveolar bone
- Reduces the difference of elasticity between fin threads and alveolar bone

Platform Switching

- Minimal inflammatory zone
- Prevention of downward progress of peri-implantitis
- Prevents marginal bone loss

Thread Pitch

- 1.1 mm Engineered to maximize bone volume and minimize thread size
- Transfers natural bone strength and stabilize the implant
- NOT self "tapping" but instead self "Threading"

📷 2.18 IBS implant

Let's see the advertisement for IBS implants here (📷 2.18). Titanium is 10 times stronger than bone, and bone volume is best formed when the bone is about 1 mm wide. However, this may reduce the size of the core and weaken the threads holding it around, thus weakening structural stability. So this implant is made of a slightly harder alloy. In addition, since the abutment has to be thin, it is basically a tissue-level implant type, and the abutment is fastened at a height farther than the bone. It can be seen as a design that reflects the ideal and reality. Basically, I do not prefer to use bone-level implants because I want to be able to perform all surgeries with just one type of implant, but I really like this design. Since the size of the implant core has been reduced, it cannot be made at bone-level, so it was made to restore like a tissue-level implant. However, the connection between the abutment and the crown is made in a slightly different form from the existing tissue level, and I know that

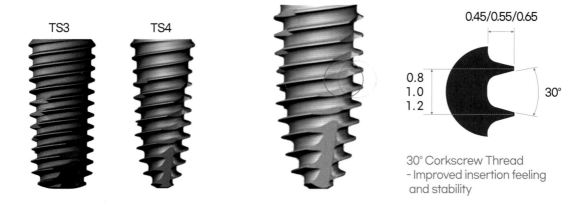

TS3   TS4

0.45/0.55/0.65

0.8
1.0
1.2

30°

30° Corkscrew Thread
- Improved insertion feeling
 and stability

📷 2.19 Comparison of TS3 and TS4 of implants   📷 2.20 Osstem TS4 thread explanation brochure

various applied products from other companies are coming out because the response is rather good. I'm also thinking about when to use it, but I haven't really started using it because I'm not doing prosthetics myself.

📷 **2.19** shows the difference between TS3 and TS4 of Osstem implants. It can be seen that TS4 increases the thread as the diameter of the implant increases. This may be for the convenience of placement while maintaining the structural stability of the implant itself. There is no big difference between TS3 and TS4 in small size, but in 5.0 you can see a big difference in threads. In addition, the overall body shape is adopted as the root type. It has good initial fixation, and good initial fixation can be obtained especially in places with poor bone quality. So, I often use this TS4 after under-drilling one size if the bone quality is poor in the maxillary molars. Also this implant type is selected in the maxillary anterior teeth where the apex may break through the buccal plate or damage adjacent structures.

Recently, as I started to be interested in digital world, my interest in immediate loading using scan bodies has also increased. In this case, TS4 is also used for maxillary premolars. Because the thread is large and root-shaped, the initial fixation is very good. In any case, you can think of it as taking advantage of the root shape in a small diameter size, and taking advantage of a large thread in a large diameter size.

As a result of using the TS4 implant for several years, there has been no case of failure yet, so I am thinking of using it in most cases in the maxillary second molars. The fixation is very good even if the bone quality is very poor. And it also has good inital fixation in immediate placement after extraction in the maxillary molar area because it is root-shaped and has a large screw thread.

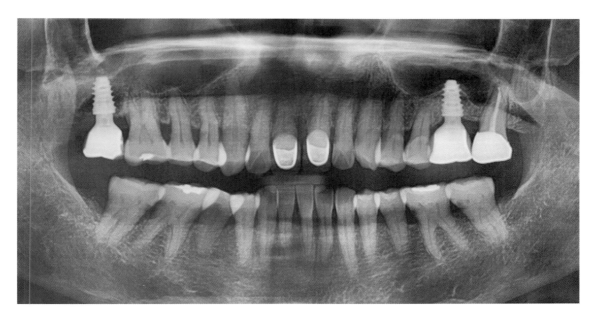

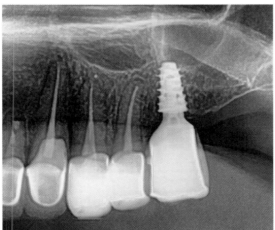
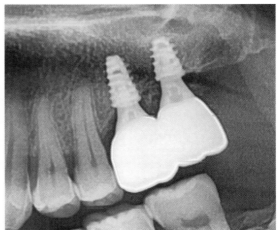

📷 2.21 **3 years after the surgery**
It can be a good choice for maxillary molars in middle-aged women who have comparably poor bone quality.

Case 1

This is a case of a middle-aged woman a while after the extraction. It looks like there is no issue on the radiograph, but at the time of the surgery, the bone was so soft that I could place initial lance drill with my finger into the bone. I figured it is not necessary to drill further, I used TS3 4.0 drill (diameter of 3.3 mm) to drill and placed 5.0×10 mm implant. I usually do not place implants that are longer than 8 mm, but because her bone density was so poor, I placed 10 mm. 📷 **2.22** shows the panoramic xray and the clinical photo of the case.

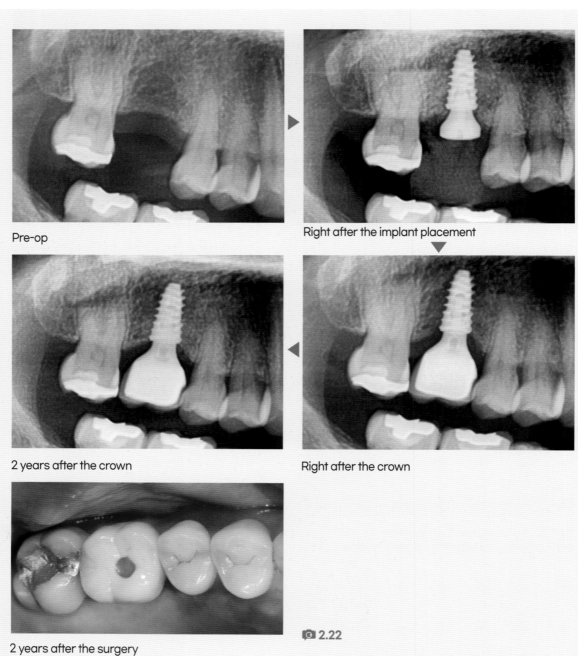

Pre-op

Right after the implant placement

2 years after the crown

Right after the crown

2 years after the surgery

📷 **2.22**

Case 2

Implant was placed with crestal sinus elevation after 1 month of extraction of the tooth that had infection (📷 **2.23**). Except for the sinus floor, there was no place to obtain the initial fixation, so without the drilling, 3.0 diameter osteotome was used to lift the sinus floor bone and after the bone graft, TS3 5.0×8.5 mm implant was placed.

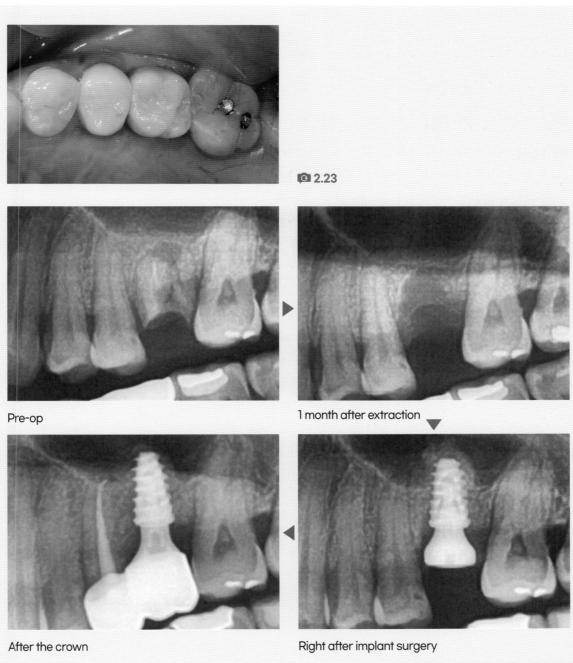

📷 **2.23**

Pre-op

1 month after extraction

After the crown

Right after implant surgery

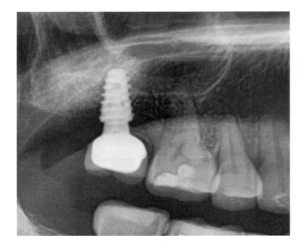

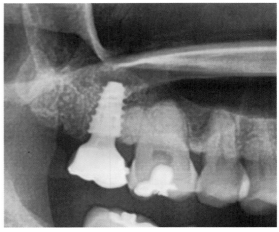

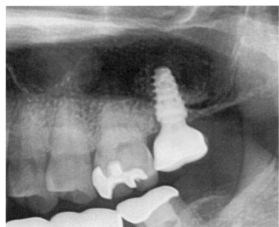

📷 **2.24** 2nd molar case with sinus elevation

The maxillary 2nd molars tend to have lower sinus, and the distance from the bone height to the opposing tooth is often narrow. Usually, when sinus elevation is performed with a crestal approach when the bone height is not good like this, it is often the case surgery is completed forgetting that the distance to the opposing tooth is not enough by focusing too much on initial fixation. Even in this case, in order to secure a minimum distance of 8 mm for the abutment and the crown (originally recommend a minimum of 10 mm, but this will be dealt with in the depth of implants in **Chapter 4-3**), I tend to place TS4 implant a little deeper after the sinus elevation (📷 **2.24**). This is because the TS4 has a large thread, so there is less chance of implant being pushed into the sinus even if the bone volume is low and the bone quality is poor.

How many threads does your implant have?

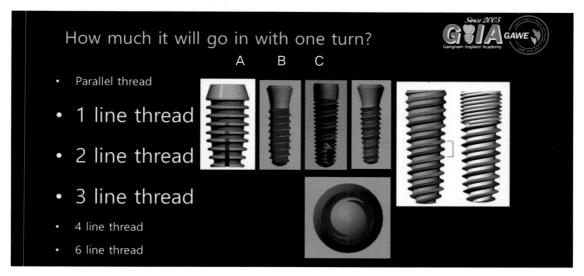

📷 **2.25** Figures showing the number of threads (my lecture slide)

The number of threads in the structure of the implant thread is a very important issue. First of all, there are parallel, non-threaded parallel screws, such as the 📷 **2.25A** Bicon. And there are traditional 📷 **2.25B** single-row screws. The single-row screw is a structure in which the threads are placed one by one when the screw is rotated once. Because it takes a relatively long time to place the implant, it is said that the position or direction can be changed during the placement process, and there is too much friction on the surface of the implant, which is said to cause damage. Also, due to a lot of friction, the bone may be adversely affected.

How about making the implants with 3 rows like 📷 **2.25C** and placing them really fast? This is a form in which three threads start and twist at the same time, and when the implant is rotated once, three threads are inserted. So, if you have the same screw size as a single-row screw, you'll be able to place three times as fast. It also reduces friction between the implant and bone. However, since the depth changes a lot even if the implant fixture is turned a little, it is not easy to adjust the detailed height when placing the implant. In addition, recently the trend is to make larger threads and longer pitches, and if these screws adopt a three-line screw, it is easy to form an implant in which only one or two turns are required. Of course, it may not be easy to adjust the height. In addition, as the diameter of the implant decreases, the angle of the thread must descend too steeply in the apex direction, which may affect the progression of peri-implantitis. I haven't thought about it much, but the more parallel the threads, the more the peri-implantitis acts as a downward barrier, so it may not be good to be too steep.

As a result, people have to think of the word "moderate" again along with the phrase "if it's too much, it's not as good as it can be", so most familiar implants these days use double-stranded screws. Again, this means that if the implant is rotated one full 360°, it will go in by two more threads. Of course, there are single row thread implants such as Anyridge, which has small thread and large core size, and Nobel Active. At the very least, it is very important to know whether the implant you are placing is a single or two-row screw.

The final height of the implant can be adjusted by the rotation angle of the implant

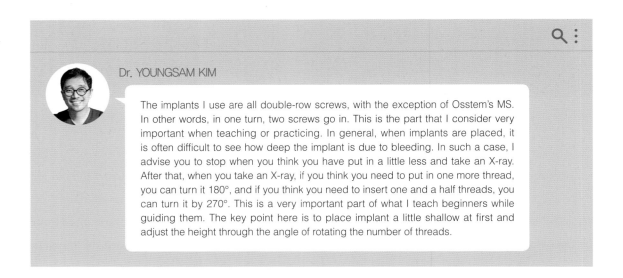

Dr. YOUNGSAM KIM

The implants I use are all double-row screws, with the exception of Osstem's MS. In other words, in one turn, two screws go in. This is the part that I consider very important when teaching or practicing. In general, when implants are placed, it is often difficult to see how deep the implant is due to bleeding. In such a case, I advise you to stop when you think you have put in a little less and take an X-ray. After that, when you take an X-ray, if you think you need to put in one more thread, you can turn it 180°, and if you think you need to insert one and a half threads, you can turn it by 270°. This is a very important part of what I teach beginners while guiding them. The key point here is to place implant a little shallow at first and adjust the height through the angle of rotating the number of threads.

How many times do you turn when you place an implant?

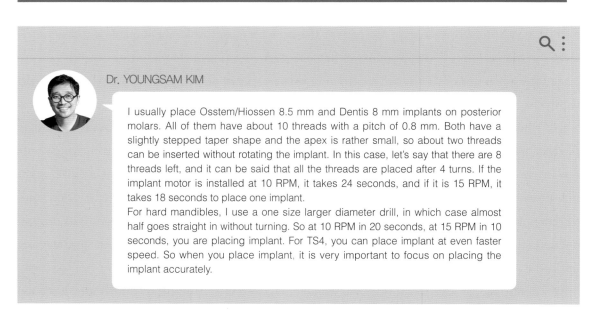

Dr. YOUNGSAM KIM

I usually place Osstem/Hiossen 8.5 mm and Dentis 8 mm implants on posterior molars. All of them have about 10 threads with a pitch of 0.8 mm. Both have a slightly stepped taper shape and the apex is rather small, so about two threads can be inserted without rotating the implant. In this case, let's say that there are 8 threads left, and it can be said that all the threads are placed after 4 turns. If the implant motor is installed at 10 RPM, it takes 24 seconds, and if it is 15 RPM, it takes 18 seconds to place one implant.
For hard mandibles, I use a one size larger diameter drill, in which case almost half goes straight in without turning. So at 10 RPM in 20 seconds, at 15 RPM in 10 seconds, you are placing implant. For TS4, you can place implant at even faster speed. So when you place implant, it is very important to focus on placing the implant accurately.

Earlier, we talked about the body shape and threads of implants. But in fact, to separate the two is difficult because the body shape and thread complement each other's strengths and weaknesses and function as an implant.

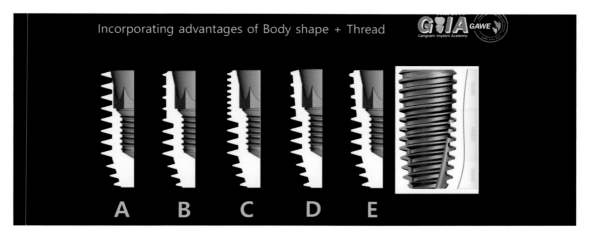

📷 **2.26** Implant body shape and thread shape (I drew it roughly with PPT so please understand how it looks)

📷 **2.26** is the change in the implant body shape and thread shape that I recently observed. The thread is a little bigger but if you make it like 📷 **2.26A**, the top part of the implant is too weak, so you have no choice but to increase the core size to make it like 📷 **2.26B**. Implantium, Dentium's first work, has this shape. Since the threads are small anyway, it is necessary to make them dense and take the form of micro-threads like 📷 **2.26C**. Osstem's GS3 is an example, and in the past, each company had this type of implant. But in Osstem's GS3, there were frequent cases of crestal bone absorption around the micro-threads for some unknown reason.

I've had this happen often too. We are talking about the normal cases with no issues in implant placement depth, abutment length, and micro-gap and movements. The excessive pressure on the alveolar bone can be considered as the primary cause. Of course, this problem can be solved like Ankylos or Astra to some extent by forming the coronal part close to the full size of the implant.

However, Osstem boldly discontinued the GS3. Probably the most I've ever placed in a short period of time was GS3. I personally liked this product. Since the cervical region is made of very fine micro-threads, there were only very few problems with implant tearing. There was no vertical tearing in one case. Of course, the vertical fracture is rare even in TS3, and you will find out later in this book. For information on vertical fracture in detail, see **Chapter 3-2 Choosing Implant Diameter**, and **Chapter 8-2 Fracture of Fixtures and Abutments**. However, I still think that the biggest reason is that the surgeon used excessive force. In addition, at that time, Osstem users were unfamiliar with bone-level internal friction type (Astra type) implants. The implants in general were relatively parallel and the size and the shape of threads were consistent which made the "feeling" of placing implant in coronal or apical consistent. However, it was different "feeling" for Astra type implants, because the cervical area became much thicker or thread became smaller which caused the torque to become suddenly much higher when implant's coronal part starts to go into cortical bone. Also another reason for failure can be that the abutment height and passive fit for internal friction type implants were not taken into consideration during surgery. Dentium's implantium is closer to 📷 **2.26D** compared to the GS3. In 📷 **2.26B**, only the coronal part is slightly thicker. And I think it is made to withstand even a little bone loss by having the implant top a bevel of 0.5 mm and with special surface treatment and threads. However, I think that GS3 may not have been given such attention to detail.

Eventually, micro-threads disappeared. Then the implant should be like 📷 **2.26D**, but if that happens, the thread in the coronal part becomes too small, so I think that the thread was increased a little more at the very top only. In fact, the sizes of OSSTEM implants are 3.7, 4.2, 4.6, and 5.1 instead of 3.5, 4.0, 4.5, and 5.0. In Detnis, OneQ implants were marked with a 0.2 mm increase, in the form of 3.7, 4.2, 4.7, and 5.2 mm. For reference, I've seen Osstem sold in foreign countries as 4.2, 4.6, 5.1 instead of 4.0, 4.5 and 5.0. Perhaps it is because the law of the country requires that the actual size to be indicated.

Anyway, implants like 📷 **2.26E** came out. Considering that the depth of hexa is about 2.8, the core is large to prevent tearing of the implant up to the depth of hexa. Below that, it takes the form of a first-order stepped taper, with a smaller core and larger threads. And since the length of the screw is about 6.5 mm, it is possible to make a step once more in the apex part that is longer than that, and the thread can be bigger. Osstem's TS3 doesn't show it very well, but it's a feature that appears clearly in TS4. I think the TS3 form is an ideal form that reflects the ideal and reality. All bone-level implants in Korea (Osstem's TS3 and TS4, Dentis' OneQ, and Shinheung's Luna) have a similar shape (only my own thoughts).

Stress reduction on crestal bone

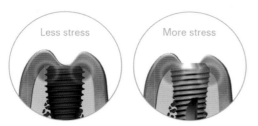

- Placing a fixture into the alveolar bone is easier to control due to the straight upper portion of the fixture.

- Crestal bone loss is minimized by reducing stress in the cortical bone.

📷 **2.27** MegaGen AnyOne implant

📷 **2.27** is an advertisement image of MegaGen Implant. The top part of implants from other companies has a slightly larger diameter as mentioned earlier, but MegaGen's AnyOne advertises that the coronal part is parallel, which reduces stress on the cortical bone and thus has less crestal bone loss. Either way, it seems to be true that giving a lot of stress at the crestal is recognized as one of the causes of crestal bone loss.

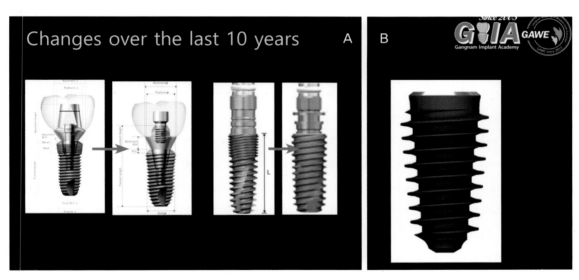

📷 **2.28** Changes overtime for Osstem and Dentium implants

As a result, implants with micro-threads began to disappear from 10 years ago (📷 **2.28A**). Even in Anyridge, there are no threads in the coronal part at all (📷 **2.28B**). Of course, I believe that this can weaken the structure and cause the implant to tear, but it is becoming certain that it is outdated idea to apply tight force and put excessive stress on the cortical bone when placing implant.

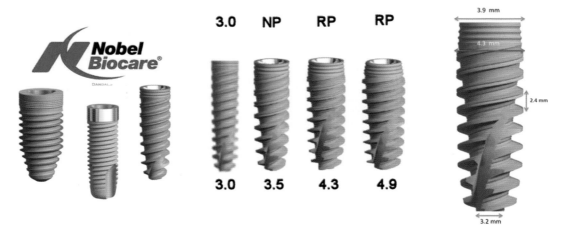

■ 2.29 Nobel Biocare Active implant

■ 2.29 is Nobel Active, the flagship product of Nobel Biocare. Among these implants, from 4.3 mm in diameter, they have a back-tapered shape in the cervical region. Of course, this often weakens the cervical strength and causes the implant to tear. Perhaps it would have been a big deal if it had been sold a lot in Korea. As Shinheung stopped selling Nobel Biocare implants, people started to use less. If a good dealer provides a stable supply, I would have used it, but it is said that they have decided to withdraw from Korea.

The same goes for Straumann's new BLX design. Now, placing "tight" to get initial fixation in the coronal bone is not a trend. So where do I get the initial fixation? It is an Ankylos method that has been passed down - **deep thread in the apical region.**

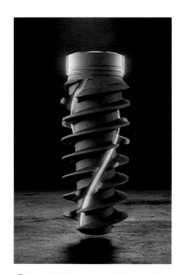

■ 2.30 Straumann BLX Poster

Straumann BLX has just been released so there is not much data yet. But Nobel Active has already been placed a lot, where you see some cases of apex fixture fracture due to thin threads at the apex. These will be revisited in **Chapters 8-2 Fracture of Fixtures and Abutments** at the end of this book.

Anyway, Straumann's BLX is a zirconium and titanium alloy called Roxolid, which has already been proven and successful in terms of strength, so I think this is why such design was adopted (**■ 2.30**). Let's think again here. The world's best implant companies and Megagen all have the same basic concept. The thread of the implant became thinner and larger, and the coronal part of the implant became smaller. Even if we don't put these implants in right now, we should be aware that those who have researched more than us think this is the best concept right now.

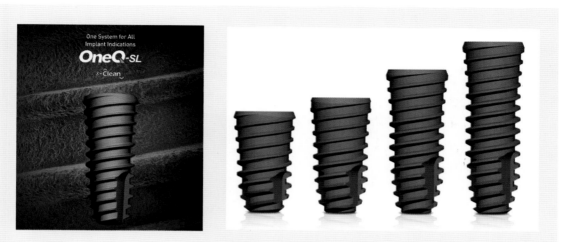

📷 **2.31** Dentis' older product called OneQ that I use the most from Dentis products

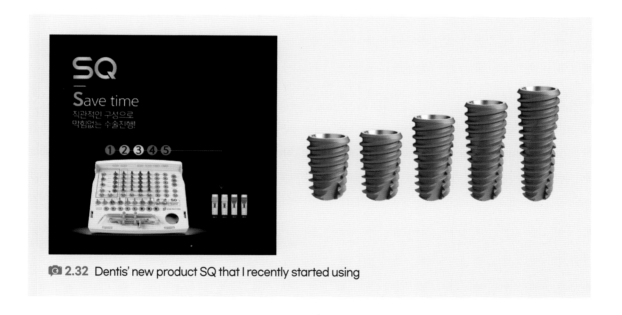

📷 **2.32** Dentis' new product SQ that I recently started using

These are the old and new products of Dentis (📷 **2.31, 2.32**). The SQ product with a reduced diameter of the crestal part was newly released. Of course, the old OneQ products are still in production and are still in use. I think it is very good to use after maxillary sinus elevation when the bone mass of the maxilla is low. At the end, it gets bigger by 0.2 mm from the crestal side, so there is less risk of being pushed into sinus, and the initial fixation is good. The thread size is generally the same. Therefore, although vertical tearing is small in the cervical region, it doesn't get initial fixation at the apical end which is quite disappointing. I would like to see a product that is an improvement from OneQ product which adds larger threads as it goes toward the apical.

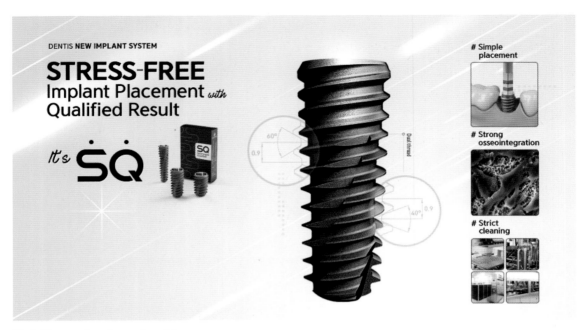

📷 **2.33** new Dentis product SQ

This is SQ's advertisement (📷 **2.33**). Stress-free is emphasized. The S-line of the crestal part, which is the core of OneQ, was boldly removed and made parallel (the overall body shape is root shaped) and as it goes toward the apex the core is smaller and the threads are thinner and deeper. It is a design that contains a typical modern concept. However, it is made smaller than the indicated size in both diameter and length. Since I am worried about the vertical fracture of the molars, I still prefer the older version of

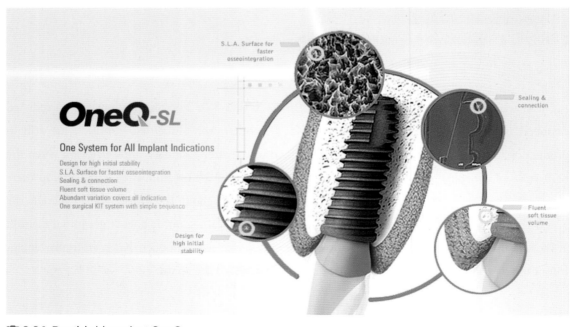

📷 **2.34** Dentis' old product OneQ

OneQ. Otherwise, an implant marked with a size larger than 5.0 should be placed in the molar area.

Compare this to the previous OneQ advertisement (📷 2.34). OneQ is emphasizing that it is designed for initial fixation. It is already known that the tapered shape is advantageous for initial fixation. It seems that the initial fixation is improved and the emphasis is placed on the structural stability of the implant as it increases in size of 0.2 mm increments. I have been using it for a long time, and even though hundreds of implants have been placed over the years at live surgery in Korea, up to this point, there is still no case of vertical fracture. In many ways, it is a product that has never caused a problem such as peri-implantitis and bone resorption.

Live surgery seminar case

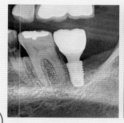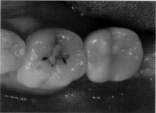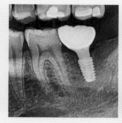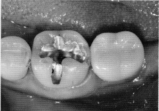

Dentis' old product OneQ 5.2x8　　　　**Dentis' new product SQ 5.0x8**

This is the size that I place the most for the posterior molars.

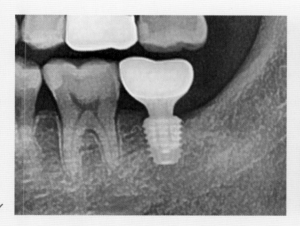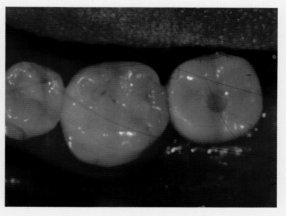

The case was finished with SQ 6.0 because 5.2 drilling was performed with the Dentis OneQ kit, but could not achieve the initial fixation because the employee gave the SQ 5.0 fixture.

These cases were done by the doctors attending the implant seminar but they are very well done. How is it so well done? You will find out when you keep reading this book.

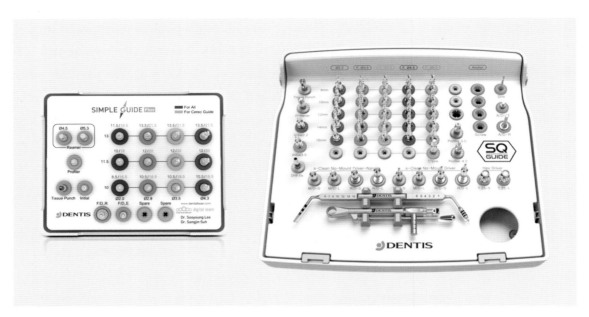

📷 **2.35** Old Dentis kit and new Denits kit

Then, why did Dentis suddenly create a new product called SQ? Is it simply to put less stress on the crestal? In this regard, it was already possible to overcome it by the operator, so each had a knack for it. Personally, I have been very satisfied with OneQ. If so, what was lacking to make SQ? I think it's because it didn't fit well with the guide system. The biggest problem with guide implants is "depth control." Because it is a little different from seeing and feeling with your own eyes, it must not have been easy for the operators to judge the bone quality. When the bone is too hard, sometimes you increase the hole size by lifting the drill a little, but it is not easy in guided surgery. I am against the idea of equating guided surgery with flapless, but the guide appeals to beginners or people who are not proficient in implants, and it is advertised as such. There must have been cases where the beginners had failures due to poor depth control. As a slang term, "stucker," has emerged because it cannot be taken out and is stuck inside. As I mentioned earlier, the tapered shape has the greatest difficulty in height adjustment, so I think that the coronal part is made in a slightly smaller shape, which is a little more advantageous for height adjustment. That is why the newly created guide system and the implant in the shape that fit it were introduced together.

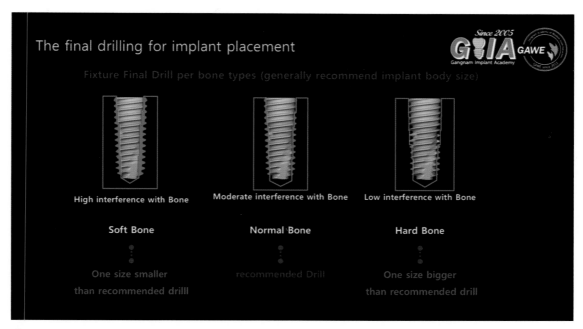

The final drilling for implant placement

Fixture Final Drill per bone types (generally recommend implant body size)

High interference with Bone — Moderate interference with Bone — Low interference with Bone

Soft Bone — Normal Bone — Hard Bone

One size smaller than recommended drilll — recommended Drill — One size bigger than recommended drill

📷 **2.36** Educational material from Osstem implant about different drilling based on the bone

📷 **2.36** is the content used as educational material in Osstem Implant.

Drilling for normal bones and drilling for soft or hard bones are illustrated. To be honest, you do not really need to think much about the soft bone here. This is because there is no problem with drilling the soft bone like a normal bone. It never fails as long as the implant is not moving sideways, under the premise that you are not putting a lot of force when placing implant. If you cannot achieve good stability and fixation you can always place a cover screw. The problem arises when it is hard bone. In the mandible, you should generally assume that it is a hard bone. The design of the implant these days is made in this kind of form, so I think it would be better for the counter sink burs or the coronal shaping burs to be slightly bigger than what they are now.

What is a countersink bur?

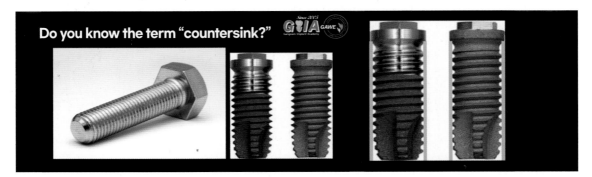

📷 2.37 Explanation of Countersink

Let's think about the word "countersink bur." (📷 **2.37**). Why do we call a bur that widens the implant coronal part a countersink bur? Countersink literally means to not sink. It was used to prevent the head screw from coming out of the general screw. If you look at the implants of Branemark in the early days, they look almost like regular nail screws.

When implants were first introduced, the emphasis was placed on mechanical stability rather than implants being ankylosed to the bone. As a result, extra bump was created on the cortical bone to avoid falling into the mandible, and this part is countersink part. If you look at the early implants, after drilling (pink color), the countersink part was formed to keep it from sinking in its exact shape for mechanical stability of the cortical bone. As a result, from there, the burs that create or expand the coronal portion were expressed as "counter sink burs." Recently, each company calls them by names such as "Coronal Shaping Bur" and "Cortical Removal Bur", but the concept should be considered similar.

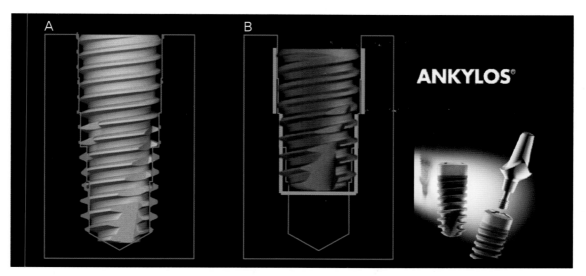

📷 **2.38** Illustration to show to reduce the initial fixation on the coronal portion

📷 **2.38A** is a schematic diagram of implant on a hard bone recommended by Osstem. The coronal part should be regarded as an implant full-size drill, and it is the same as the ankylos method, which obtains fixation only in the apex. However, the problem is that the ankylos method is good, but placing short implants are more of the trend now. No matter how good the bone is, I do not place implants that exceed 8 mm (8.5 mm for Osstem). Since the implants are shorter, there is comparably less portion of implant that can obtain the initial fixation. I wish that the companies can make the shorter implants with the thinner and larger the thread as it goes toward the apex, as long as there are no structural problems. Anyways, the basic concept is the same for short implants. The coronal part should be drilled in full size so that the implant does not move sideways, and **the fixation is obtained from the lower thread in the apex rather than the cortical bone as much as possible.**

2-3

Classification and Understanding of Abutments

Mastering dental implants

Abutments and Screws

Although most modern implant abutments have a hex structure that is separate from the screw (two-piece abutment), this is surprisingly a relatively recent development. While the external hex implants always had the anti-rotational feature separate from the screw, the internal friction type implants have only implemented the two-piece abutment in recent years. Straumann's tissue-level implants introduced the anti-rotational octagon feature in 1999, and they were made available in Korea only after 2000. In the early days, the abutment and the screw was a singular, fused component; most companies still produce one-piece abutments with the screw and abutment being a single component. Therefore, it is critical to know and understand the onze-piece abutment as we see patients with existing implants. The one-piece abutment does not include an anti-rotational hex and it is often susceptible to unwanted rotation and loosening of the abutment, particularly for single crowns.

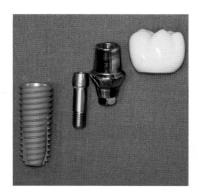

📷 3.1 Hexagonal abutment and separate screw; the most common type in recent years

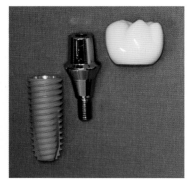

📷 3.2 One-piece abutment without anti-rotational hex

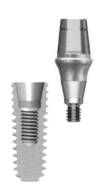

📷 3.3 One-piece abutment (non-hex) fixture and abutment from Osstem. Currently in pro-duction

If a patient complains of a mobile implant placed at a different clinic, the first thing that should be checked is if the abutment and screw are separate. It is often determined by looking carefully at the radiograph. If you were to drill a hole through the crown to find the screw with the intention of re-tightening, you would not be able to find it if a one-piece abutment was used. In this case, the crown is not separated from the abutment as it moves; the entire crown needs to be drilled away to remove it from the abutment (like a traditional crown), or rotate the entire crown to remove the one-piece abutment from the fixture. This is a relatively rare situation but is important to know nonetheless.

A non-hex fixture is still in production from Osstem. Someone must be placing those implants, so that patient may turn up in my office one day. In my 20 years' experience of practice ownership, this happened three times. One was a tissue-level solid abutment rotating along with the crown, and other two were one-piece abutments on Astra Tech-type implants. The first case was especially a huge struggle as I was creating a hole towards the fixture but the screw hole was nowhere to be seen. I kept trying until I ended up drilling away the entire crown, only to find out the screw and abutment were one-piece. Back then, gold was the material of choice for a crown, as opposed to zirconia which is more commonly used these days. Removing the abutment from a zirconia crown would be much more difficult compared to a gold crown. Non-hex abutments are in fashion thanks to its larger surface area, but if you were to use one, I strongly suggest using a two-piece system where the screw and abutment are separate.

What if a one-piece abutment crown is mobile?

Many years ago, the internal friction type implant abutments often implemented a one-piece system. The use of such abutments are decreasing because once the screw loosens, the entire crown becomes mobile, and it is much more difficult to re-tighten the screw as opposed to a two-piece abutment. Despite the infrequent use in recent days, they have been the norm for a period of time, and there are still clinics that routinely use such implants. Hence, it is important to understand the structure of the one-piece abutment. For bridges, a one-piece abutment without an anti-rotational feature is not an issue as it is not subject to rotational forces. However, for a single crown, I recommend using a two-piece abutment, especially for the terminal molar. Let's have a look at the case below.

If a dentist who wasn't aware of the one-piece abutment attempted this case, they would have a hard

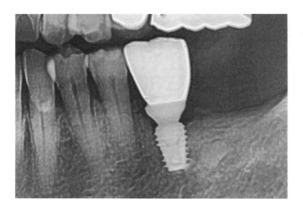

Implant crown with one-piece abutment

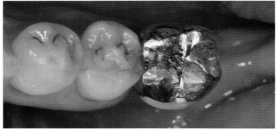

Implant crown with one-piece abutment

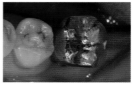 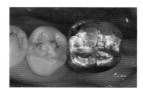

The implant crown is rotating with the abutment. The crown is rotated 90' to the left and 180' to the right, anti-clockwise. The 35 is preventing further rotation.

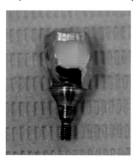

Crown and one-piece abutment removed

time, to say the least, by drilling the entire crown to remove it from the abutment. One-piece abutments saw widespread use at some point and are more common than one may think. It is especially common in tissue-level implants; the radiograph should always be scrutinised prior to creating a hole in the crown to find the screw hole.

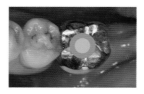 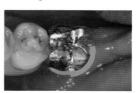

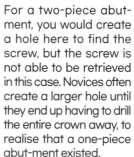 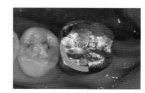

For a two-piece abutment, you would create a hole here to find the screw, but the screw is not able to be retrieved in this case. Novices often create a larger hole until they end up having to drill the entire crown away, to realise that a one-piece abut-ment existed.

The mesial portion of the crown was removed to allow full rotation and removal of the crown.

The terminology, 'bone level' and 'tissue level' were commonly used to categorize types of Straumann's implant in the past, but nowadays these concepts can be applied to most of all implants. When ITI (Straumann) and Branemark (Nobel biocare) were two biggest competitors in implant market in the past (even though they still are now), Branemark focused on placing implants at bone level followed by external hexa type abutment for crown whereas ITI had an single piece tissue level implant that included 2.8 mm height of abutment with smooth surface for crown. However, as complications of tissue level implant arise, Straumann started to focus on bone level implant and it became their main product in the modern days

New companies that came after ITI and Branemark, based a lot on their bone level and tissue level concepts, producing both types of implant system, which is why terminology bone level and tissue level can be applied to most of all implants nowadays. Afterwards, as complications of the external hexa type of bone level implant started to surface, implant companies developed their main implant system to bone level with Astra Tech's internal friction type. Here are some examples of bone and tissue level implants from Osstem.

📷 **3.4A** is bone level, 📷 **3.4B** is tissue level implant. Tissue level implant has direct contact from implant to crown. Abutment type is normally solid abutment (single piece abutment) and places a crown on top of it. The problem with the tissue level implant was that the height of the smooth surface that contacts with gingiva was fixed to 2.8 mm for all. This was not always ideal for anterior

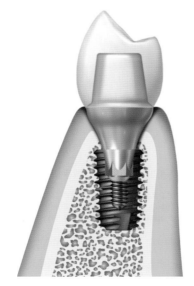 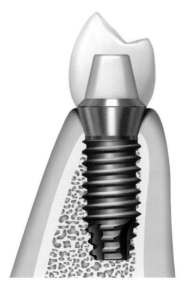

A. Bone level imlpant   B. Tissue level implant

📷 **3.4** Comparison between Bone level imlpant and Tissue level implant

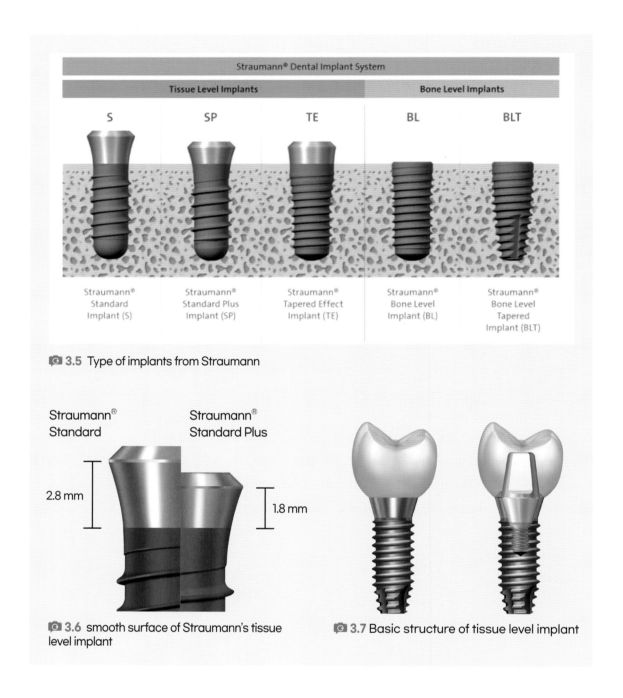

3.5 Type of implants from Straumann

Straumann®
Standard

Straumann®
Standard Plus

2.8 mm

1.8 mm

3.6 smooth surface of Straumann's tissue level implant

3.7 Basic structure of tissue level implant

cases requiring aesthetics, and later the company developed another type of implant called 'Standard Plus' ,with only 1.8 mm height of smooth surface for anterior and premolar teeth (**3.6**).

Even though it was not perfect, it could be used well by adjusting depth of implant placement. I used to mostly use External hexa type initially, however, because implant price was becoming cheaper among practices, the fact that bone loss was inevitable and hefty lab fee for gold abutment from UCLA, it was difficult to use External hexa type. Ever since then I started to use mostly SS2, Tissue level implant from Osstem for posterior areas.

Tissue level implant case 1

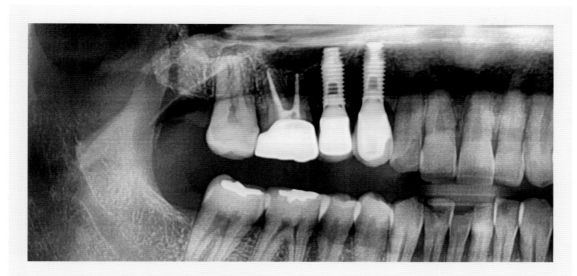

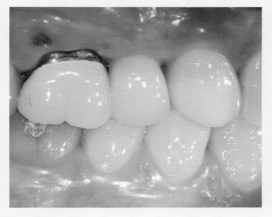

Buccal View
16 Showing crown margin due to gingival recession over time. On the other hand 13 14 tissue
level implant crowns show to maintain a better
gingival aesthetics than 16.

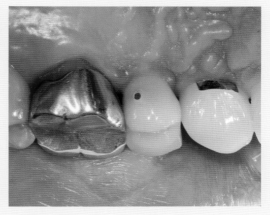

Palatal View
Palatal side shows gingiva is better main-tained
with tissue level implants on 13 14.

📷 **3.8** Tissue level implants of 13 14 (Osstem SS2) placed in 2005. 15 years later

Photo 📷 **3.8** represents a case of tissue level implant placed on 13 14 sites on a 30 year old patient.
It shows great stability on gingiva and bone as the depth was carefully calculated and placed, causing
almost no bone resorption. Next is a referred case from another dentist due to a difficult situation -
patient requiring an implant to replace mobile upper maxillary anteriors.

Tissue level implant case 2

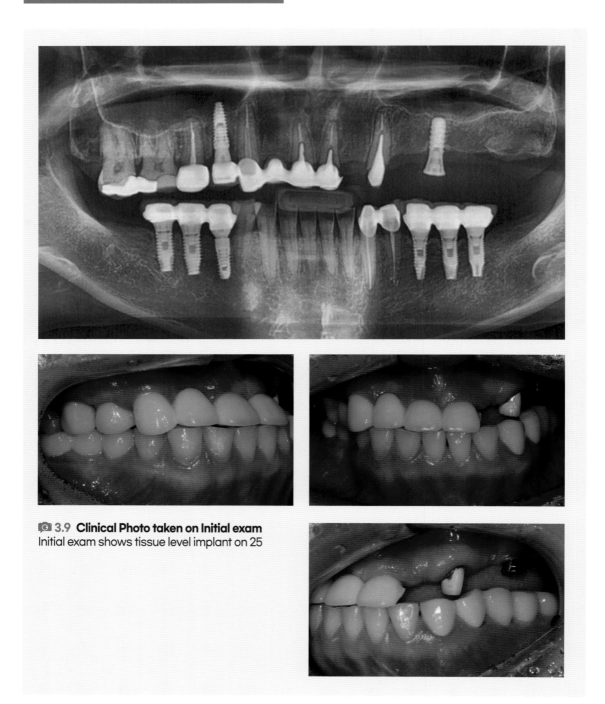

📷 **3.9 Clinical Photo taken on Initial exam**
Initial exam shows tissue level implant on 25

In 2016, a 35 years old female patient represented failing post crowns with secondary caries in the upper anterior region. Additionally, the patient also had poor occlusion making the situation worse. We have convinced the patient to get orthognathic surgery to correct the jaw and bite relationship in order to place the implant in a better position (📷 **3.9**).

Now have a look at the 25 tissue level implant that was done a long time ago. It was more like a white elephant. As the patient's occlusion was not stable yet and that bone around 25 was also fragile, we decided to keep the existing 25 implant and work the whole treatment plan around it. 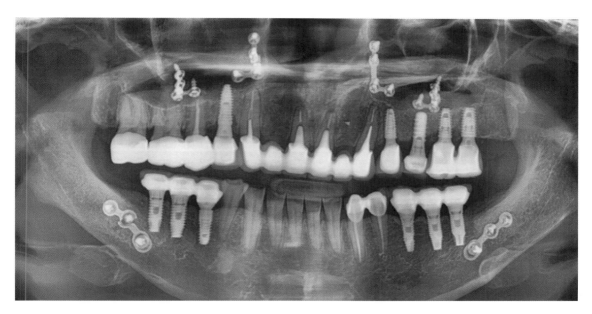 **3.10** represents post-operative treatment.

25 left as a fly in an ointment. That single implant spoiled the perfect rehab case that could have been so pleasant. There has been a gingival recession and bone resorption around 25 implants over years, where now the metal frame of the implant is exposed. I mean it would have been placed at the

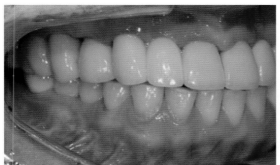

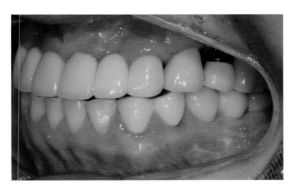

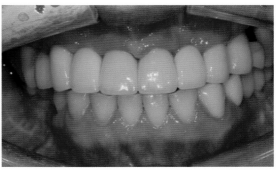

📷 **3.10 Photo and OPG after rehab and surgery**
The metal frame of tissue implant on 25 is quite visible.

Cases of restoration of anterior region with posts

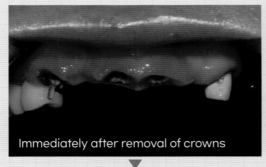

Immediately after removal of crowns

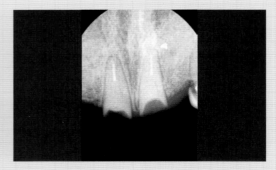

▼

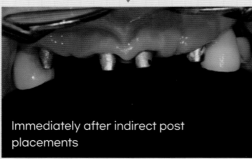

Immediately after indirect post placements

📷 3.11

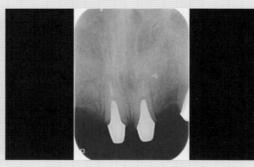

▼

📷 3.12 I don't normally do general treatments nowadays, but when I used to, I always tried to avoid using posts, and if I would ever use it, it would always be indirect posts. I had to see this patient as no associate wanted to treat this patient.

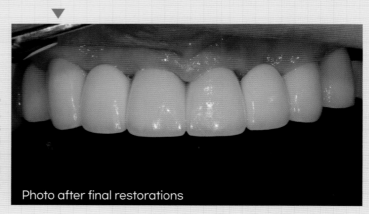

Photo after final restorations

I have decided to do bridge on anterior teeth after learning that the patient's occlusion has been much more ideal after orthognathic surgery. I realized again that nothing can beat natural teeth, even if it's a great implant. Also advised the patient that her bite condition was not quite stable as it was not long after orthognathic surgery was performed and therefore, advised to come back for regular occlusion check, as slightest amount of bite change could hugely impact on the anterior bridge. In similar cases like this, we must ensure to eliminate overloading on the anterior region, especially if all molars are implants.

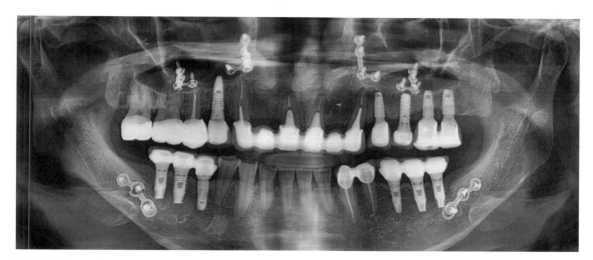

📷 **3.13** OPG after 6 months later

correct gingival level back when it was first placed, but now this is very unpleasant to see, especially considering when the patient is a young female. Therefore, we must pay more attention to placing implants at the correct height when it comes to areas with high aesthetic standards.

This is a panoramic X-ray taken 6 months later of the same patient (📷 **3.13**). Even if we advised to come back for a regular occlusal check, she only showed up for the first time in 6 months. Her dentition was reasonable then, but she never showed up afterwards. I wish to believe something more important was keeping her away, but generally there are lots of patients who don't listen to the dentist's advice.

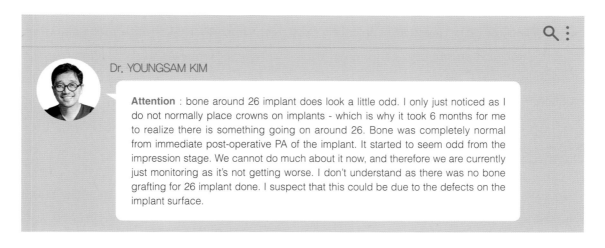

Dr. YOUNGSAM KIM

Attention : bone around 26 implant does look a little odd. I only just noticed as I do not normally place crowns on implants - which is why it took 6 months for me to realize there is something going on around 26. Bone was completely normal from immediate post-operative PA of the implant. It started to seem odd from the impression stage. We cannot do much about it now, and therefore we are currently just monitoring as it's not getting worse. I don't understand as there was no bone grafting for 26 implant done. I suspect that this could be due to the defects on the implant surface.

It's good to avoid tissue level implant as it is hard to predict gingival shape and height. Moreover, when you are using a tissue level implant, you always need an extra step in the surgery or restoration stage to check how the gingival height is going to be. This is quite a nuisance and very annoying as you are required to keep a lot more implant stocks for various sizes per different gingival height. Moreover, sometimes you end up doing two stages due to weaker primary stability, which then also forces you to have bone level implants as a backup. And again this is another kind of stock. By then,

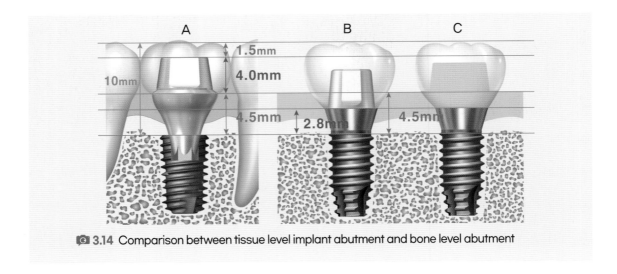

3.14 Comparison between tissue level implant abutment and bone level abutment

you just think "I should just stick to the bone level implant". Around that time, many have found how to maintain good gingival stability with the bone level implants. With its simplicity, bone level implants have become a trend among dentists over tissue level implants.

3.14A represents the ideal height of the bone level implant for a single placement. **3.14B** picture is drawn based on the method that we tend to place an extra 1 mm below for bone level implants. In reality, there are often times where the top margin is positioned in the middle of the gingiva even for 2.8 mm tissue level implant, in cases with thicker gingiva or times where we place implants even deeper on purpose to gain ideal distance from the opposing tooth. In this kind of scenario, most tissue level implants use extra abutment between the fixture and crown **3.14C**, which makes almost no difference to bone level implant. This is quite ironic for tissue level implant, as the biggest advantage of using tissue level is the use of solid abutment. This is another reason why bone level implants could become a trend, as it has one-piece abutment from bone to gingiva without any margin.

Tissue level implant case 3

Use of solid abutment is the biggest advantage of tissue level implant as it allows simplifies crown restorations. Please be mindful that the cases I have are quite old as it has been more than 10 years since I have used a tissue level implant.

As seen from **3.15** case, one simply takes an impression and restores crown at the gingival level. Downside is that you can see extra cements stuck between crown and fixture immediately after. This patient still uses this implant strongly, however he does not come for a check up as he has a son-in law in a rural area who can check for him. Recent photo is from the son-in law dentist.

It is common to see crown loosening from tissue level implant, as the size for solid abutment is relatively small.

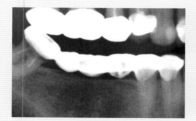

Initial pano (07-04-2005)

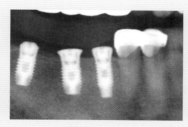

Immediate post op (14-04-2005)

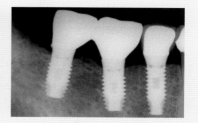

Immediate post restoration
(22-07-2005)

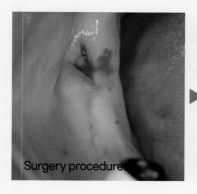

Surgery procedure

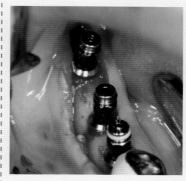

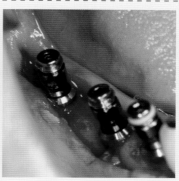

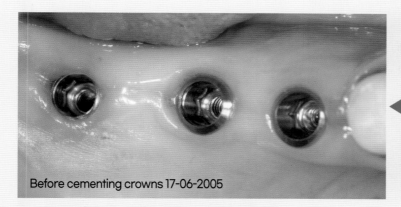

Before cementing crowns 17-06-2005

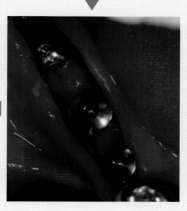

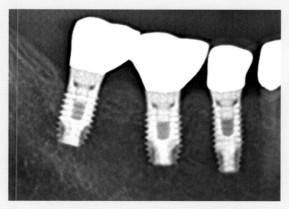

Most recent photo after 15 years of placement from
son-in law dentist

📷 3.15

Tissue level implant case 4

Now let's take a look at a case with a problem. 📷 **3.16** shows the bridge loosening case of an implant that is only four years old; the implant was placed in 2007 and the bridge fell off in 2011. I cannot estimate how many single crowns would've come loosened when even a bridge can become loosened this easily.

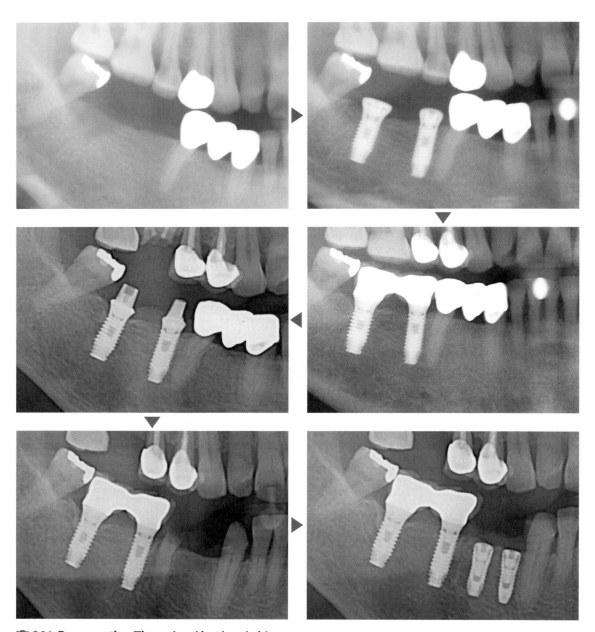

📷 **3.16 Recementing Tissue level implant bridge**
PA shows 45 is solid abutment, 46 is normal abutment where abutment and screw are seperated. Come to think of it, this type of abutment is not great for making a bridge. If you have to tighten 45 screw due to crown loosening, the stopping position is not going to be constant everytime when it's tightened, meaning the crown may not fully fit.

Tissue level implant case 5

📷 **3.17** also shows a case that was done in 2007. Solid abutment crown came loose and dislodged. The crown was replaced by using a custom abutment. There was only one option for wide neck type abutment (ø 6.0 mm) from Ostem, and it was not convenient to have a single height option of 2.0 mm (not 1.8 mm or 2.8 mm) from gingival height perspective. This becomes a problem especially when you have to place an implant at a deeper level because you don't have enough prosthodontic distance for a crown from the opposing tooth. Photo shows the implant with healing abutment that is not fully fitting. It is a shame to not be able to follow up this patient in the clinic as the patient is currently overseas. It is very important to be aware of this tissue level ø 6.0 mm wide neck SS2 as there are many of this placed in South Korea.

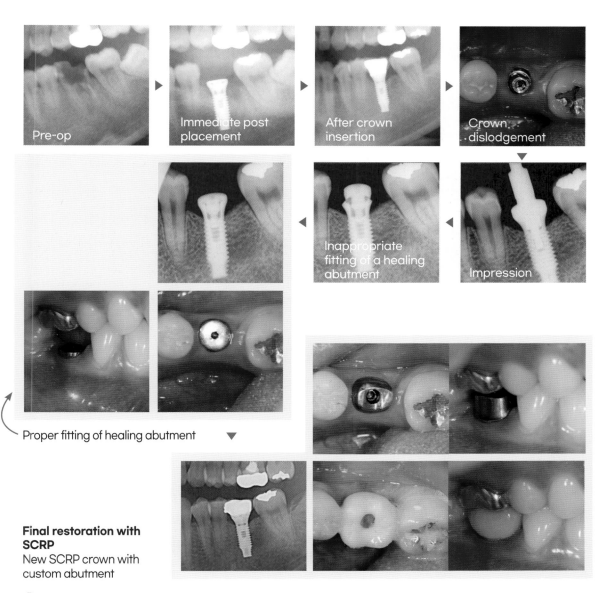

Pre-op

Immediate post placement

After crown insertion

Crown dislodgement

Inappropriate fitting of a healing abutment

Impression

Proper fitting of healing abutment

Final restoration with SCRP
New SCRP crown with custom abutment

📷 **3.17**

Two cases above have been saved due to collegue's good old habit. Crown loosening problem limits the clinicians to use solid abutment as it happens quite commonly.

However what's worse is when a solid abutment comes loose with the crown still intact. In this case, the crown and abutment is slightly moving but cannot fully rotate 360 degrees due to neighbouring teeth, and therefore cannot be retrieved. This can become a big problem for a beginner who has little knowledge about a solid abutment crown, when they try to look for a screw hole in the crown that does not exist. There was even literature published to explain why this happens so commonly. For single crown cases, clinicians now rarely use solid abutment in posterior regions. In order to retrieve the loosened solid abutment, you would have to remove a lot of crown surface as solid abutments were normally small in size. This was quite stressful for many clinicians, but it was still doable back in old times when gold crowns were predominant, which is relatively softer than zirconia or PFM crowns that are mostly used now. As zirconia and PFM crowns become more dominant, removing solid abutment screw has become one of the most difficult things to do for a clinician.

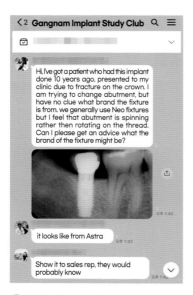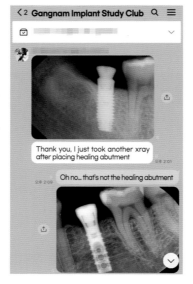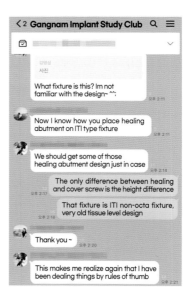

📷 **3.18** Kakao talk

In 📷 **3.18**, one questioned how to restore a crown on a tissue level implant that was done by someone else. One advised that it seems to be Ossem SS2, but nobody can know in reality. One replaced the old crown and placed a healing abutment. One must make sure to cover all the margin for tissue level implant, so that when crown is restored, there would be no gap between an implant and crown. You never know when you will encounter this type of tissue level implant case. There are already millions of tissue level implants in South Korea. You must be familiar with basic structure.

Tissue level case 6

In 2004, we used to always place SS2 tissue level implants for patients with good bone quality (📷 3.19). I remember an interesting case with this special patient. The patient has severe bipolar disorder. When the implant was placed, the patient's behaviour was very compulsive, and when time came to restore the crown, the patient was very depressed and suspicious. She mentioned that "google says it takes two surgeries before crown insert. Why do you only perform a single surgery before placing the crown" and she refused to have the crown put. It is quite a sad story but it also reflects how generalized it was to do two stage implant using external hexa type among the clinicians.

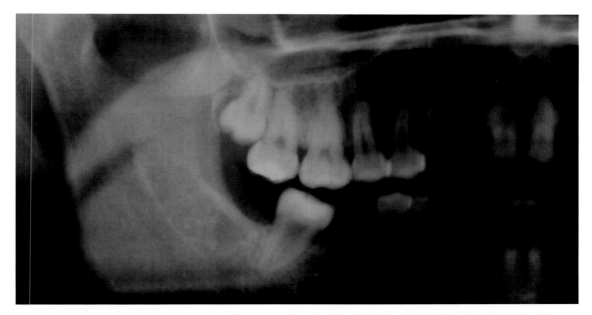

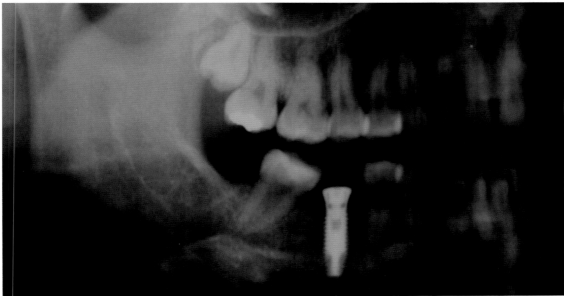

📷 **3.19** 2004 patient refused to put the crown on tissue level implant

Tissue level case 7

A 60 years old patient came in due to a fistula around 25 (📷 **3.20**). It was decided to remove 26 pontic by sectioning 25 distal and 27 mesial, followed by root canal treatment on 25 and periodontal treatment on 27. However it was found that the root on 27 had fractured during periodontal treatment phase (📷 **3.21**). It was then replaced with an implant over two stage surgeries (📷 **3.22**).

A

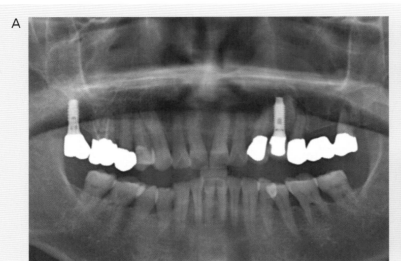

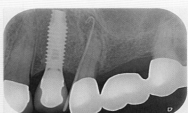

Initial PA showing fistula tracing with GP point

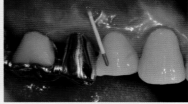

Fistula tracing with mirror

Pre-op Panorama, 2011/04

📷 **3.20** 2011.04.25 Patient presented with cc being sinus perforation

B

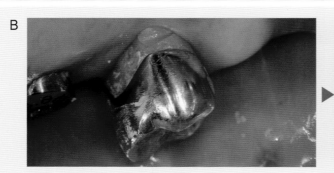

📷 **3.21** 27 fractured root visible

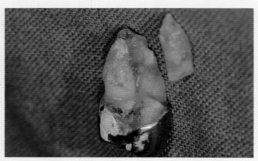

📷 **3.22** Extracted 27

C

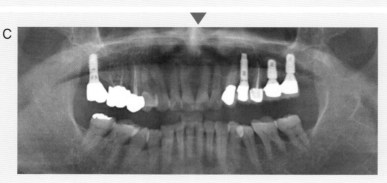

📷 **3.23** post op after final restorations on implants on 26 27

Dr. YOUNGSAM KIM

P.S I made sure that fistula was from 25 by tracing with GP point. I then advised the nurse to take a photo of the GP tracing while I was seeing another patient briefly. When I came back, I started doing root canal on 15. Patient then asked "why are you doing it on the right hand side?". I realized that the photo was reversed as it was in the mirror. It was the first time in 12 years since graduating that I performed root canal treatment on the wrong tooth. I begged for forgiveness and that I will do anything for him if he lets me continue other work. I have finished doing RCT on the hurting tooth, 25. Later, he told me that he had already been to another clinic before coming to mine. He thought that I was an honest dentist as I wanted to save 25 whilst he was advised to replace 25 26 27 with implants, which made him forgive me and continue treatments. Ever since then I treat this patient as if I owe him my life.

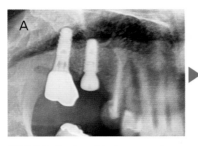

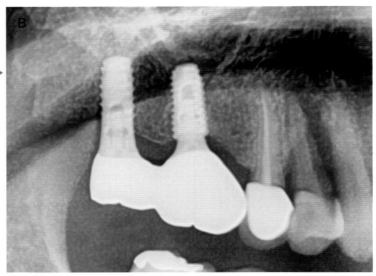

📷 3.24 Post op 16 placement

Note : The crown shape does not look too great on 17. If I can defend on this, 15 temporary crown was too wide and 17 implant was placed slightly tilted on the distal side. I admit that I was not taking many xrays to check pathways, which I believe to cause this problem. If there is a temporary crown around where you are going to place an implant, make sure to check pathways from X Rays, not judging from temporary crowns.

After 4 years, the 16 tooth was replaced with an implant in 2015. The 17 crown on tissue level implant often came loose and caused food impaction between 17/16. I removed the 17 crown and placed a bridge between 16-17 when I was restoring the 16 implant. I used SCRP this time so that it can be fixed and repaired easily. The main reason that we are discussing this case in this chapter is to emphasize again, that this **tissue level implant patient can come to you anytime and that patient can become a very important person to you.** This patient means a lot to me, and therefore I will fix anything for him if the 24 implant becomes problematic as well. Hence, **you must be familiar with characteristics of tissue level implant and how to make crowns for it.** Moreover, I even did a gold crown for him on the 16 and 17 with the bottom of my heart and respect in the eras of cheap zirconias. We later also did another implant for him on the tooth 14, as it had a vertical root fracture.

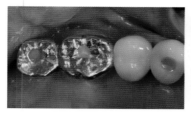
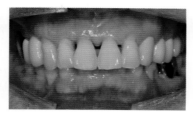
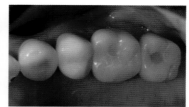

📷 3.25 2021/04
In 2016, the 14 implant was placed. All implants shows nothing significant, they are all going well. Even the teeth 15 and 25 with RCTs doing well

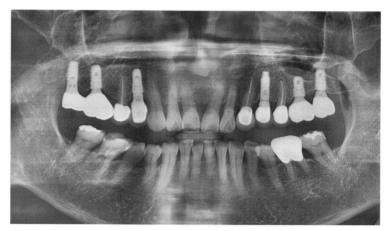

This is a panorama taken in 2021/04, after 10 years since the initial visit (📷 **3.25**). I am still ashamed of the 16 implant pathway as it's not perfect. If i was to make an excuse, the temporary of 15 was too wide, 17 was too distalized and opposing for 16 was also buccally tilted, making it very difficult to estimate perfect pathway. I will explain why it was so difficult later in the upcoming clinical book. There is nothing I like about the 16 implant placement and even the 26. I always consider the central groove of neighbouring teeth and opposing tooth, but this becomes confusing and inaccurate for guiding implant pathways when the patient has a severe crowding or occlusion issues. Even when I was placing the 26, the 27 crown's mesial surface has been trimmed off, and the 25 was also wide on distal like the 15 temporary that I discussed above. However, you can see the 14 implant has a good pathway as it did not have anything interfering like the 16 or the 26. You can also see the 15 and 25 RCT teeth are also doing good.

In addition, buccal emergency profile is very important for upper premolar regions. Both the crown on the 24 tissue level implant (that was done 15 years ago) and the crown on bone level implant on the 14 (that was done 5 years ago) have a well formed emergence profile. Also with great oral hygiene care, the patient's perio status has been very stable, even around implants.

What is more important than choosing bone level or Tissue level? It is the implant abutment connections. Let's take a look at them in detail.

A
External Hex   Iternal Morse taper   Internal conical seal

B

C

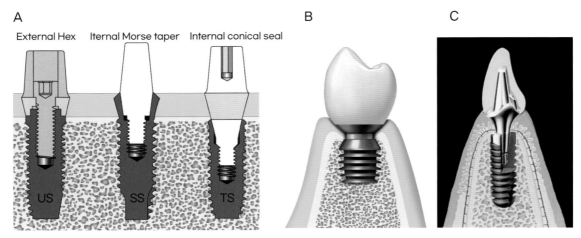

📷 3.26 **Different types of implant abutment connections**

📷 **3.26A** shows a diagram of implant abutment connections of the Osstem implant that I normally use. This shows and almost can say that it includes most of the important characteristics of famous implants around the world. The US system I that I have used for the first time is based on the external hexa system of the Nobel biocare implant. The SS system of the Osstem implant has 8° internal taper fundamental from Struamann's Tissue level implant, and the TS system of the Osstem has 11° internal taper fundamental from Astra Implant. Aforementioned, the Osstem implant carries most similar fundamentals from famous implant companies among the world except that it has different anti rotational octa and height of the hexa. Therefore, it is compatible for those healing abutments and cover screws without octa and hexa. Later with the change from the Astra implant, where it changed the entire internal hexa system to their own, we normally name the TS system of the Osstem, 'Old Astra type'. Regardless, **the most of the implants from South Korean companies are the 'Old Astra type' that has slightly different size and height of the hexa to Astra implants.** The first company to create the 'old Astra type' was Dentium even though they had slightly different hexa system to Astra; this maybe due to patent issue, later on Osstem created the system that is very close to the 'old Astra type' and that it is almost compatible with Astra implants. Moreover, most latecomer companies in South Korea started to create a system that is also compatible with the Osstem company as it is the most popular implant company in South Korea Osstem. With this reason, most of the implants from South Korea are very similar to Astra implants, as they are almost identical to 'old Astra type' implants. Because

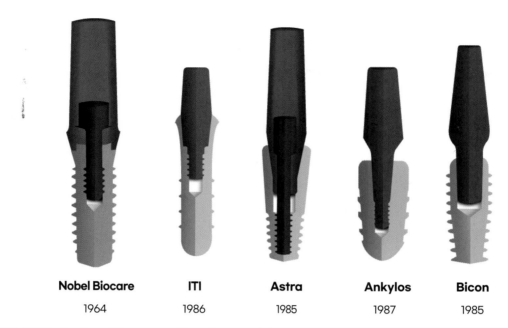

Nobel Biocare	ITI	Astra	Ankylos	Bicon
1964	1986	1985	1987	1985

📷 **3.27 Mechanics of the tapered interference fit in dental implants**

Source: Journal of Biomechanics Volume 36, Issue 11 , November 2003, Pages 1649-1658.

of this, implants from newborn company DIO and ShinHeung are almost compatible with Osstem implants. However, I still think that you do not have to necessarily mix them as they will have different levels of error and skills in the production phase. Anyhow, Dentium has become a company with the most unique internal hexa system that is not compatible with the other implant as they did not follow the Osstem implant. 📷 **3.26B** shows a Bicon implant system in which you literally smash implants into the bone and abutments into implants, and that has an internal taper of 1.5° (true morse taper). 📷 **3.26C** represents the Ankylos system with 5.74° internal taper. There are various types of implant abutment systems around the world, however the types that have been long lasting are seen on 📷 **3.27**.

📷 **3.27** shows the basis of the modern implants that I believe is very important to know. This picture shows all implant abutment connection types. Rest of the connection types that are not alike from the picture 📷 **3.27**, came from any of these roots. Of course there are other forms of implant abutment connection and some unique types that are still being used. However, you will soon realize why those cannot become popular, and most major companies do not make replicas of them.

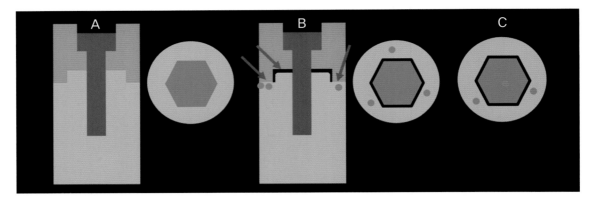

⊙ 3.28 Diagram of external hexa type implant (referenced from my lecture)
A: Ideal fitting, **B**: Realistic fitting. Better fitting at the red arrow is more important than the blue arrow. Realistically speaking, it is safe to say there would be only three points (green dots) of contact made to fit, rather than all surfaces of the screw being connected at the red arrow margin **C**: If there is an interference inside the screw, there could be less than three contact points at the abutment fitting surface margin.

First of all, let's take a look at external hexa type abutments (⊙ **3.28**). External hexa type of Branemark implant system has a hex with 0.7 mm height as a default. This external hex structure is created only to serve an anti-rotational and slipping purpose, not supporting connection. In fact, the implant and abutment is only relying on the small screw, which makes higher prevalence of screw fracture amongst other existing problems. This can be slightly improved if the hex had a higher height, but then it loses the benefit as bone level implant, as higher hex height will then be exposed outside gingiva like tissue level implant. Moreover, if implant and abutment connection is a butt joint, it will eventually cause many complications regardless whether it is external or internal type

Generally, the male part of the screw is smaller than the female part, in order to increase fitting surfaces even in a state without occlusion. Let's throw a hypothesis here. Can a metal with low ductility like a titanium can fit surface to surface? Even for a chair with four legs we normally use, we know that only three legs would be in contact with the ground in a stationary state, and the other would be floating, unless there is a force putting down. As a result, there will be a gap at the fitting margin between implant and abutment because there will only be three points of contact. In addition if there is a fitting contact point on the screw between implant and abutment, there would be only one or two contact points at the margin, meaning increased gap at the fitting margin. This is why it is inevitable to have a gap at a butt joint connection. If the marginal gap is less than 20 μm, it is said to avoid bacterial proliferation. I thought this literature report was from a modern study, but it turns out to be referenced from a few decades old studies related to perio and prosthodontics. Surely there can be modern findings related to this, but I have not seen one yet. Just so you know, when the size of streptococci is around 2-5 μm, I believe it is still possible for them to infiltrate and proliferate in the 20 μm marginal gap. However, also knowing that streptococci tend to herd, 20 μm space is perhaps considered insufficient for them to colonize in my opinion.

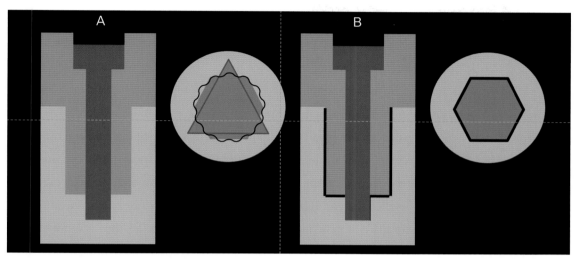

📷 3.29 Diagram of internal fit type
A: Ideal connection, **B**: Realisting connection

Let's take a look at internal fit type (📷 **3.29**). The reason this type is not categorized as 'internal hexa type' is that there are various shapes of internal type from flower to triangle. Internal hexa type has internal connection, unlike with external hexa that has external connection which can be visible from gingiva. This allows for internal hexa type to have deeper connection surface area, normally more than 1.5 mm which is almost twice the amount of external hexa type. However, it generally has butt joint connection, where you can expect a marginal gap even on unloading state and on loading state, this gap can be greater. Moreover, internal fit type can have less prevalence of screw fracture as it rotates internally, but it can sometimes have implant tear problems.

The most common method to reduce marginal gap for crown or inlay is placing a bevel on the margin. This is why few internal fit type implants have a bevel around the margin and some companies still

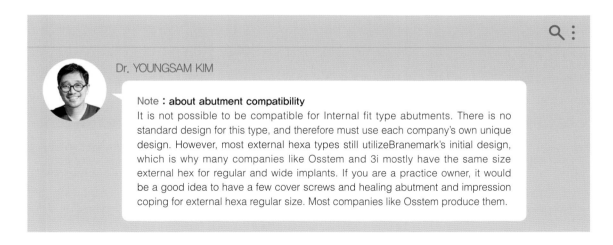

Dr. YOUNGSAM KIM

Note : about abutment compatibility
It is not possible to be compatible for Internal fit type abutments. There is no standard design for this type, and therefore must use each company's own unique design. However, most external hexa types still utilizeBranemark's initial design, which is why many companies like Osstem and 3i mostly have the same size external hex for regular and wide implants. If you are a practice owner, it would be a good idea to have a few cover screws and healing abutment and impression coping for external hexa regular size. Most companies like Osstem produce them.

utilize this design. However, I personally do not think it is an ideal design. You can see most of this type of implants are made with alloy rather than CP titanium, in order to avoid fractures at bevel margins. Also it is required to consider some spacing internally in order to increase fitting at the bevel surface. As a result, you can expect a smaller marginal gap at fitting surface due to beveling effect, but it is not possible to limit a gap expansion from forces of moving occlusion. The main reason companies consider extra spacing inside is intended for more smooth and better fitting of implant and abutment, ultimately reducing chances of misfit and preventing larger gaps. Imagine even if an implant is produced with perfect measurements and technology, nobody can predict and control the amount of contraction and expansion of the metal depending on different patients' internal oral temperature, micro deviations in inserting angle of the implant and more. Above examples explain why it is not possible to have both perfectly calculated internal fitting and fitting at bevelled margin. Realistically, it is always going to be one or the other, not both fitting if there was no extra space. If bevelling surface misfits and internal fits then it is not too bad but if internal fit is interfered, then it would have the worst case scenario - abutment not fully integrating with implant and being stuck in halfway, causing open gap between implant and abutment. Surprisingly this has happened quite often, which is why companies are forced to create extra space in the internal hex in order to facilitate clinical convenience. Moreover, there is a tendency to have small internal taper degrees in this type of implant (normally 1-2°) for clinical convenience (ex. Zimmer's Tapered Screw-Vent).

In summary, even if bevelling margin creates a smaller gap at the connection margin, it is not possible to minimize gap expansion occurring internal hex once loaded, and therefore, the benefit becomes meaningless after all.

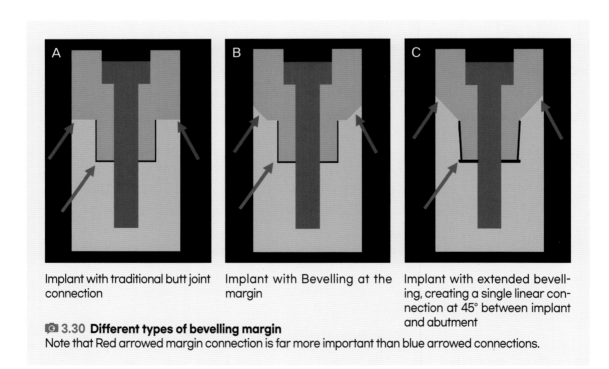

Implant with traditional butt joint connection

Implant with Bevelling at the margin

Implant with extended bevelling, creating a single linear connection at 45° between implant and abutment

📷 **3.30 Different types of bevelling margin**
Note that Red arrowed margin connection is far more important than blue arrowed connections.

Following diagram shows an example of an internal friction type implant, which is Struamann's Tissue level implant that has a morse taper of 8°. I will briefly discuss the concept of morse taper as tissue level implants have been covered a lot above.

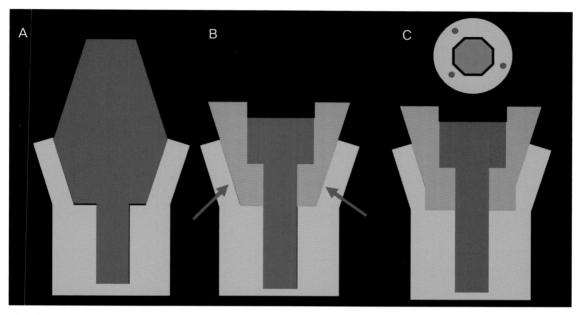

📷 **3.31 PPT slide made by me for lectures**
A: Diagram of solid abutment where abutment and screw were connected as one body, **B**: Diagram of two body system where abutment and screw are seperate. This type of internal friction type needs to ensure there is minimal gap on red arrowed points. **C**: Diagram of an implant that has external octa as anti-rotational purpose

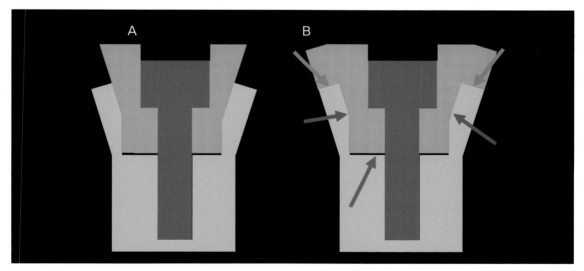

📷 **3.32 A**: Diagram of when crown margin conjuncts tissue level implant margin , **B**: Diagram of when another abutment conjuncts with tissue level implant margin. In this case, green arrow points must have the highest fitting surface, meaning there would be inevitable gaps in the red and blue arrowed area.

Definition of 8 degrees from Straumann

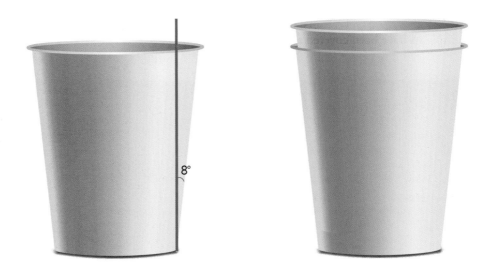

📷 3.33 Actual measurement of taper angle of paper cups used in our practice. It was the same 8 degrees as Straumann's implant.

If a metal conjuncts another metal at a taper of 6-8°, it is known that the conjunction between two metals is stable with minimal gap and also it is easily retrievable. This is why this taper angle is often utilized on assembly of metals, especially upon insertion of metal into the internal surface of another metal. Let's take a look at the example of paper cups even though they are not metal (📷 3.33). Normally paper cups have 8° taper. When paper cups are inserted into each other, you can see they can fit very closely without gaps at the margin, with almost no shrinkage and most of all they are easily separable from each other. Imagine if this was applied on metals, the concept of fitting well when integrated together without a gap and also being easily retrievable. This is a very important concept for an implant. Not only should abutments not have marginal gaps and micro movement, but it also should be easily retrievable and that this should be repeatable without an error - surfaces fitting at the exactly same location. This is why morse taper is highlighted. The other examples shown above not only have bigger marginal gaps than the one with morse taper, but also these marginal gaps become greater when loaded, due to constantly changing micro movements.

As aforementioned, referring to diagrams shown 📷 3.31, the history of internal fit type abutments starts from solid abutment, evolves into two-body type and eventually with anti-rotational octa feature. Then we started to get abutments covering implant top margin in order to raise crown margin as much as gingival height. Most of these abutments include bevelling systems in order to minimize the gap-creating another internal gap to facilitate bevelling systems - meaning more internal micro movement upon loading. After all this loses the benefits of morse taper.

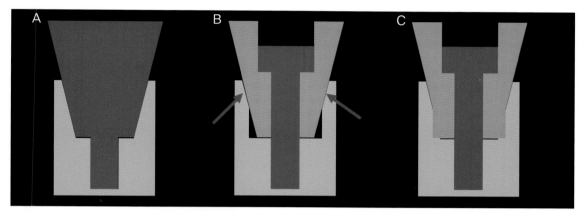

📷 **3.34 Diagram of Astra implant types**
A: Solid abutment , **B:** Two-body abutment, **C:** Two-body abutment with anti rotational hexa

Finally, we will discuss Astra's implant with 11° (📷 **3.34**). If one was not to differentiate tissue level or bone level, we would have categorized both early Straumann implants and Astra implants as an internal friction type. Likewise with Straumann's implant, Astra implants evolved from type A to B and then C (📷 **3.34**). Most historical changes of Astra are the same with Straumann.

The difference of the bone level of Astra to Tissue level of Straumann would be that there is a **micro gap exist at the connection between implant fixture and abutment for bone level.** However, bone level implants has an advantage that it can manipulate gingival heights with abutment height. But many denied that Astra's 11° morse taper form is not true morse taper form (6-8°) in the past. However, even if it was not true morse taper, Astra has proven its successful clinical applications with 11° especially on reducing biological problems like micro gap issues and also on great mechanical engineering aspects.

Straumann, who insisted that 11° is not a true morse taper, eventually created an internal friction type bone level implant with 15°, even 4° higher than Atra's implant. I will discuss pros and cons of different degrees of internal friction later on.

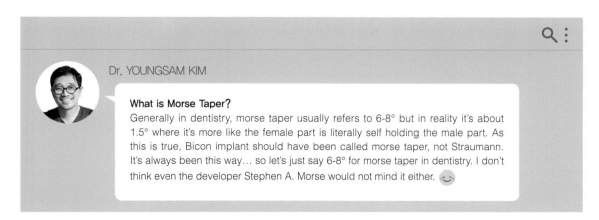

Dr. YOUNGSAM KIM

What is Morse Taper?
Generally in dentistry, morse taper usually refers to 6-8° but in reality it's about 1.5° where it's more like the female part is literally self holding the male part. As this is true, Bicon implant should have been called morse taper, not Straumann. It's always been this way… so let's just say 6-8° for morse taper in dentistry. I don't think even the developer Stephen A. Morse would not mind it either. 🙂

Often the term platform switching is used to describe these Astra type implants, but this is not a right description. Platform switching refers to when an abutment is narrower than an implant fixture, not just Astra implants (📷 **3.35**).

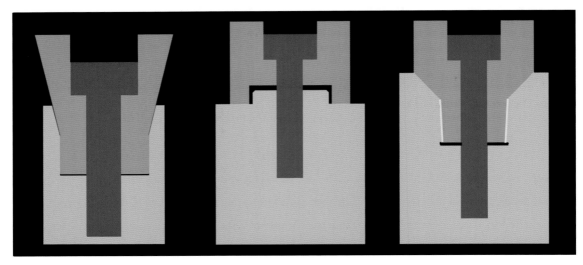

📷 **3.35** Different types of platform switching

Platform switching can be applied to any type, not just internal friction type, even for external hexa and bevel type as long as the abutment is narrower than implant fixture.

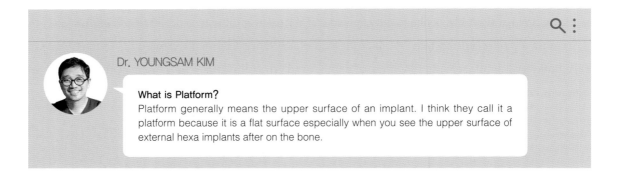

Dr. YOUNGSAM KIM

What is Platform?
Platform generally means the upper surface of an implant. I think they call it a platform because it is a flat surface especially when you see the upper surface of external hexa implants after on the bone.

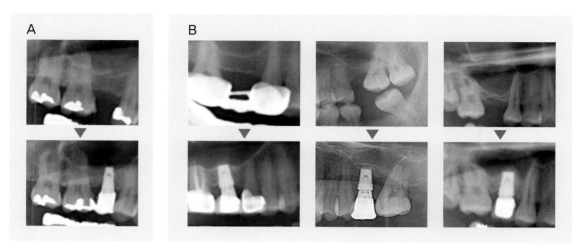

📷 3.36 **A**: External hexa type endopore 4.1 regular size integrated with regular size abutment, **B**: 5.0 wide size implant integrated with 4.1 regular size abutment

📷 **3.36** is an endopore implant case that I often use in my book where the abutment is external hexa type from Nobel Biocare. First case represents 4.1 regular implant with 4.1 abutment, it is noted that fitting between two is very smooth. However, the second case with 5.0 wide implant with 4.1 abutment shows 0.45 mm platform switching. This not only reduces micro gap and movements but also it allows occlusal loading into the internal surface. Increased length from gingiva to implant and narrowed abutment allows thicker gingiva help to prevent bone resorption. These four endopore cases in 📷 **3.36** are well over 10 years old and they have not reported failure yet, unless they went to a different dentist.

Come to think of it, I've been less appreciative about how important a narrow abutment is for platform switching. If the benefit of platform switching was mainly focused on that it allows occlusal loading to the internal surface of an implant, I think it would not be too bad to emphasize the benefits from having narrower abutments in the future.

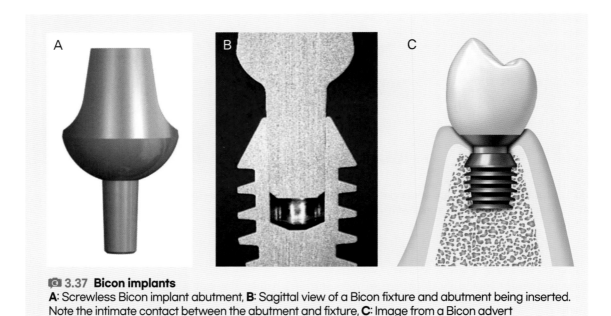

📷 **3.37 Bicon implants**
A: Screwless Bicon implant abutment, **B**: Sagittal view of a Bicon fixture and abutment being inserted. Note the intimate contact between the abutment and fixture, **C**: Image from a Bicon advert

Finally, I cannot refrain from mentioning the Bicon implant system. Bicon implants not only "shove" the implant body in, but also the abutment. The abutment has a 1.5° angulation. Bicon suggests that a true cold-welding occurs between the abutment and implant which means that there are no micro-movements or gaps in the margin. This is true, to a certain extent. If the angulation is small, the abutment and fixture are contacted more intimately, but the abutment will be more difficult to remove (self-holding). Furthermore, the real issue arises with height adjustment during initial implant placement.

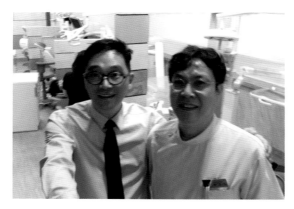

📷 **3.38 A senior dentist I have a lot of respect for. He has been using the Bicon system for a long time.** Not only is he talented and friendly, he is also very good-looking but unfortunately the camera was unstable.

However, due to the ease of placement, dentists familiar with using the Bicon system tend to prefer it to other systems, which is a testament to the advantages of the system. In the past, you would place the abutment and prep it accordingly. Recent developments allow us to take an impression at the fixture stage and send it to the lab to mill the required abutment. This was shared by a senior dentist that I massively respect. He is a specialist prosthodontist with an excellent understanding of occlusion, as well as his renowned preparations thanks to his exceptional hand skills (📷 3.38).

In his case, I believe the Bicon system might be great because of his expertise in abutment preparation. However, a mallet is required, and an accurate height adjustment is difficult to execute. It is unfortunate that this system is getting a little outdated in the world of modern digital dentistry.

Micromovement based on abutment types

- **Summary**
- https://youtu.be/Ek-7vpf-IUE

- **Full videos - Part 1 & 2**
- https://youtu.be/AhsjiYjmTLE
- https://youtu.be/-z5jXFAtfZc

If you watch the videos, you will understand why you need an Astra-type abutment. I have summarized the causes for crestal bone loss in the table below.

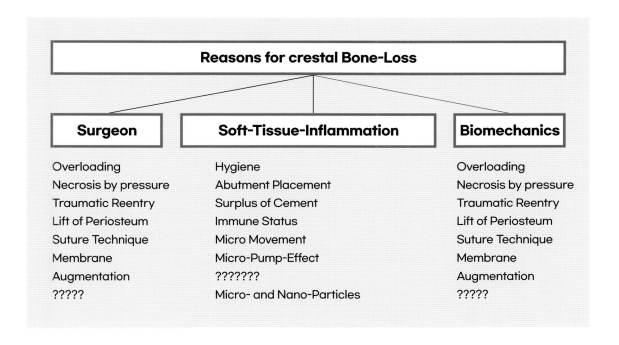

Reasons for crestal Bone-Loss		
Surgeon	**Soft-Tissue-Inflammation**	**Biomechanics**
Overloading	Hygiene	Overloading
Necrosis by pressure	Abutment Placement	Necrosis by pressure
Traumatic Reentry	Surplus of Cement	Traumatic Reentry
Lift of Periosteum	Immune Status	Lift of Periosteum
Suture Technique	Micro Movement	Suture Technique
Membrane	Micro-Pump-Effect	Membrane
Augmentation	???????	Augmentation
?????	Micro- and Nano-Particles	?????

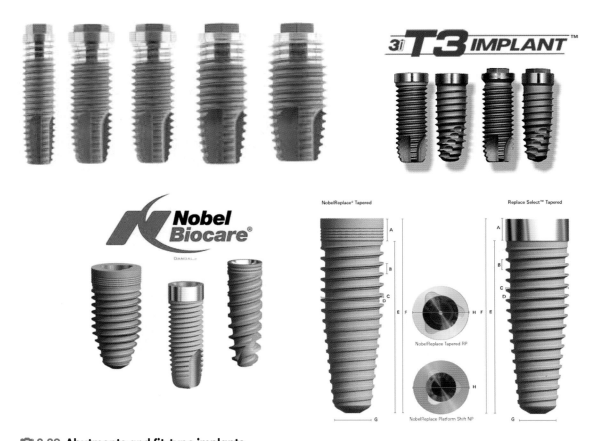

◎ 3.39 Abutments and fit-type implants
Such implants cannot avoid bone loss. Therefore they typically have a smooth surface of at least 1 mm from the abutment connection.

Fit type implants, as opposed to internal friction type implants, have gapped margins and micro-movements which lead to crestal bone loss. When the rough surface of the implant is exposed out of the bone, this will exacerbate peri-implantitis; hence the reason for having a smooth surface for 1.5-2 mm from the abutment connection level. However, this means the length of the osseointegrated portion of the implant is reduced, which reduces stability and defeats the purpose.

Let's dive into internal friction type implants.

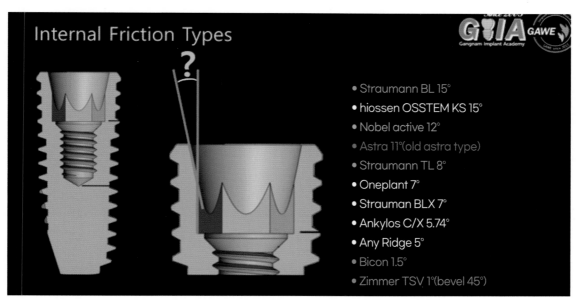

Internal Friction Types

- Straumann BL 15°
- hiossen OSSTEM KS 15°
- Nobel active 12°
- Astra 11°(old astra type)
- Straumann TL 8°
- Oneplant 7°
- Strauman BLX 7°
- Ankylos C/X 5.74°
- Any Ridge 5°
- Bicon 1.5°
- Zimmer TSV 1°(bevel 45°)

📷 **3.40** Angulation of an internal friction type implant (from my presentation slides)

What is the optimal internal angulation for an internal friction type implant? I have listed the different internal angulations from each company above. Among the different internal friction type implants (with an internal hex structure), **Straumann has the largest angulation at 15°, and AnyRidge the smallest at 5°.** There are some implants that do have 30°- 45° internal angulations but they are typically not categorized as internal friction type implants.

Advantages of a larger internal friction angle

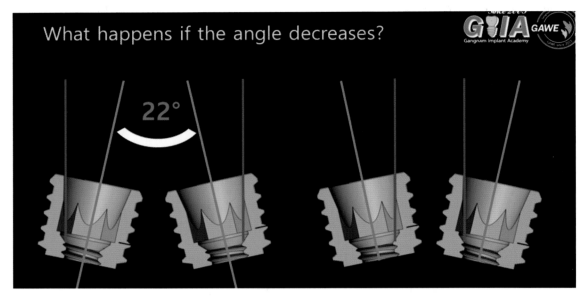

📷 **3.41** An illustration of why it is more difficult to construct a bridge the larger the discrepancy in angulation of two implants (ignoring the internal hex part)

So what are the advantages of a larger internal angulation? The biggest advantage would be the ease of surgery. A smaller angulation means the implant needs to be as parallel as possible to adjacent teeth, and the same applies in the case of multiple implant placements. From impression coping to abutment or crown insertion, a smaller angulation will be more tedious to work with. With larger angulations, you have more freedom in this regard. However, a larger angulation means there is less surface for friction between the implant and the abutment. Hence, the benefit of a larger angulation is the ease of implant placement while sacrificing a degree of intimacy in implant to abutment connection. This is a conclusion that I made personally.

Straumann bone-level implants, often regarded as the best implant in the world right now, is an internal friction type implant with a 15° angulation. In my opinion, the reason why Straumann is regarded as one of the best is not only because of its internal structure, but also because of their Roxolid alloy, excellent surface treatment, and exceptional accuracy. There is no reason to be too fixated on the 15° angulation.

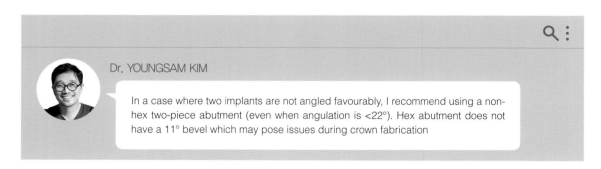

Dr. YOUNGSAM KIM

In a case where two implants are not angled favourably, I recommend using a non-hex two-piece abutment (even when angulation is <22°). Hex abutment does not have a 11° bevel which may pose issues during crown fabrication

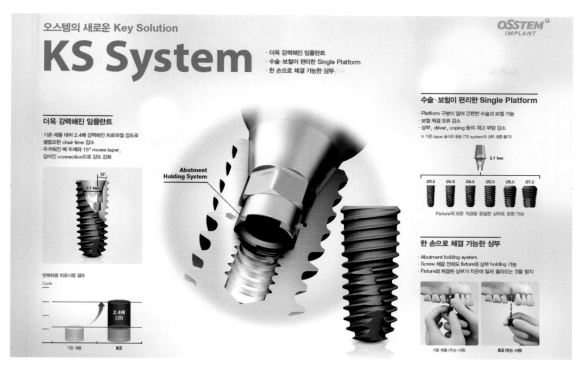

📷 3.42 Advert for the new KS system from Osstem

As seen in 📷 **3.42**, Osstem started producing a product similar to the Straumann bone-level implant. It is probable that the reason for the increased angulation (to 15°) is to reinforce the thickness of the internal implant structure that comes into contact with the abutment. I had no intention to use this new KS system until recently. However, while I was writing this book, I had a few cases of fixture tearing, and have decided to implement the KS system from 2022 if the reviews are favorable. I will be discussing fixture tearing in the final chapter of this book, so let's discuss further on internal friction angles.

Advantages of a smaller internal friction angle

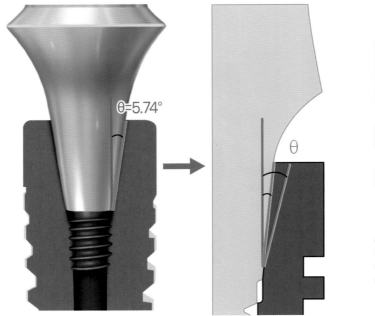

Ankylos implant with an anti-rotational feature. Still boasts a superior contact surface area.

📷 **3.43** Illustration of the Ankylos implant system

On the contrary, what are the advantages of a smaller internal angle? It is the wide and long contact surface area which provides almost a cold-welding like effect. As seen in 📷 **3.43**, there is a very intimate implant-to-abutment contact in the Ankylos implant system, thanks to its 5.74° internal angle. This is why Anyklos did not implement anti-rotational features into their implant system for a long time. They have only recently added an anti-rotational feature into their implants. Among Korean implants, Any Ridge has the smallest internal angle at 5°, and OnePlant has a 7° internal angle.

With a smaller angle, the abutment will have a more intimate contact with the implant, reducing micro-gaps. This is a big advantage. However, if one was to combine multiple implants for a long-spanning prosthesis, the path of insertion becomes an issue. Furthermore, the abutment is more prone to "sinking" into the implant structure. While there are multiple solutions to the path of

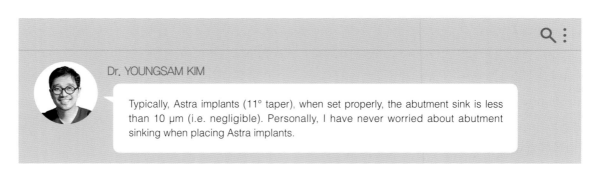

Dr. YOUNGSAM KIM

Typically, Astra implants (11° taper), when set properly, the abutment sink is less than 10 μm (i.e. negligible). Personally, I have never worried about abutment sinking when placing Astra implants.

insertion problem, abutment sinking is a difficult issue to tackle.

The biggest issue with abutment sinking is the decrease in occlusal height. In a sense, the abutment contacts the implant body more intimately, reducing micro-gaps and movements. However, this means that the removal of the abutment becomes very difficult. If abutment sinking continues, the fixture is at risk of tearing.

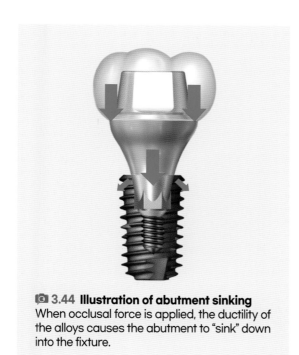

📷 **3.44 Illustration of abutment sinking**
When occlusal force is applied, the ductility of the alloys causes the abutment to "sink" down into the fixture.

Any Ridge, the implant system with the smallest internal angle at 5°, named their abutment "EZ Post". It really does look like a post you place after root canal treatment. With a small internal angle like this, the abutment and fixture will have a greater contact surface area, but there are numerous other disadvantages. We've discussed the advantages enough so let's dive into the disadvantages of a smaller internal angle. Often, I find that the implant mount is difficult to remove. Perhaps the implant mount is cold welded too? But I imagine you could see why this could be a common occurrence. Dr. Hee-gyeong Jeon, the dentist who placed the most amount of Any Ridge implants in the world, mentions that handpiece damage occurs frequently as excess force is applied from the handpiece in removing the mount drivers. Another issue is that the occlusal height of the crown decreases due to abutment sinking. He stressed his efforts in finding a feasible solution to this problem, such as retightening. However, the greatest issue was the fracture of implants and abutments. He placed over 20,000 Any Ridge implants so far, and he had to remove over 300 in the early days.

So what was the issue? As aforementioned, Any Ridge implants have large threads that are made of Grade 4 CP titanium (not titanium alloy). A larger thread means the "body" of the implant is smaller. So even when you place a 5.0 mm fixture on a molar site, the core diameter of the fixture is only about 3.3 mm, which is roughly equivalent to a 4.0 mm fixture for other companies. Furthermore, the threads do not continue to the cervical portion of the implant, which decreases its strength against tearing. Placing a 5.0 mm Any Ridge fixture in a molar site leads to a very high risk of implant fractures. Then, what happens if you use a larger core size, like 4.0 mm or 4.8 mm? That will lead to abutment sinking followed by fracture. If you place a 5.0 mm fixture in a molar site, the fixture breaks; if you use a 6.0 mm or greater to increase the core size, the abutment gives. There are reported cases of abutment fractures from other implant systems.

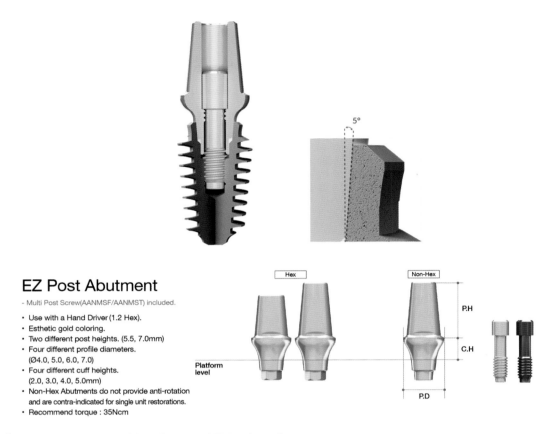

EZ Post Abutment

- Multi Post Screw(AANMSF/AANMST) included.

- Use with a Hand Driver (1.2 Hex).
- Esthetic gold coloring.
- Two different post heights. (5.5, 7.0mm)
- Four different profile diameters.
  (Ø4.0, 5.0, 6.0, 7.0)
- Four different cuff heights.
  (2.0, 3.0, 4.0, 5.0mm)
- Non-Hex Abutments do not provide anti-rotation
  and are contra-indicated for single unit restorations.
- Recommend torque : 35Ncm

📷 **3.45** Megagen Any Ridge abutment (EZ Post) catalogue

A stacked paper cup is easily removed. Even fractured Astra abutments, thanks to its 11° internal angle, are removed without too much hassle. On the other hand, Any Ridge abutments are almost impossible to remove when fractured. This means the fixture must be removed as well in most cases. That is why Dr. Hee-Gyeong Jeon had to remove almost 300 implants. Thanks to his specialist training in oral surgery, he was able to remove the osseointegrated fixtures; most general dentists will have a much harder time removing them. Any Ridge implants really struggled through these issues in their early days.

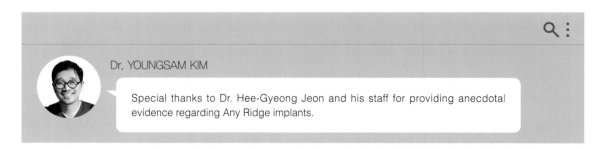

Dr. YOUNGSAM KIM

Special thanks to Dr. Hee-Gyeong Jeon and his staff for providing anecdotal evidence regarding Any Ridge implants.

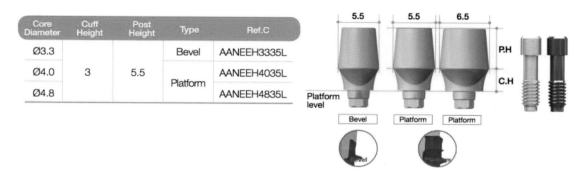

Core Diameter	Cuff Height	Post Height	Type	Ref.C
Ø3.3			Bevel	AANEEH3335L
Ø4.0	3	5.5	Platform	AANEEH4035L
Ø4.8				AANEEH4835L

📷 **3.46** Extra EZ Post, developed by Any Ridge in collaboration with Dr Hee-Gyeong Jeon

Dr Hee-Gyeong Jeon introduced me to the Extra EZ Post, which he developed for the Any Ridge implant system. A wing-like platform was implemented to cover the implant core, preventing abutment sinkage. This is somewhat a similar structure to the Zimmer implant system (45° bevel, 1° internal taper). However, since Any Ridge has a 5° internal angle rather than 1°, the abutment is set without complete locking. Micro-gaps and movements are minimised with a small internal taper, then a stopper is used to prevent abutment sinkage. I think the degree of precision will either make or break this system, as the implant needs to be set properly to work. According to Dr Hee-Gyeong Jeon, the results are outstanding. Eliminating cervical bone loss by decreasing micro-gaps and movements, as well as eliminating abutment sinking and fracture by implementing a stopper, resulted in him not having to witness any more implant fractures since then.

All in all, **I still prefer the Astra system with 11° of internal friction.** Easy fabrication of prostheses, minimal abutment sinking and biologically acceptable levels of micro gaps are its advantages.

For Astra-type implants, proper placement location and abutment seating is critical. These two factors are obviously very important in other systems as well, and these will be discussed multiple times throughout this book. In conclusion, **if proper implant placement and abutment placement can be achieved, the Astra implant system gets my highest recommendation.**

BLX

Let's have a look at Straumann's BLX, introduced in 2019. The BLX's abutment has an important feature, and that is the 7° internal angle. To my knowledge, OnePlant from South Korea has been using the same 7° taper for a long time. It's a good middle ground, given that the Morse taper is 6-8°. As explained before, the smaller the angle, the higher the risk for abutment sinkage. Straumann had actually implemented Any Ridge's "Extra EZ Post" system (where a platform is used to prevent the abutment from sinking). They could've gotten the idea from somewhere else, but being a Korean myself, I like to think that Straumann took some inspiration from a Korean product. The shape of the fixture is also very similar to that of an Any Ridge implant. This makes me quite proud.

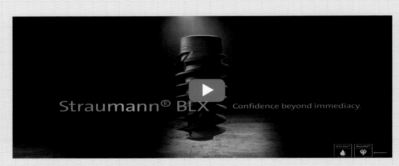

Introduction to Straumann BLX

https://youtu.be/sGnBskcVNuM

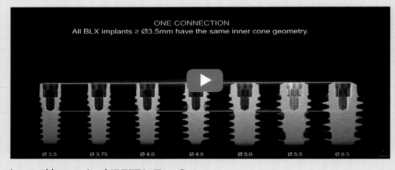

BLX abutment concept

https://youtu.be/JB7F76gTowQ

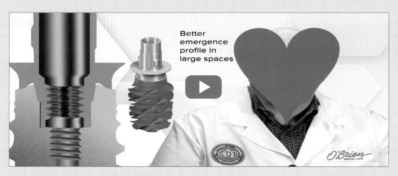

Explanation of the BLX system

https://youtu.be/7JcMvsnXMeY

Culmination of BLX cases

I hope to one day place an Any Ridge implant on a maxillary posterior site and place a crown using the "Extra EZ Post" system. However, my staff would not be too delighted at the thought of implementing yet another implant system, so this makes me a little bit hesitant. I have been giving lectures about wisdom teeth extraction in various countries at the moment, and I hope to show the world the power of Korean implant dentistry one day. This is why I have been predominantly using Straumann implants. I have been using their BLT system for a while, but I have decided to try the BLX system on molar sites. Although I am not too familiar with the BLX design, there is nothing quite like their Roxolid alloy in terms of tensile strength, so I think I should be able to get great success with the BLX system. I am still "trialing" the BLX and am in the process of observing outcomes; it was only made available in Korea in December 2020.

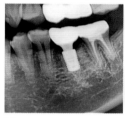
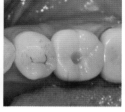

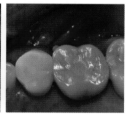

BL case
The first Straumann bone-level implant, introduced in 2007. Each thread is quite tiny.

BLT case
Bone-level tapered implant introduced in 2015; similar thread size as BL. Threads look too small when placed in the maxillary arch.

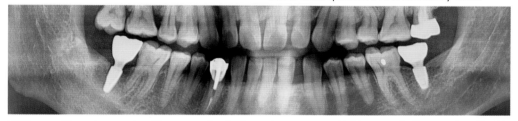

BLT case. I have been using Straumann implants as they are most highly regarded internationally; this helps me in presenting my cases on an international level. Because of the almost nonexistent threads, there is a certain lack of "feel" when placing the fixture, as opposed to other systems like Osstem or Dentis. I think that is something Straumann took into consideration when developing the BLX system. The threads are larger and there are blade-like structures implemented in the fixture, facilitating placement especially in hard cortical bone. The "feel" with these BLX implants is outstanding.

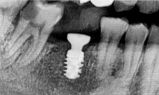

During fixture placement ▼

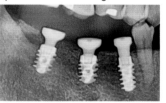

Immediately after fixture placement ▼

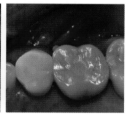

Immediately after fixture placement ▼

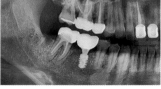

Post-operative

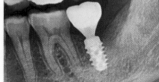

Post-operative

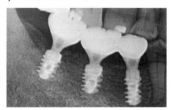

Post-operative

After reading this chapter, you will conclude that bone-level internal friction type implants are the way to go. Now let's talk about hex and non-hex implants. I am not suggesting that you use one or the other; I want to explain and illustrate what each are and their differences. There is value in studying both types in detail.

In the early days of implants, both bone-level and tissue-level internal friction type implants did not have anti-rotational features (hex or octagonal internal structures). The internal friction was enough to keep the abutment in place. However, anti-rotational features were developed and implemented over time to prevent unwanted rotation.

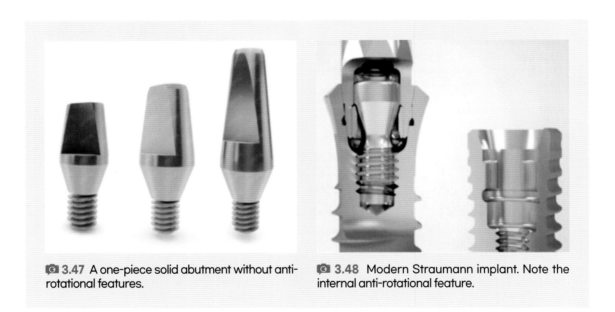

3.47 A one-piece solid abutment without anti-rotational features.

3.48 Modern Straumann implant. Note the internal anti-rotational feature.

Non-hex crown remake case

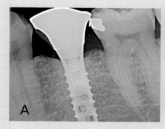
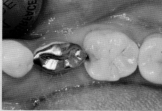
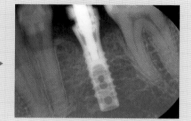

After final restorations
Mobile crown on a one-piece abutment

Crown removed and impression taken

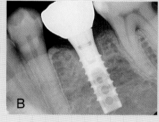
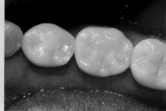
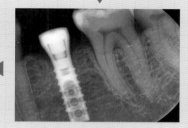

Healing abutment and crown placed

After final restorations
Two-piece abutment placed

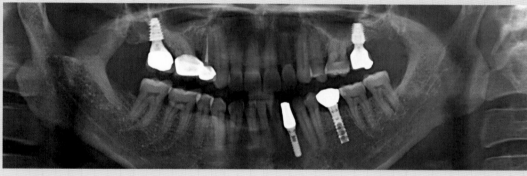

Final panoramic radiograph

📷 3.49

This is a case from my friend's sister (from **Part 1**). The existing crown of an implant placed in 1996 was mobile and was removed. Caries on the adjacent tooth were removed as well. If you look closely at 📷 **3.49A**, the original implant placed in 1996 had a non-hex one-piece abutment. The only ways to remove crowns on such abutments is to either rotate the crown and abutment out anticlockwise or drill the entire crown away. As illustrated in 📷 **3.49B**, a non-hex two-piece abutment was used to replace the original abutment. This was because of the rotational issues that come with solid (one-piece) abutments. When the abutment starts rotating with the crown, removal of the crown is quite difficult with solid abutments. Hence, a two-piece abutment was used and a SCRP (screw cement retained prosthesis) crown was used. When this new implant starts having issues, it is possible to remove the crown easily and attach a new one. I wanted to use an official Straumann abutment, but used a similar product from Osstem instead as Straumann had quoted me many months of waiting time to receive the required abutment piece. Parts are typically compatible unless an octagonal abutment is needed. A zirconia crown was placed which unfortunately resulted in the radiographs showing slight marginal discrepancies between the crown and the implant body.

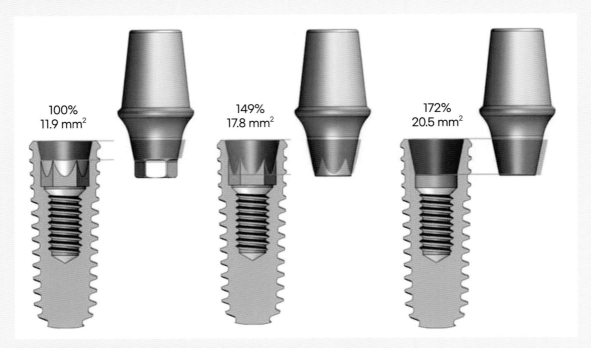

100%
11.9 mm²

149%
17.8 mm²

172%
20.5 mm²

📷 **3.50** Advantages of non-hex fixtures and abutments

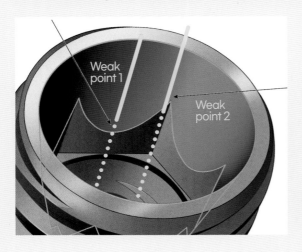

Weak
point 1

Weak
point 2

📷 **3.51** Illustration of two "weak points" of an implant, where it is most susceptible to cracks and eventual tearing

As seen in 📷 **3.50**, the increase in contact surface area improves the structural stability of the implant. 📷 **3.51** illustrates the two locations where a crack will start in an implant, which eventually leads to fixture tearing. This is further discussed in **Chapter 8-2 Fracture of Fixtures and Abutments**. In my opinion, while the contact surface area and structural stability of the fixture are important, minimizing micro gaps and movements by accurate placement and setting of the implant is far more critical.

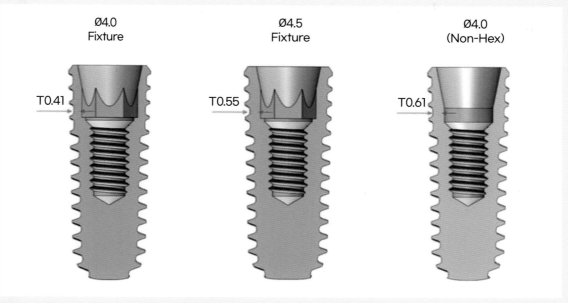

Ø4.0
Fixture

T0.41

Ø4.5
Fixture

T0.55

Ø4.0
(Non-Hex)

T0.61

📷 **3.52 Comparing the internal wall thickness of hex and non-hex fixtures**
Non-hex fixtures have no structural weak points, and the internal wall thicknesses (where the abutment contacts the fixture) are greater, which improves their strength. Osstem continues to produce non-hex implants as many dentists very much prefer them for such reasons.

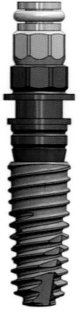

📷 **3.53** image of non-hexa fixture with the mount equipped on top

It's useful to think about why anti-rotational features were implemented in implants in the first place. Non-hex abutments are difficult to place without a mount, and hence cannot be placed using a guide. Because there are no anti-rotational features, the prosthesis cannot be made digitally prior to the surgery.

One could argue that non-hex implants are structurally more stable once placed, whether it be a single crown or a bridge. However, other issues may arise in the long-term. Because I do a lot of wisdom tooth extractions, I place implants in the lower second molar region frequently. For terminal molar sites, prevention of crown rotation is extremely important; non-hex implants only rely on the screw to achieve this. This is a compromise in structural stability.

In the case of a bridge, there is no need to actively prevent rotation, and one could think that a non-hex implant would be only advantageous, but unless a screw-type bridge or SCRP is used, replacing the bridge may be difficult.

If you attend lectures and seminars regarding implants frequently, you would be familiar with this graph.

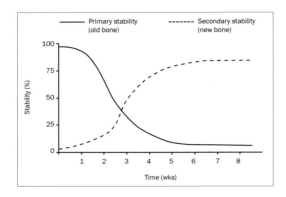

📷 **3.54** Graph from "Early Wound Healing Around Endosseous Implants: A Review of the Literature",

Source: INT J ORAL MAXILLOFAC IMPLANTS, 2005. pp.425 -431.

A graph introduced in "Early Wound Healing Around Endosseous Implants: A Review of the Literature" (INT J ORAL MAXILLOFAC IMPLANTS, 2005). I mentioned that back in 2005, I used to discuss journal articles on implantology with other Korean dentists in Toronto. This is an article I published myself. I never knew this article would become this popular.

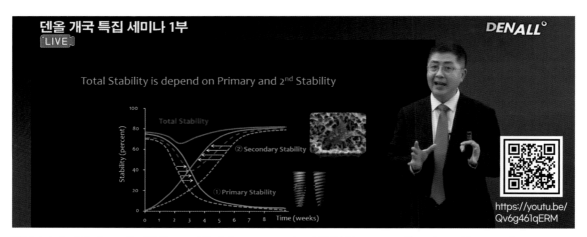

📷 **3.55 A slide from Dr Gi-Seong Kim's lecture on DenAll TV (Korean online dental lectures)**
Uses the graph from the above study. I recommend watching this lecture on YouTube.

Nowadays, almost no-one argues against the success rates of dental implants, unlike back in 2005. Most lectures focus on how to improve the total stability of the implant (as with Dr Gi-Seong Kim's lecture above). If the total stability is greater, early loading is possible, which decreases the length of total treatment period. This is why I included this chapter in this book. The total stability of an implant can only be maximized by improving both primary stability (choice of implant body and threads, accurate placement) and secondary stability (choosing implants with superior surface treatment).

"It's not important that I'm right,
but it's more important that
we are happy together."

● Haemin Sunim ●

Dr. YOUNGSAM KIM'S
CLINICAL NOTES

EASY SIMPLE SAFE EFFICIENT

MASTERING DENTAL IMPLANTS

The Essential Elements for Success in Dental Implants

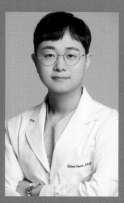

Dr. GiTae Kwon

Instagram - @tooth.stagram
Faculty of GIIA - Gangnam International Implant Academy
DDS - New York University College of Dentistry

Dr. Gitae Kwon has been a faculty member at GIIA since 2019. He is a perfectionist and has an insatiable passion for dentistry, including wisdom teeth extraction and dental implant surgery. You will be able to find him on Instagram (@tooth.stagram) or in person with Dr. Youngsam Kim for the GIIA live surgery seminar held in Tijuana (Mexico).

Choosing Implant Fixture

Your choice will last a lifetime

3-1 Choosing Implants Length

3-2 Choosing Implant Diameter

3-1
Choosing Implants Length

M a s t e r i n g   d e n t a l   i m p l a n t s

Implant Fixture Length

Let's discuss implant fixture length. Jumping to conclusion, **"Never place long implants"** As for myself, I (almost) never place any implant fixtures that are longer than 8 mm (8.5 mm HiOssen / Osstem). If a longer implant fixture must be placed, it is only for increased initial stability, not for long term stability. Generally speaking, when a 8 mm fixture is deemed sufficient, sometimes I even place a 7 mm fixture. This will be discussed in further detail later in this chapter.

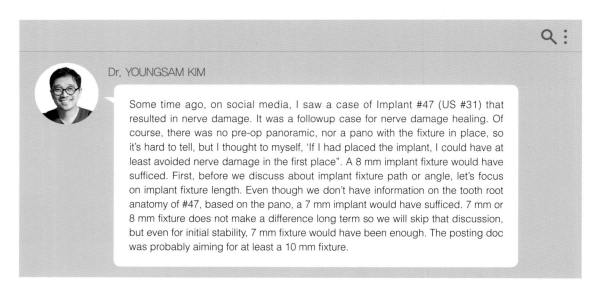

Dr. YOUNGSAM KIM

Some time ago, on social media, I saw a case of Implant #47 (US #31) that resulted in nerve damage. It was a followup case for nerve damage healing. Of course, there was no pre-op panoramic, nor a pano with the fixture in place, so it's hard to tell, but I thought to myself, 'If I had placed the implant, I could have at least avoided nerve damage in the first place". A 8 mm implant fixture would have sufficed. First, before we discuss about implant fixture path or angle, let's focus on implant fixture length. Even though we don't have information on the tooth root anatomy of #47, based on the pano, a 7 mm implant would have sufficed. 7 mm or 8 mm fixture does not make a difference long term so we will skip that discussion, but even for initial stability, 7 mm fixture would have been enough. The posting doc was probably aiming for at least a 10 mm fixture.

First, lets discuss the cons of a long implant. First, the longer the implant, the more dangerous the surgery.. The fixture may penetrate the IAN. Second, surgery becomes more complex. This is because there are many cases where excessive bone grafting is required to place a long implant. Currently, short implants are the trend, and you can understand what follows only when you know that there are no

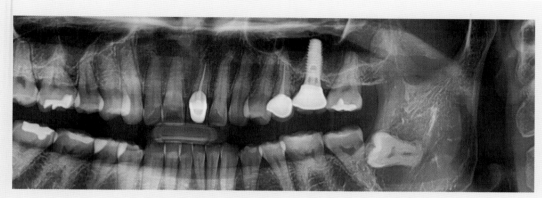

📷 **1.1** A 48-year-old female patient, Zimmer implant that I placed 18 years ago

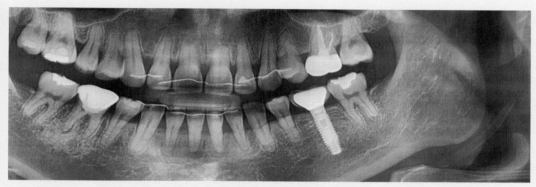

📷 **1.2** This is an Osstem SS2 tissue level implant that I placed 18 years ago for a 37-year-old female patient.

problems with the longterm prognosis of "short" implants.

📷 **1.1** and 📷 **1.2** are implants placed by myself in 2003. These patients are still returning for the regular recalls. Every time they return for their pano, I get goosebumps. Why did I do that? And if this becomes problematic, what do I do? My very first implant that I placed in May 2002 was either 13 or 15 mm, and until 2005, unless the fixture was EndoPore, I always tried to place the longest possible implant fixture.

📷 **1.1** This case, I placed the implant shortly after extraction, and there was bone in the palatal area, so I placed the longest possible fixture in the area. It is probably at least 12 mm, and possibly 14 mm. The CT reveals that the fixture is tenting the sinus membrane. I can't believe that I placed such long implant even though there was good bone in the palatal root area. Thinking about it now, it's really sad.

📷 **1.2** This case implant looks like at least 13 mm, possibly 15 mm. Back then, they used to make 15 mm implant fixtures. Looking at it now, it's pretty terrifying. It's almost like I was looking for the IAN, and placing it right above it. The patient was a high school girl at the time, what do I do if there is a problem with this implant now? Removal of implant fxiture may have caused nerve damage.

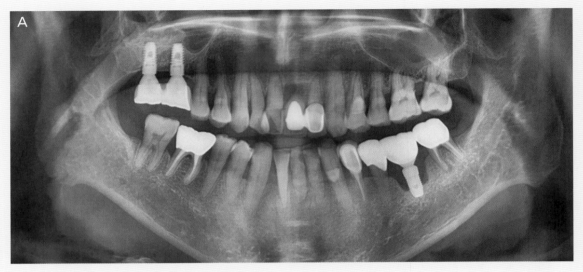

Implant #36 (US #19), 7 years after placement

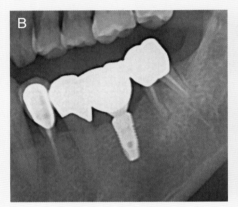

3 year followup pano

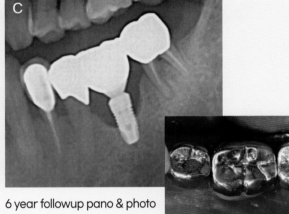

6 year followup pano & photo

📷 1.3

This is a picture of the patient's father with a long implant in the mandible as mentioned above (📷 **1.3**). To illustrate the extreme case, let's look at implant 36. 📷 **1.3A** This is from 2015, a 7 year post-op pano of an implant that I had placed in 2008. The patient works overseas, so he couldn't get routine care, but there was zero bone loss until July 2011. But we can see that he had almost 50% bone loss when he came back next tie in 3 years, some time in 2014. The patient was mostly overseas, so we couldn't provide the necessary care, until the next year when he was available for a month in Korea. This treatment and followup will be discussed in **Chapter 8-1**.

The problem is that the patient doesn't feel any discomfort at all. Although the implant fixture must have been in this state for at least a year, the implant had no mobility and there was no problem in functioning.. So the patient didn't understand the necessity of treatment.

Let's compare it with the patient's daughter's implant. This implant only has the apical 3-4 mm embedded in bone, hence very poor crown-to-root ratio. But there was absolutely no problem functioning. It could have been a problem if the bone loss advanced further, but seeing this made me think, 'contrary to popular thoughts, maybe implant length isn't the issue'. Then, if implant fixture is in good position and in normal occlusion, can we worry less about implant fixture length? Now, let's talk about the implant fixture length.

First, let's discuss Bicon & Endopore, which have traditionally pushed for short implants. Until 10 years ago, when you Googled "short implants", these two were the only ones available. What happened to them now?

Bicon Implants have been around for over 30 years. Those doctors that got used to using Bicon system continued to place mostly Bicon implants, so there were lots of copies around the world, and in Korea, there are many Bicon copies too.

What made Bicon survive for over 30 years? Is it because of the "cold welding" between implant fixture and abutment, minimizing microgap and movement? Other implants are the same. Thus, we can come to the conclusion that Bicon didn't succeed as a short because it had other special properties. Short implants from other companies were completely functional, we as clinicians just decided to use long implants with the belief that long implants were better.

What about another famous short implant brand, Endopore? I took a seminar in June of 2002, when South Korea & Japan were hosting the 2002 World Cup, and started placing Endopore implants. I continued to learn from books and seminars, and in 2005, I even had more in-depth education from University of Toronto, under the doctor that created the Endopore implant. I probably placed hundreds of Endopore implants, and the most recent one in 2009.

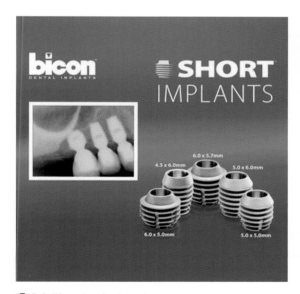

📷 1.4 Bicon Implant poster

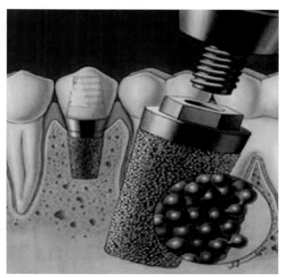

📷 1.5 Endopore Implant poster

But Endopore implants are no longer manufactured. The company was taken over by a US based company around 2008, which also declared bankruptcy soon after. Since then, they are no longer imported in Korea. Back in 2006 when I had visited Endopore symposium in Taiwan, Endopore was the biggest company in the Taiwanese market share. But this implant quickly disappeared into history. But not because it was a short implant. Now, let's analyze what lead to the failure of Endopore implant, and using this as a lesson, let's learn from it what we can, and trash what lead to its failure.

Endopore Implant emphasized short implant from the beginning. If you look at its design, its surface is very rough that even though it's short, it appears that it will function well. Early Endopore advertisements also compared placing your palm on a flat surface vs. holding onto a ball like a handle, to describe that Endopore implants can integrate to the bone, three-dimensionally. So even a short implant works well. But just short would have been sufficient. As long as it wasn't the old-skool machined surface or weird surface treatment, just short was sufficient.

Back then, dentists believed that long implants were the better implants and also predictable, we used to do large surgeries to place long implants. The doc that invented Endopore implants recommended in his lectures, books and papers to utilize short implants and minimize the surgery. His book is titled 《Minimally invasive dental implant surgery》.

Most of which focuses on success of short implants placed in patients with poor overall health or poor bone quality. His papers also discuss that short implants were utilized to avoid unnecessary bone grafts. I was able to master crestal sinus elevation thanks to Endopore implants. It is a natural result as I have been placing implants utilizing crestal sinus elevation technique since 2002. But he hasn't published any more papers since 2008. It is rumored that he sold the company for a large sum around that time, made a big donation to University of Toronto, and retired.

During my time at University of Toronto, half of his lectures were about Endopore implants. The other half were emphasis on short implants. Probably it is because without belief in long term success of short implants, he would not have used Endopore implants. Overall, his lectures were positive things about short implants, but I do remember one excerpt: He showed us a photo of an implant with apical hole, and asked us if we knew why they don't make implants that design anymore. The apical holes could be frequently

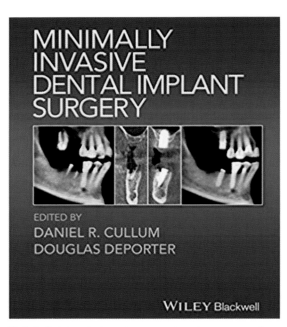

📷 1.6 《Minimally invasive dental implant surgery》

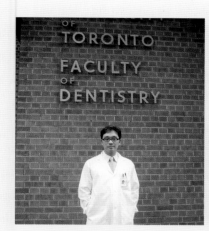

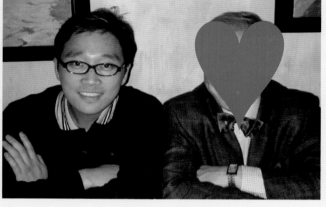

📷 1.7 Fall 2005, University of Toronto 　📷 1.8 December 2005, with Endopore developer

found in old implants. But nowadays most of them have disappeared with the exception of Zimmer, which stays persistent to its old designs. Why? According to the professor, if the implant is fixed too strongly at apex, it decreases pressure to the crestal area, and eventually lead to crestal bone resorption.

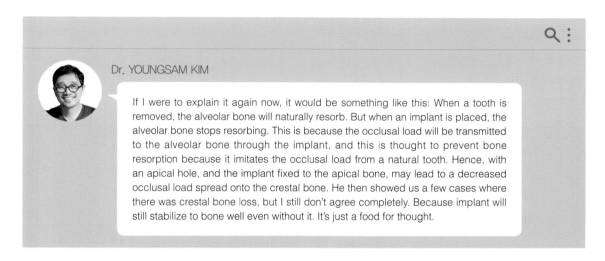

Dr. YOUNGSAM KIM

If I were to explain it again now, it would be something like this: When a tooth is removed, the alveolar bone will naturally resorb. But when an implant is placed, the alveolar bone stops resorbing. This is because the occlusal load will be transmitted to the alveolar bone through the implant, and this is thought to prevent bone resorption because it imitates the occlusal load from a natural tooth. Hence, with an apical hole, and the implant fixed to the apical bone, may lead to a decreased occlusal load spread onto the crestal bone. He then showed us a few cases where there was crestal bone loss, but I still don't agree completely. Because implant will still stabilize to bone well even without it. It's just a food for thought.

One may ask why suddenly Endopore implants are discussed in this chapter, but Endopore implants gave me a lot of confidence in short implants. Except, the reason Endopore implants didn't work is because it was an external hex type, and too rough of a surface. Now let's revisit this point. Because we can learn more from these failures.

First, let's consider how we place Endopore implants. Just like Bicon, we prepare the osteotomy to the prepared fixture size, and we fit the "trial fit gauge" of the desired fixture shape & size. If the gauge fits well, we then place the implant fixture and hit with the mallet a few times. Bicon implant is similar in concept. Thus, both implants are made of tough titanium alloy. Also, because of the use of mallet, it is favored in the Maxilla then the Mandible.

To place an implant in the Maxilla, there was a special type of osteotome (Summers Osteotome), which had a relatively sharp and concave tip. As short implants were recommended, the implant company recommended crestal elevation. Thus, I have been using this osteotome for crestal sinus elevation technique since 2002, and even to this day, I use this technique for other implant systems. If you see advertisements on Dentphoto (korean dental equipment sale website) buying osteotome, it's probably me. I also use osteotome from Osstem too, which is relatively inexpensive, which is mainly to teach my live surgery course attendees.

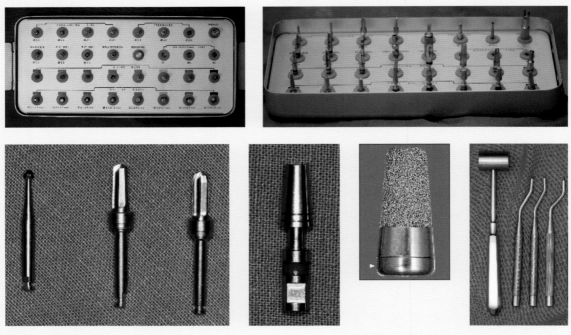

📷 1.9 Endopore implant & surgery kit

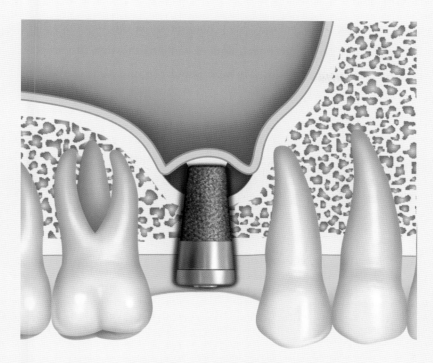

📷 1.10 Endopore implant placement using crestal approach

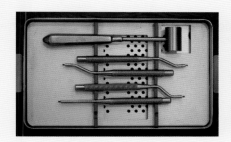
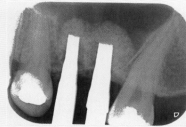

Endopore osteotome head can be detatched to take xray to evaluate osteotomy & bone graft

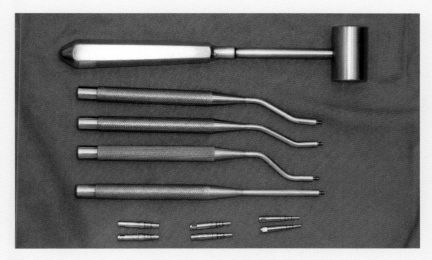

📷 1.11 Osteotome from Endopore implant allows the osteotome head to be detatched for xrays, which I use to check implant path as well as bone graft.

Chapter 2-3 Endopore implant cases (📷 1.12). I've been doing sinus elevation this way since 2002, so I lost interest in lateral sinus elevation. The surgery technique is same to this day, just implant fixture brand has changed from Endopore to other brands. My most popular lecture is the crestal sinus elevation course.

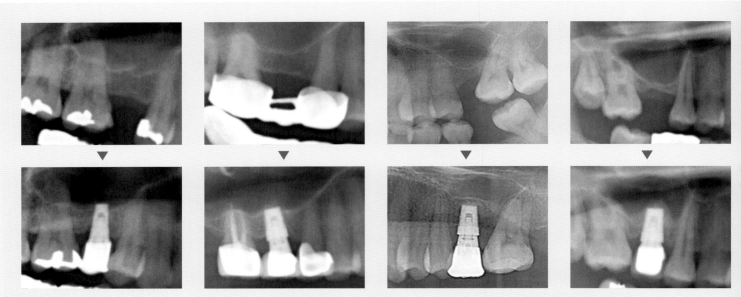

📷 **1.12** These Endopore implants are cases I use to explain "platform switching". Even though existing bone height is minimal, I use the same crestal elevation technique for all these cases. It looks quite normal now, but others used to say that it was magic.

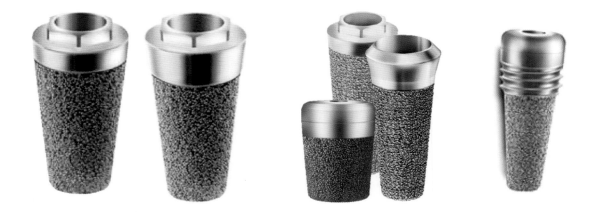

📷 **1.13** Different types of Endopore implants

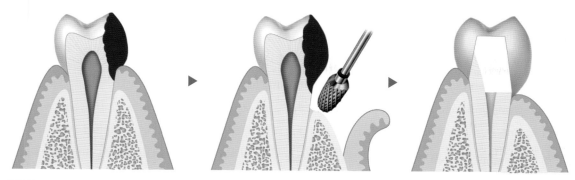

📷 **1.14** Crown lengthening procedure

So why did endopore implants disappear? Let's revisit Crown Lengthening procedure. We were taught that we need to remove 2 mm of bone from the crown margin. This is basically to achieve 2 mm of gingival height, because without that minimal 2 mm, our body will resorb at least that amount of bone to protect our body. For this reason, for a tissue level implant, where the crown margin touches the implant, the lowest gingival height is 1.8 mm. Nobel Biocare's external hex type implants, which has the same abutment connection as Endopore, 1.5 mm bone loss in the first year and 0.2 mm bone loss each following year, wasn't even considered failure, according to their guidelines. At least for the early designs of external hex type implant fixtures, the implant surfaces were machined, so it wasn't weak against inflammation. But lets take a close look at Endopore implants. There are 2 types of implants with the smooth machined surface at the top part (SCR): 1 mm SCR or 2 mm SCR

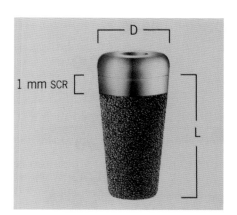
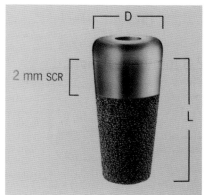

📷 **1.15**

What happens when we place the 1 mm SCR implant? Immediately after placing the crown, due to micro gap and movement, our body will cause bone resorption to create the necessary biological width. During which, if we have 1 mm bone loss, the tissue will meet the extra rough implant surface. This will result in uncontrolled inflammation. One by one, Endopore implants began falling out.

In the Autumn of 2005, the professor that invented Endopore, emphasized to me that I must

place only 7 mm implant with 2SCR (rough surface 5 mm). 2 mm is for healthy gingiva, and 5 mm is sufficient for bone attachment. It is almost the same as the basic philosophy of implants nowadays. But this was after millions of Endopore implants had already been placed worldwide. Even in Korea, I heard that a few hundred thousands Endopore implants had been placed. So I asked him, "If we don't need long implants, and if long implants are weaker against cervical bone loss, why did you invent 12 mm implants in the first place?" His answer was that it was just for FDA approval. I asked again why he made 1SCR, but didn't get a clear answer. Perhaps he didn't know that external hex type implants suffer bone loss, and when inflammation meets rough surface, how quickly it can progress. The conversation ended with him recommending UCLA gold abutment over Endopore prefab abutments.

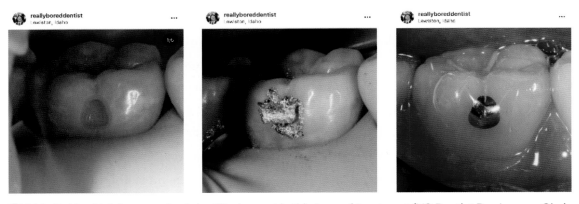

📷 1.16 Gold, which has excellent ductility, is used in this type of treatment (US Dentist Dr. Jaewoo Cho's instagram)

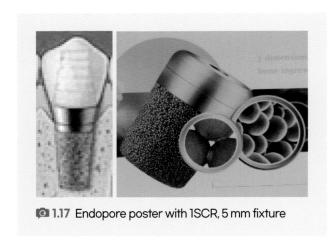

📷 1.17 Endopore poster with 1SCR, 5 mm fixture

As you can see from my earlier implant cases, Gold has good compatibility and ductility, so it has minimal microgap and mobility. As he said, if we had used 2SCR 7 mm implant with UCLA gold abutment, there are almost no issues. But it was too late at that time. He probably didn't know either.

If you see the above poster, it is a 1SCR 5 mm fixture, with Endopore prefab abutment. I am open to using Endopore implants if they are available in the market. I believe that if they are used exclusively in the certain areas, they can function very well. The professor has contributed in so many ways to dentistry, It's too bad that one or two blind spots were overlooked. Still, I would like to remember the professor who developed Endopore as a great revolutionary clinician.

Harvard ITI Course

CourseAs I was staying in Toronto and started to become open toward short implants, there was a ITI (Strauman) implant seminar at Harvard Univeristy. Along with a few other Korean dentists, we decided to drive down for a quick trip. Those that came with their family took a plane for family trip prior to the seminar. Just so happened that at my host house, a last year resident was at University of Tortonto for a month. The two of us decided to drive down to Boston, MA. The seminar was held from Monday through Wednesday, and we left Toronto Sunday at 6PM with a rental car. We took turns at the wheel and we finally made it to Harvard University Monday morning at 9:30 AM. We did arrive 30 minutes late, but we were allowed in for the seminar. I guess I was young back then.

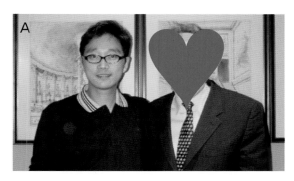
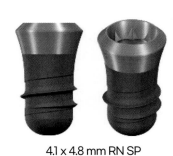

4.1 x 4.8 mm RN SP

📷 1.18 **A**: November 2005, with professor at Harvard University, **B**: Strauman Regular size 6 mm Standard Plus (smooth surface 1.8 mm) Implant

During the seminar, a professor at Harvard University performed a live surgery on a patient, but maybe there was a sinus perforation or something while placing implant on upper 1st premolar, they ended up finishing the case with a 4.1 by 6 mm, smaller size than the original treatment plan. As you can see from 📷 1.18, Strauman 6 mm implant is almost cylindrical with almost no threads. Moreover, since the surgery site was a 1st premolar, a standard plus fixture with a 1.8 mm machined surface was for esthetic results. That makes it even close to a cylindrical implant with almost no threads. Anyways, the surgery ended with "Short implants are OK, and functionally perfectly fine". I don't know what they were going to do with the prosthetics part, but to me it was a refreshing shock that they were able to talk about short implants like that in public.

Following that, I didn't immediately start placing short implants. I just tried to avoid excessively long implants. Soon, I learned that 8.5 mm or 7 mm implants have no problem, and I could become more aggressive with short implants. After assessing that 4.5 by 8 mm single implant functions well in posterior areas with thin alveolar bone, I started placing 4.5 by 7 mm implants, starting with bridge then moving on to single implants.

UCLA Periodontics

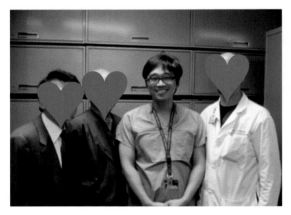

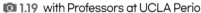
1.19 with Professors at UCLA Perio

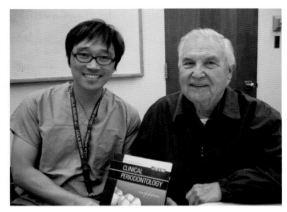
1.20 Jan 2008, Professor Carranza at UCLA

Then again, from the fall of 2007 to the spring of 2008, I went to the UCLA Department of Periodontology as a preceptorship for about a year. The Department of Periodontology atUCLA was the home of Professor Carranza, one of the two great masters of periodontology, and was one of the most prestigious in the field of periodontal treatment. Of course, the actual facility or interior was not big and flashy compared to its reputation, but size doesn't necessarily equal the quality of the program. Professor Carranza had already been retired, but when he visited the clinic for treatment, I visited him for a photo. When you consider that the two of the greatest clinicians of periodontology, professor Carranza and professor Lindhe are still alive (Professor Lindhe passed in 2019), one can understand how short history of dentistry is, compared to medicine. Implant surgeries were supervised by a younger professor. Professor X, who is now retired, lectured residents, and a Korean professor who is also well known in Korea also lectured as a adjunct professor on Fridays.

My impression on UCLA periodontology team's implant style could best be described conservative, or a bit outdated. Perhaps because they are an institution teaching residents, they had to focus on the theoretical aspect more, but because I had already placed a lot of implants already, I learned more about the cultural differences than theories on dental implants. Perhaps it was because the professors provided guidance and lectures only, and the actual treatments were provided solely by residents. At this point, I had the feeling that implant dentistry (both treatment and education) wasn't really far behind the education in the United States. I recall that even at UCLA, the Korean adjunct professor had the quickest and best hands. Generally speaking, at UCLA back then, when the patients had good bone, they opted to place longer implants over short implants.

For example, their go to implant fixture of choice was over 10 mm for posterior, and 12 mm for anteriors.

Short implant example 1

1Let's dive into one of my cases. This is from March 2009, back when I used to place a lot of GS3 implants. My brother introduced to me one of his very important business partner. It was a gentleman in his late 50s, from a large corporation executive, who had been using a lower RPD for many years (📷 1.18). But as you can see from the photo, abutment tooth #44 (US #28)was a complete goner, and his chief concern was that he wanted to stop using dentures, and transition to implants. According to the patient, other dentist had said that he would need a big GBR, possibly grafting from the hip. The patient had found that to be too extreme, when my brother introduced him to my clinic. Back then, I had started to use short implants as my go-to implants, so I decided to place short implants on this patient. I used to believe that for posteriors we need to place at least 5.0 mm diameter, but because of the thin alveolar bone and thin keratinized gingiva, I finished the case using a 4.5 mm by 7 mm fixture. The patient was satisfied that the surgery was simple, and I was satisfied as well.

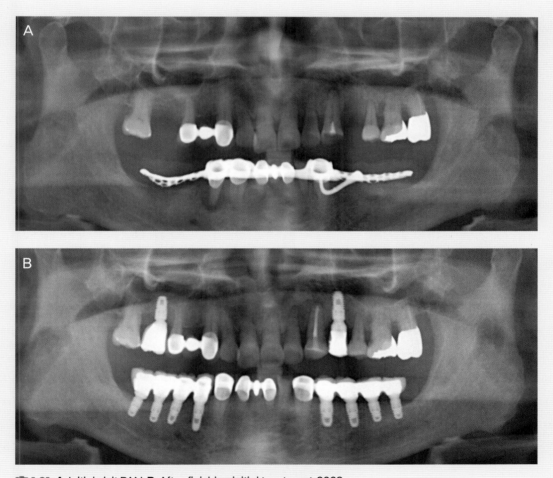

📷 1.21 **A**: Initial visit PAN, **B**: After finishing initial treatment, 2009
Although the cervical bone loss of #16 (US #3) is a bit disappointing, I think it was partly because of my imperfect surgery technique and also a GS3 implant was used, which had a lot of controversy at the time due to cervical bone resorption.

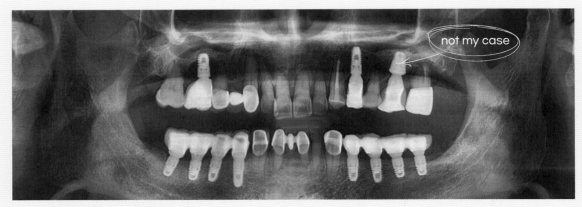

📷 **1.22** 2017 followup

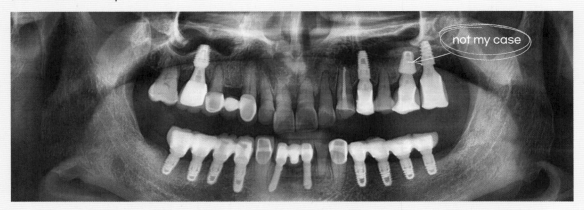

📷 **1.23** 2019 followup. Recently completed everything, including lower anteriors using onebody implant.

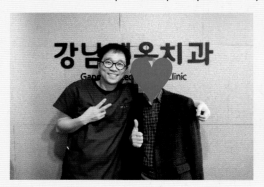

📷 **1.24** with the patient

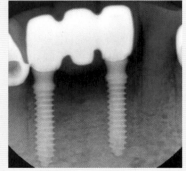

📷 **1.25** On the PAN, it appears that the lower anteriors are off-angle, but it is because of discrepancy, and actually they are placed very parallel.

*The patient came back 8 years later (📷 **1.22**). He had since retired and left Soul, and had found a dentist there with whom the patient had one implant. The patient wasn't completely satisfied with that result, and wanted to return to me to continue the other treatments. Thus, in recent 2-3 years I had been replacing a few problem ones, one at a time (📷 **1.23**). Since the crown was placed on implant #16 (US #3) there was some bone loss around the cervical microthread of the implant, but because the implant fixture used was an Osstem GS3, I just took the result and replaced the implant as I do normally. Because the patient lives far from Seoul, he made his own decision to visit local dentist for an extraction when problem occurred, and returned to see me when he decided that it was 'sufficient healing time'. Therefore, some treatment had to be done even though the healed site was far from ideal. In regards to implant #16, patient returned shortly after the explant, I had to place a thicker implant in a deeper position.*

Short implant example 2

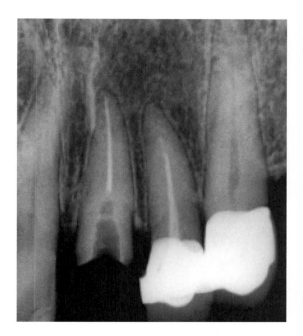
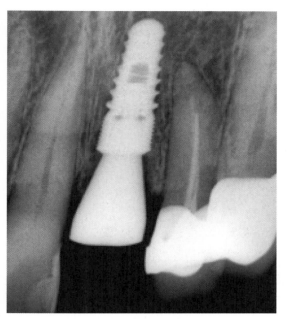

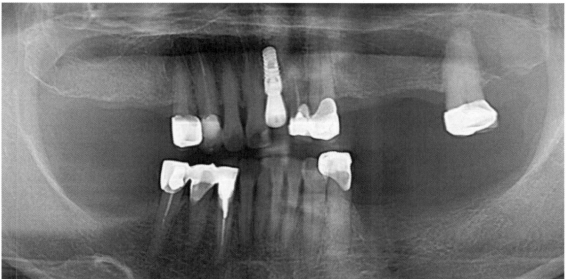

📷 1.26 Pano taken immediately after placement of implant #11 (US #9)

This case is something I am dying to forget. In 2012, my highschool friend's mother-in-law visited to have an implant placed in #11 (US #9). The treatment plan included a conversion from RPD to implants, starting with the incisor. Pano was taken after implant #11 was placed. For some reason, I don't have any initial pano or other xrays.

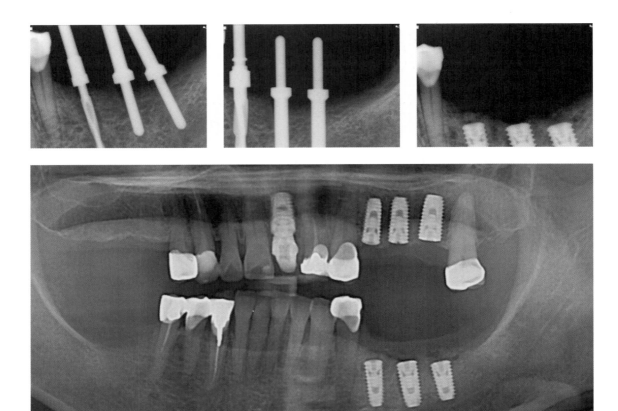

📷 **1.27** PAs of implant placement step-by-step & immediate post-op pano

Panoramic xray immediately after placement of lower left 3 implants (📷 **1.27**). The top left implants are all 10 mm length, and for the bottom, it is as follows: 10 mm (#35), 10 mm (#36), 8.5 mm (#37). As most others, when one is distracted by something else, big mistakes happen. Worse comes to worst, the periapical xrays have all missed the apices. I think I was too focused on the implant path and angle over the IAN. The drills that were used for this surgery were from a very simple kit where the drills had no stopper, and had just simple line. Up to 4-5 years ago, I used just the simple drill kit with no stopper. When implants are usually placed in such proximity to IAN, patients usually express some degree of pain, but this patient had no symptoms during the surgery. The implants appear to be very close on the panoramic, but the patient had zero discomfort so I finished the surgery. Most implant surgeries are finished in 1 stage with the healing abutment placed on the spot, but because the patient wanted to continue to use the existing partial denture, I decided to do the surgery with a second stage planed. Nowadays I would still have placed the healing abutment, but when one thing goes wrong, it's because I'm doing something different from my norm. The following day patient returned for the surgery dressing but still didn't mention anything. Then suddenly after a week, patient reported paresthesia. When I asked why it wasn't mentioned in the beginning, it's because the patient's friend had suffered paresthesia following dental implants, so the patient thought that paresthesia was normal.

So first, I removed the 2 implants to the front that were placed too deep. Patient's symptoms hadn't resolved even one month later, so I removed #37 as well (📷 1.28).

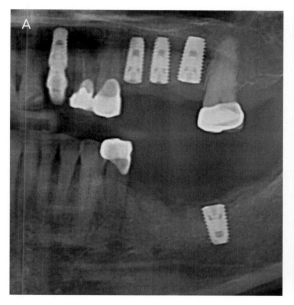 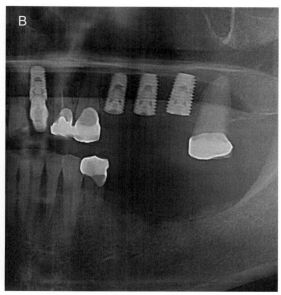

📷 1.28 **A**: after initial implant removal, **B**: 1.5 month later, #37 removed too

My Paresthesia cases

I have 2 paresthesia cases, related to dental implants. First was 10 years ago when I was working evening shift, urgently placing implant in lower premolar area. The extraction socket hadn't fully healed so I should have waited longer, but I was too aggressive, and due to lack of initial stability, I used a longer implant that impinged on the nerve. Also I was falling behind so I skipped the interim xrays, and though to myself 'this should be enough'. The second case is the above case. For both cases, I did the surgery in some different manner and environment from my norm. I feel like when something goes wrong, I was a totally different person performing the procedure.

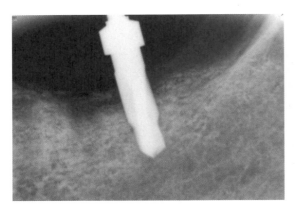

Final drill depth check

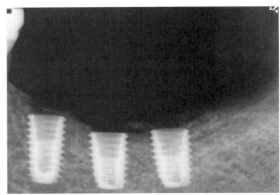

Implant not placed to full depth to check proximity to IAN

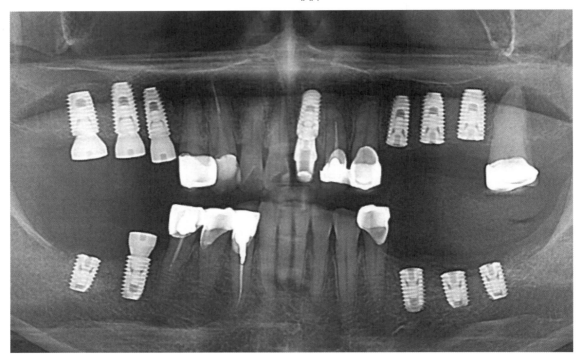

Final

📷 **1.29** **6 months later, implants placed in the opposite 30's sites, and final pano**

We were planned to place implants on both sides, so we decided to place implants on the contralateral side first, then revisited this side 6 months later (📷 **1.29**). This time, I chose 8.5 mm (#35), 7 mm (#36), 7 mm (#37), and took xrays each step like always. Looking back now, I think, 'Why didn't I do this in the first place?' Especially because they were going to be splinted, not singles. From this day, I have made my mind to try to avoid unnecessarily long implants when possible. However, I sometimes do get an urge to place longer implants when there is excess bone. But now I think like this. If one feels an urge to place long implants where it is not necessary, it could be because of one's lack of competency. Resisting such urge is skills.

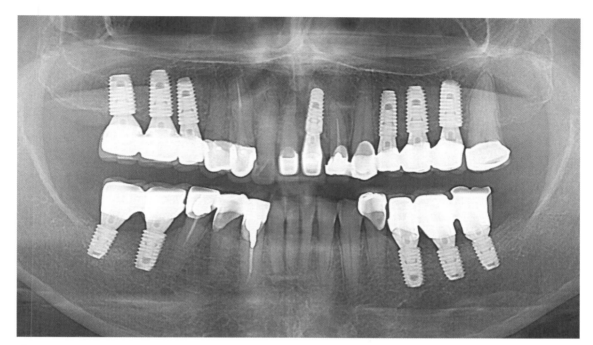

📷 **1.30** May 2014, after final prosthesis

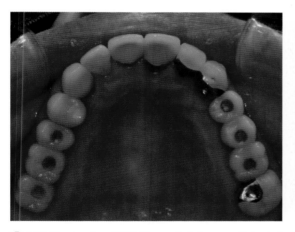
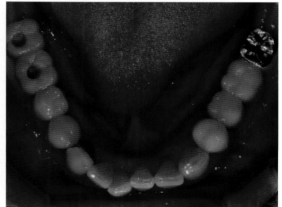

📷 **1.31** September 2015, 16 month followup clinical photos

I had placed this patient placed on temporary crowns for a while and finally finished the case in February 2014 (📷 **1.30**). Then, when the patient returned for reacall, patient complained of discomfort on lower lips, to which I replaced the abutment crowns for bridge. From the clinical photos from September 2015, you can see that everything has been changed except for 22=23 bridge (splint) and #27 crown (📷 **1.31**). When the patient came back most recently, the porcelain on #27 was so worn down and I really didn't like the esthetics of #22, but since it was splinted to 23, I decided to leave it for now. Then, patient returns with complains of discomfort on lower lips on a rainy day. so I am considering replacing 22=23 for the patient at no charge.

There is one interesting episode related to this patient. 5 months after the implant crown on #21 was placed, patient fell and broke the two front teeth as shown in the photo below (📷 1.32).

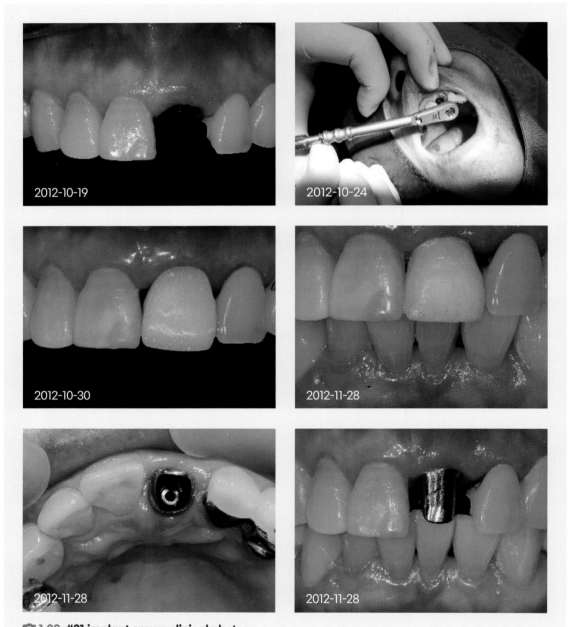

📷 1.32 **#21 implant crown clinical photos**
The metal showing under #22 was esthetically displeasing to me, but the patient declined treatment.

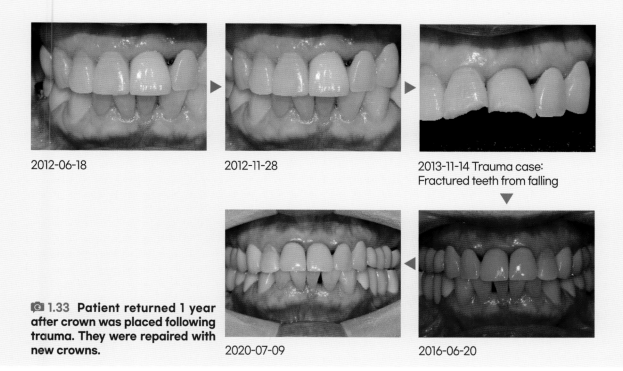

2012-06-18

2012-11-28

2013-11-14 Trauma case: Fractured teeth from falling

📷 **1.33 Patient returned 1 year after crown was placed following trauma. They were repaired with new crowns.**

2020-07-09

2016-06-20

I was really surprised to find out that the 1 year old implant fixture was fine even after a trauma like this (📷 **1.33**). Procelain from PFM broke off, but the implant was fine. Anyway, I ended up fixing the front two teeth with crowns. 22=23 splint crowns are still displeasing to see, but it is about 8 years old and is functioning fine.

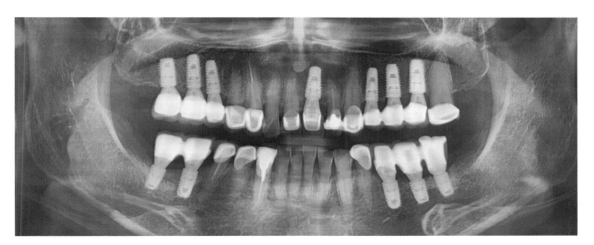

📷 **1.34** July 2020 pano

The implants are about 7 years since placement, and patient is functioning with them with no problem (📷 **1.34**). Why was I obsessed with long implants back then? Now lets discuss step-by-step why short implants are good.

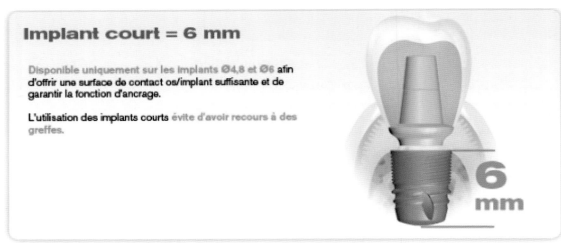

Implant court = 6 mm

Disponible uniquement sur les implants Ø4,8 et Ø6 afin d'offrir une surface de contact os/implant suffisante et de garantir la fonction d'ancrage.

L'utilisation des implants courts évite d'avoir recours à des greffes.

6 mm

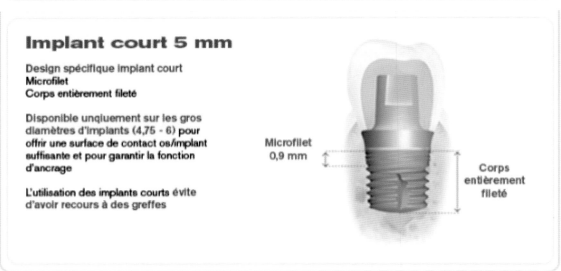

Implant court 5 mm

Design spécifique implant court
Microfilet
Corps entièrement fileté

Disponible uniquement sur les gros diamètres d'implants (4,75 - 6) pour offrir une surface de contact os/implant suffisante et pour garantir la fonction d'ancrage

L'utilisation des implants courts évite d'avoir recours à des greffes

Microfilet
0,9 mm

Corps entièrement fileté

📷 1.35 Short implant Euroteknika (EKT) from France

These days, most implant companies make short implants. 📷 1.35 is the French implant Euroteknika used on patient's tooth #21. This company already makes such short implants. Once upon a time, we used to believe that short implants were only possible for wide implants with diameter 6 mm or more. But now they make regular diameter (4.0 mm) short implants as well.

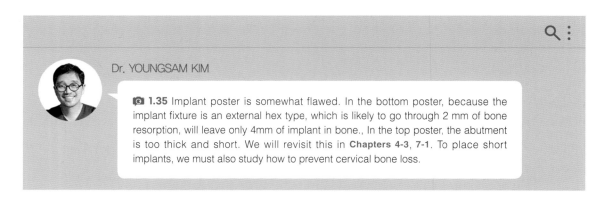

Dr. YOUNGSAM KIM

📷 1.35 Implant poster is somewhat flawed. In the bottom poster, because the implant fixture is an external hex type, which is likely to go through 2 mm of bone resorption, will leave only 4mm of implant in bone., In the top poster, the abutment is too thick and short. We will revisit this in **Chapters 4-3, 7-1**. To place short implants, we must also study how to prevent cervical bone loss.

Defining "short" implant

ImplantThere is no official definition of short implants. Maybe we can say that the definition has changed over time? The definition varies from each study, as the experimental group and control group is different in all studies. Once upon a time some old papers define long as 15 mm or longer, and short as 10 mm or shorter. We no longer necessarily define it as such, but I believe that **for molars, 10 mm or longer should be defined long.** (The reason I specified "for molars", is because for anteriors, long implants are sometimes preferred to fabricate immediate prosthesis (temporary crown), which is irrelevant to long term prognosis. Of course, posterior teeth can also be immediately loaded too. For molars, I think that 5 mm or shorter should be considered "short implant", but since there are more dentists preferring long implants, I will compromise and **definite short implants to be 7 mm or shorter.** The Korean FDA considers 7 mm or shorter to be a short implant, and must pass extra regulations and tests to get an approval. According to current regulations short implants with 5 mm or wider diameter can be approved as short as 6 mm without additional tests. Osstem manufactures 6 mm implants but with different surface treatment on the cervical area to make actually 4 mm or 5 mm length short implants. Few short implant posters from Korean implant brands (📷 1.36).

Osstem

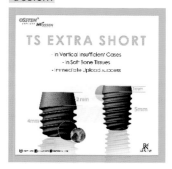

Dentis

▼ **SQ SHORT**

1. 3 options are available by selectively applying the surface treatment, according to the amount of availble bone height: 4/5/6 mm

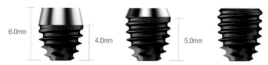

2. Clear demarcation of machined collar improves visibility and increases safety of depth control during implant placement, and also helps against peri-implantitis and prevents bone resorption by stablizing soft tissue response
3. Aggressive apex design helps improve initial stability and aids in self-tapping

Neobiotech

구분	IS-II active Short				IS-III active Short		
이미지							
직경(Ø)	Ø5.0		Ø5.5		Ø5.0	Ø5.5	Ø6.0
길이(mm)	7.3mm				6.6mm		
Bioseal(mm)	2.3mm	1.3mm	2.3mm	1.3mm	-		

▲Short Fixture 라인업

Dentium

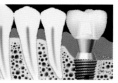

MegaGen

"Special 7mm" essential for special case

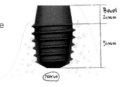

For Irregular Ridge

This 'Special 7mm' fixture can be used for non-uniform bone loss case with limited available vertical dimension.
Ø4.5, Ø5.0, Ø6.0, Ø7.0

 7mm Implant

📷 **1.36** Short implants from many companies

The reason short implants are still 6-7 mm and not shorter

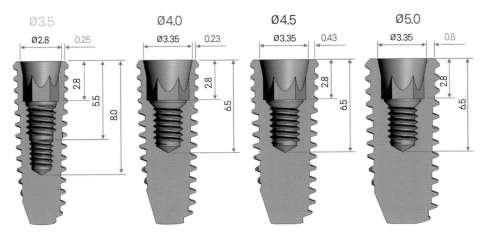

📷 1.37 Cross section of Osstem implant

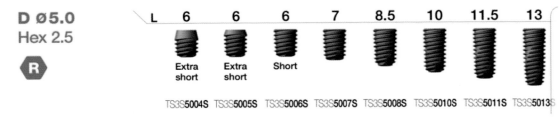

📷 1.38 Diameter 5.0 wide implant shape and total length

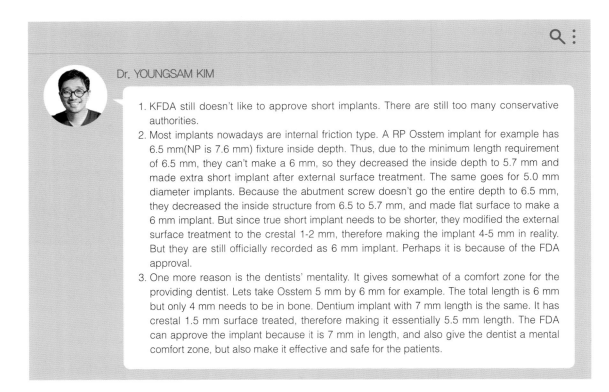

Dr. YOUNGSAM KIM

1. KFDA still doesn't like to approve short implants. There are still too many conservative authorities.

2. Most implants nowadays are internal friction type. A RP Osstem implant for example has 6.5 mm(NP is 7.6 mm) fixture inside depth. Thus, due to the minimum length requirement of 6.5 mm, they can't make a 6 mm, so they decreased the inside depth to 5.7 mm and made extra short implant after external surface treatment. The same goes for 5.0 mm diameter implants. Because the abutment screw doesn't go the entire depth to 6.5 mm, they decreased the inside structure from 6.5 to 5.7 mm, and made flat surface to make a 6 mm implant. But since true short implant needs to be shorter, they modified the external surface treatment to the crestal 1-2 mm, therefore making the implant 4-5 mm in reality. But they are still officially recorded as 6 mm implant. Perhaps it is because of the FDA approval.

3. One more reason is the dentists' mentality. It gives somewhat of a comfort zone for the providing dentist. Lets take Osstem 5 mm by 6 mm for example. The total length is 6 mm but only 4 mm needs to be in bone. Dentium implant with 7 mm length is the same. It has crestal 1.5 mm surface treated, therefore making it essentially 5.5 mm length. The FDA can approve the implant because it is 7 mm in length, and also give the dentist a mental comfort zone, but also make it effective and safe for the patients.

Most implant companies manufacture 7 mm length implants. As mentioned before, most don't even define7 mm as short implant anymore. Osstem has started to manufacture "extra short" implants which are less than 7 mm length. If you look at the shape of the extra short implant, the total length is still 6-7 mm, and have a different surface treatment on the cervical area. There's a few reason for this.

Short implant & Crown-root ratio

However, there are still people who have doubts about short implants. I will mention a peridontology textbook. Let's take a look at professor Carranza's book. I studied the 8th version of this textbook. I got professor's signature in February 2008, which was the 10th version. According to the book, crown-to-root ratio is very important for a natural tooth's long term prognosis, 1:1.5 is ideal and 1:1 is clinically acceptable. He also mentions that as the fulcrum goes down to the apex, the force in the form of class 1 lever increases, leading to increased lateral force, causing bone loss. I'm sure everybody learned that in dental school. Maybe it's just common sense.

Carl Misch's book published in the same year 2008 《Contemporary implant dentistry》 mentions that the crown-to-root ratio in implant must be considered in a completely different manner from natural tooth. In addition to that, in implant, as opposed to natural tooth, there is no rotational movement nor the implant length play a factor on mobility. Also, it is stated that implant length

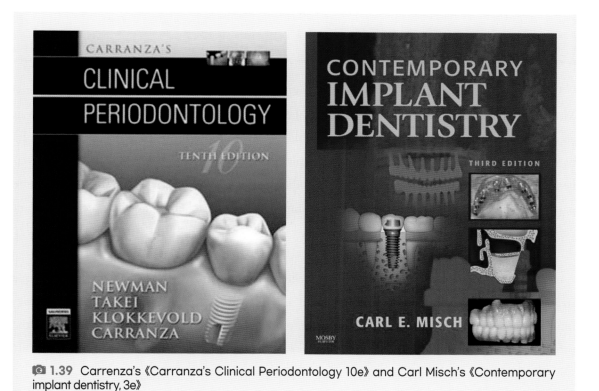

📷 1.39 Carrenza's 《Carranza's Clinical Periodontology 10e》 and Carl Misch's 《Contemporary implant dentistry, 3e》

doesn't make a difference in resistance against lateral forces. Let's look at published paper about crown-toroot ratio in implants. They all have the same conclusion.

- **An Assesment of crown-to-root-ratios with short sintered porous-surfaced implants supporting prothesis in partially endentulous patients (2005) (International journal of oral and maxillofacial implants)**

  This paper compares single 9-12 mm implant vs. 5-7 mm splinted implants, and the conclusion is that the 5-7 mm splinted implants have less crestal bone loss. They do mention that it could be only in their study sample, but the results say that implant crown-to-root ratio is insignificant in measuring crestal bone loss. Also, the study concludes that sometimes splinting may decrease stress to the bone, and may actually have negative effects on crestal bone.

- **High Crown to Implant Ratio as Stress Factor in Short Implants Therapy (2016) Balkan Journal of Dental Medicine)**

  This paper concentrates on Bicon implants, and the conclusion is that implant crown to root ratio is irrelevant to crestal marginal bone loss.

- **Crown-to-Implant Ratios of Short-Length Implants (2010) (journal of oral implantology)**

  This paper studies implants with crown-to-root ratio of 2:1, and the conclusion is that crown-to-root ratio is irrelevant to implant success.

There have been many studies to evaluate the success and long term prognosis of short implants. Most of the papers conclude that there is no significant clinical success or failure of short implants in comparison to more traditional implants. In addition, a few papers claim that short implants actually have less crestal bone loss compared to long implants or implants with splinted crowns. However, because most studies conclude that there is no significant difference, perhaps we can presume that those papers which claim favorable prognosis of short implants may have been funded by certain implant companies.

In conclusion, there is no scientific evidence behind crown-to-root ratio in implants, but the same standards in natural tooth may not apply and it is a topic of its own. It is evident that further studies must be made to study the true crown-to-root ratio limit in implants. For reference, I recall that the professor who developed Endopore implants believed that a crown-to-root ratio of 2.5:1 is clinically OK.

Short implant case 3

Let's take a look at my cases. I placed a 7 mm implant in #46 (US #30) area (📷 1.40). Firstly, even though #17 is a 7 mm implant, but because it is splinted, we will not consider it a true short implant. Also when it is placed in between existing teeth, I won't consider it short. 📷 1.40C, D are cases from my associate dentist. All of my associate dentists are required to take my seminar to be hired as an associate dentist, so I presume that they became more open toward short implants after my lectures.

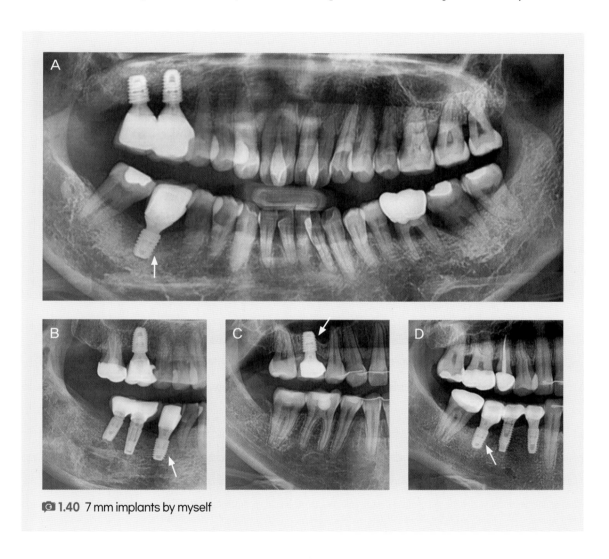

📷 1.40 7 mm implants by myself

Short implant case 4

Another case by myself (📷 1.41). I placed two 7 mm implants in #25, 26 area. These were placed at different times, and the crowns are not splinted. First, I placed a 4.5×7 mm in #25, then I placed another implant in #26 area because of the failing rootcanal from the patient's previous dentist. The front crown is an SCRP as well, but I decided not to splint. Perhaps in the past I would have felt an urge to spint the two crowns.

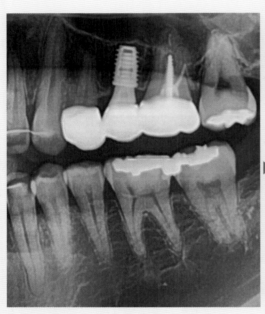

7 mm implant on #25 done 2 years ago

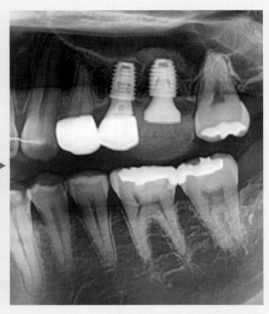

Immediately after implant #26 was placed. Pt had pain in #26, but after unsuccessful retx rct with endodontist, #26, was recommended for extraction

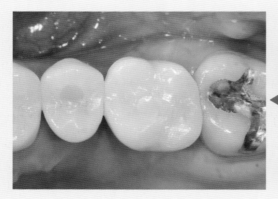

Final clinical photo. Note the position of screw hole, we can appreciate that implant is well positioned bucco-lingually.

📷 1.41 **Single crowns**

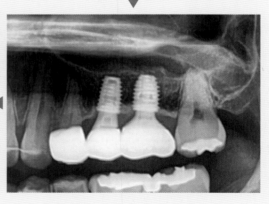

Immediately after implant crowns delivered

Helpful tips when placing crowns on short implants

A few days ago on a national holiday, I was organizing patient photos at my clinic getting ready to publish this book, when a patient urgently called the office. The patient had visited another dentist, who told the patient that the implant will have to be removed. Even though it was a national holiday, because I was in clinic, I told the patient to come over right now. The next steps are as following (📷 1.42).

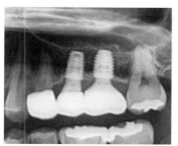

pano from 1 year ago (2 years after crowns placed). Everything appears OK

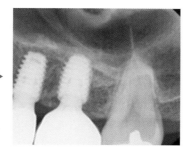

Periapical X-ray taken when pt arrived. #26 crown had mobility, but with no bone loss was visible, so I suspected screw loosening.

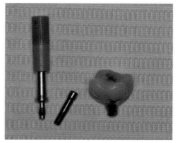

Just to be safe, I measured ISQ after crown removal. It came out normal, and measured 87.

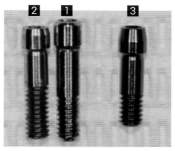

I changed the screw to (2), but there was still tilting. Next, I tried the short prefab screw (3) from Osstem, and now the abutment was able to be seated and screwed in completely

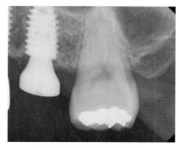

Suspecting abutment deformation or strip fracture in implant, I placed a healing abutment, and everything was normal here too.

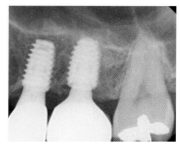

So I re-torqued to 35 NCm, but the crown was still tilted, and even on the PA you can clearly see the gap between implant and abutment.

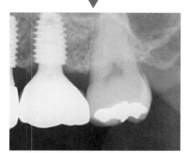

Final PA of abutment and crown in place What happened is, excess occlusal load caused pressure on the screw, leading it to be elongated, and finally it got to the floor of the implant. The implant is Shinhung luna 5.0x7 mm, and the abutment is custom designed from Myplant company that specializes in custom abutments. Anyway, because the dental tech doesn't know what implant fixture is placed, so this problem could occur. But let's focus on the implant length once more. Even after such mishaps, the two single implants are functioning well on their own. Don't forget that once an implant becomes osseointegrated, implant length doesn't matter anymore..

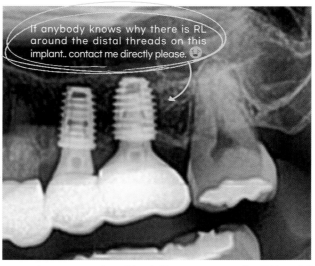

If anybody knows why there is RL around the distal threads on this implant.. contact me directly please. 😊

pano after crowns placed back (3 years post-op for #25, and 4 years for #24)

📷 1.42

Splint? or Singles??

Some dentists believe that is standard to make crowns on posterior molar multi units as single/single crowns. When asked why, most don't have scientific evidence and have illogical reasonings. In the long term perspective, most implant failures are due to mechanical fracture, so I make these multi unit prosthesis splinted SCRP. Splinting is not to spread the force on the implant fixture, but to prevent rotational torque at the abutment level. Thus, I don't believe that 2 vs 3 is much of a difference, but 1 vs 2 can have a major impact.

So, When I am placing 4 implants in 4=5=6=7 position, I would group two and splint 4=5, and 6=7. When I am placing 3 implants in 5=6=7 position, 5 is placed single and 6=7 is splinted. But since I have been practicing only wisdom teeth extractions and implant surgeries, I haven't finished crowns in recent years. Most patients ask me to finish everything, but I am very stern and leave the prosthetics to my prosthodontists.

Short implant case 5

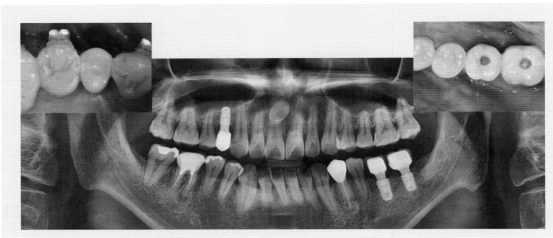

📷 1.43 7 mm placed in #37 position has quite a large crown, but I didn't necessarily splint it with #36. If the porcelain fractures in the future, I may consider splinting it to #36.

This patient is a brother of one of my favorite staff, a healthy male in his 30s (📷 1.43). I placed a 4.0× 7 mm in #14 position. I started with #36 implant after distally pushing #37 as it had mesially inclined following loss of #36. He eventually needed #37 removed, so implants #36 and 37 were placed at two different occasions. As a result, #36 has a small crown like a premolar on implant 5.0×8.5, and #37 has a large crown on implant 5.0×7 mm. I thought about removing the crowns and making new ones splinted to improve the esthetics but I am postponing for now. They may not look very esthetic, but functionally stable. Perhaps in the past, I would have splinted out of concern about the implant in #37 position.

Short implant case 6

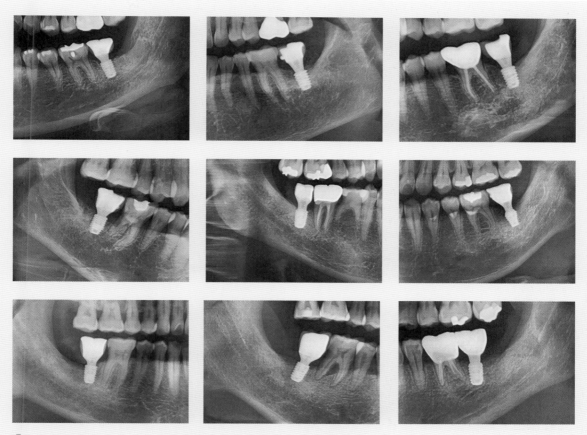

📷 1.44 7 mm single implant placed on lower second molar position

Because I do a lot of wisdom teeth extractions, I end up placing many implants in the 7s position. In many occasion following extraction of 8s, there is a significant bone loss. Especially when the 8s leading to loss of 8s and 7s, due to the bone loss, it can become nearly impossible to place a long implant. Thus I frequently place short implants in lower 7s position. I think that it can only be considered a short implant when implant is placed in lower terminal tooth position (7s, with no posterior 8s). The above cases are my cases from my lecture on implant length back in 2017, so they were placed before 2017. Up to this date, there hasn't been a single case that has turned out to be problematic. Even more, there hasn't been a peri-implantitis case either, so I am beginning to think that there are more pros than cons. 😊

Short implant cases 7 (7 mm implant in upper terminal tooth position)

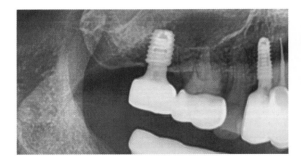

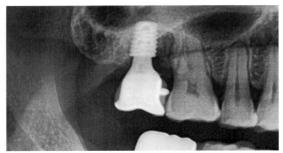

📷 **1.45** 1 year after implant crown was placed on #27, #26 needed to be removed and was replaced with an implant. Crowns are single/single. Both implants were placed with crestal sinus elevation, but used different bone graft materials. The patient is a distant family member so I used some bone I got from sales rep as samples.

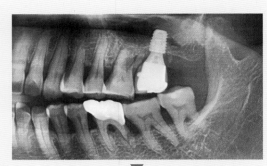

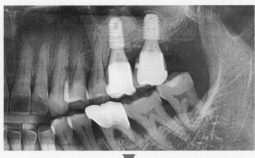

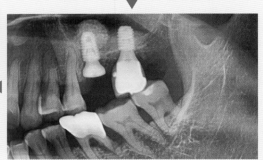

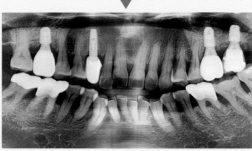

Pano 2 years after crowns placed. Implant crowns are in good condition. For reference, #16 implant is also a 7 mm implant. Actually, the long implant in #13 position placed 6 years ago is a total eyesore. If I were to do it now, I would decrease the length and place it 2 mm deeper to achieve a S curved emergence profile. I thought the implant was placed deep enough when I was placing it, but it ended up with some marginal bone loss.

I place single 7 mm implants in upper terminal 7s as well, with no failure. Just like the case from lower mandible, #27 is a 7 mm implant as well, but even though #26 may need an implant as well, #26 and #27 are not necessarily splinted (📷 **1.45**). Single/single vs two splinted is a big difference, so when the implants are placed simultaneously, it's best to splint the crowns. But when the implants are placed separately, single/single long term prognosis is fair, and doesn't necessarily require splinting.

Short implant case 8

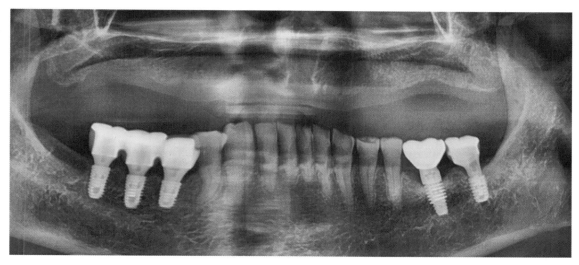

📷 1.46

📷 **1.46** You can see that #37 and #45 have 7 mm implants. Generally speaking, I place equal or shorter size implants in the back compared to the one in front. This case is from Dr. Pyun, the co-author of this book and owner partner of my clinic, Gangnam Leon Dental. I think he placed a short implant in #45 to avoid the nerve. Perhaps it would have been even better if he had placed 7 mm implant in 46, 47 position too.

I think that Dr. Pyun is a very skilled dentist. He is great at extraction of wisdom teeth, but is also a master in placing dental implants. He is so good that sometimes I mistake his cases for mine. ☺

After multiple times of offering partnership at my clinc, he has finally accepted my offer and became my partner. Even when I am nagging him, he takes it open-mindedly. Maybe that's why his clinical skills are so great...

Short implant case 9

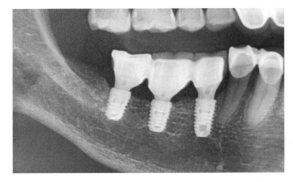 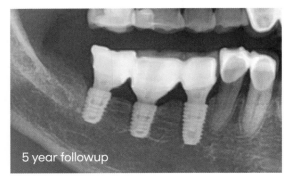

5 year followup

📷 1.47

4.5×6 mm placed in #46, 47 position (📷 **1.47**). The three units are splinted together with no problem. If I were to do the prosthesis, I would have made the 5s a single, and splint 6=7.

📷 **1.48** is a pano from the same patient. Both side implants were placed in 2015. Back then, I thought I was placing short implants, but now they look perfectly normal. Actually, the long implants in the 30s (Lower left) make me feel somewhat uncomfortable. Why is that?

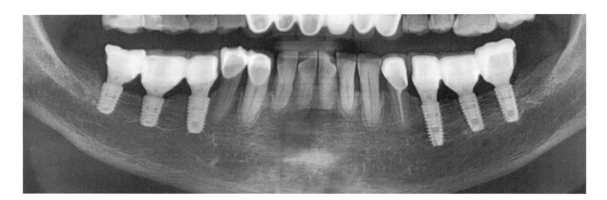

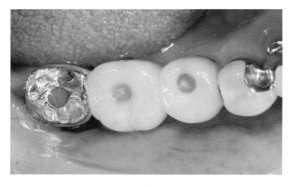 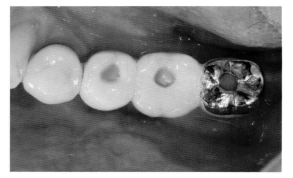

📷 1.48 **Occlusal photo.** I have been making SCRP crowns for a long time now.

Single terminal molar using 6 mm implant

Short implant case 10

Recently, if a 6 mm implant is splinted, they aren't even considered a short implant. Perhaps a 6 mm implant placed single in the terminal molar position can be considered a short implant. I have many cases like the ones below, with zero failures. If it fails in the future, it's probably not due to the length, but due to other factors that may lead to implant failure in general.

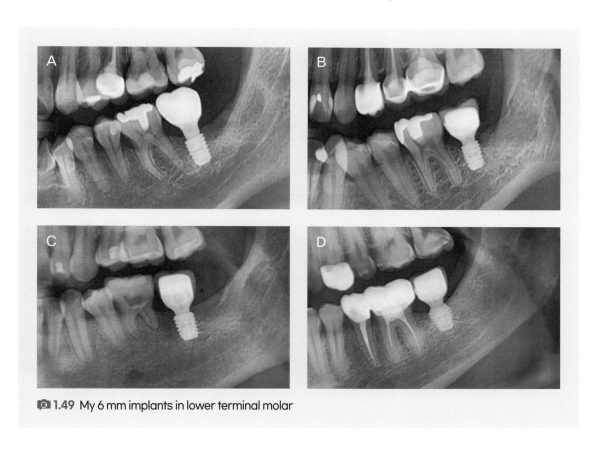

📷 **1.49** My 6 mm implants in lower terminal molar

Short implant case 11

📷 **1.50** This case was a 55 y.o. female patient. Bridge was removed and an implant was placed in 46 position. single crowns were placed in 45, 46, 47. 2 years later, 47 had to be removed due to mobility. Was the occlusion the problem? I placed a 5.0×6 mm implant 6 weeks after extraction of 47. As mentioned earlier, because the implant length doesn't play a factor in long term success, I decided to keep single crowns for 46 and 47 instead of splinting.

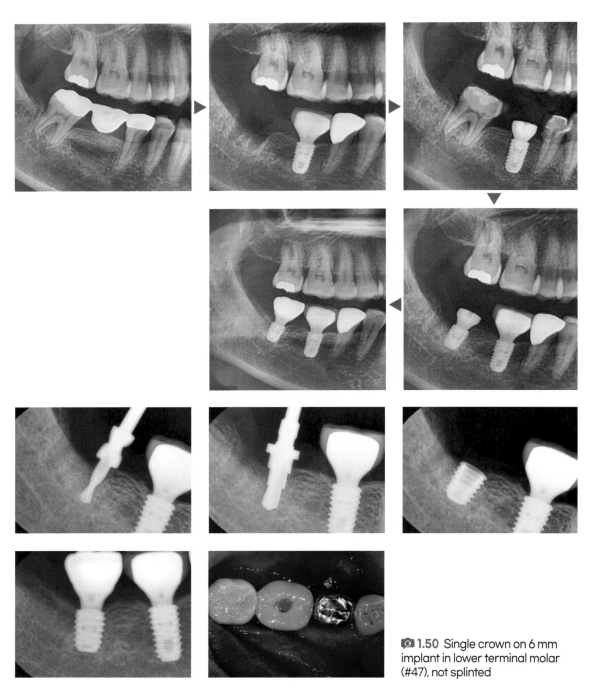

📷 **1.50** Single crown on 6 mm implant in lower terminal molar (#47), not splinted

What do some popular lecturers think about implant length? I had a chance to discuss this topic with a few other lecturers from Osstem.

Dr. Yongjin Kim is a very popular lecturer known for his skills and personality (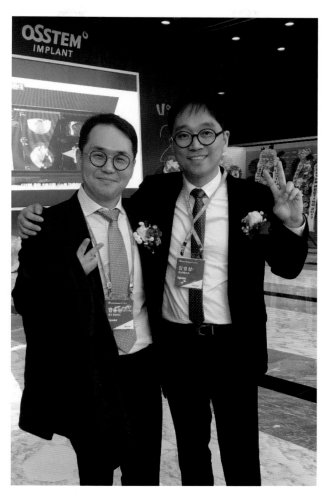 1.51). He shared his own original powerpoint, and told me, "**There is absolutely no consensus that long implants are better than short implants, and there are more papers supporting short implants. Also, there is no need to favor wider implants**". We will discuss about implant width in the next chapter. Next is my mentor and also the best implant instructor in all of Korea, Dr. Yongseok Cho. Recently, one who took Dr Cho's seminar told me that during the seminar, Dr Cho mentioned that 3 mm implant is sufficient. I had to ask Dr Cho so I sent him a text. He replied to me that he would even use 3 mm, but 4 mm are the shortest implants currently manufactured.

1.51 with Dr. Yongjin Kim

There is a post on Dr Cho's facebook account on 2 implants, which is rumored that he placed himself in his own mouth with a mirror. There is sufficient bone, but he placed 5.0×4 mm on a upper 6s, and 5.0×5 mm on a lower 7s. He has commented that he has been using it well for many years already (1.53). I don't need any implants yet, but when the day does come, I wish to follow on my mentor's footsteps sometime in the future.

Dr. Cho is a true master of implant surgery, and I would like to introduce another master: Dr. Kisung Kim (1.54), a master of prosthesis and genius lecturer. In his seminars, Dr. Kim claims, "**Anyone who places a 13 mm or longer implant in molar position is nuts**". What he is saying is the longest implant to be placed in molar position should be 11.5 mm at most, but really, someone that places 11.5 mm in a molar position might not be totally nuts but perhaps still abnormal.

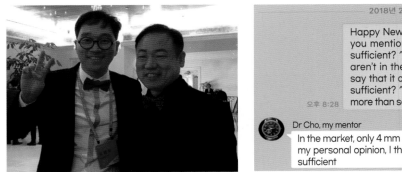

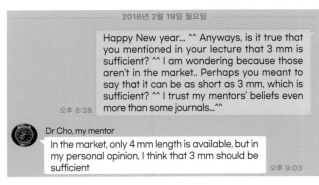

2018년 2월 19일 월요일

Happy New year... ^^ Anyways, is it true that you mentioned in your lecture that 3 mm is sufficient? ^^ I am wondering because those aren't in the market.. Perhaps you meant to say that it can be as short as 3 mm, which is sufficient? ^^ I trust my mentors' beliefs even more than some journals...^^

오후 8:28

Dr Cho, my mentor

In the market, only 4 mm length is available, but in my personal opinion, I think that 3 mm should be sufficient

오후 9:03

📷 **1.52** Dr. Yongseok Cho, my mentor

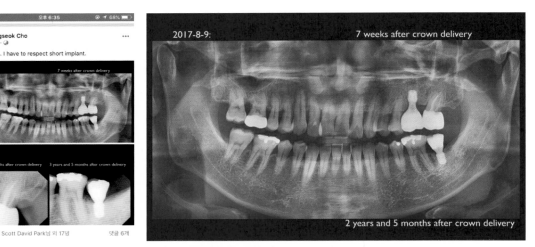

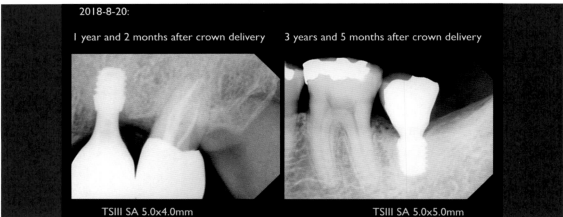

📷 **1.53 From Dr Cho's facebook account**
He has kindly approved me to publish his post in my book. I appreciate it once again.

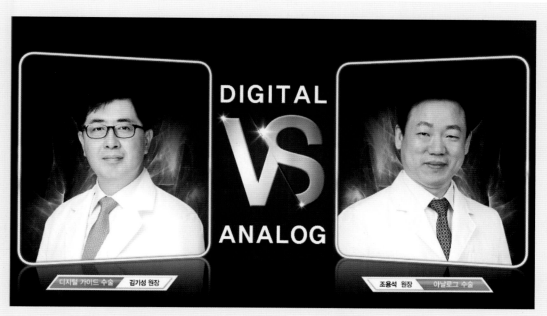

Dr Kisung Kim vs. Dr Yongseok Cho. Dr Kim's skills are on par with Dr Cho.
Both are true masters of implant surgery, possibly the two best in all of Korea.

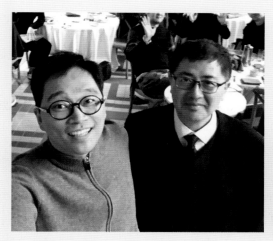

📷 **1.54 Genius lecturer Dr. Kisung Kim**
When I have any questions on prosthesis Dr
Kim already has a seminar prepared. He must
have some special abilities...

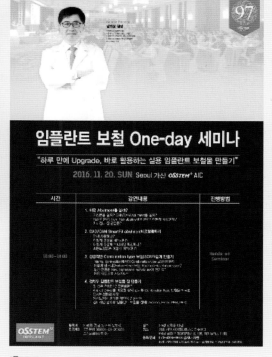

📷 **1.55** Dr. Kim's seminars

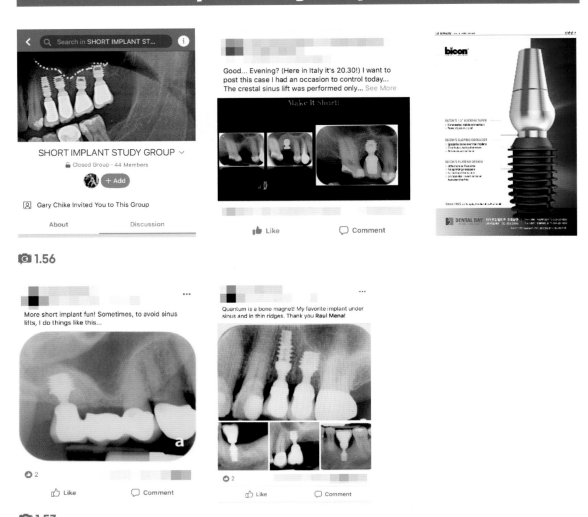

1.56

1.57

I had uploaded a few short implant cases on my facebook page, and I was soon invited to a facebook group 'Short implant study group'. The facebook group was founded sometime in Septebmer 2018, so I qualified as a founding member. As I am writing this book in May 2021, there are over 8,700 members in the group. Most of the members there usually place Bicon or Bicon replicas, but I guess because I place short implants, I was invited to the group. I don't place Bicon, so I won't comment on the implant system.

Anyway, there are cases of many different short implant manufacturers. A famous implant clinician from Toronto, Dr. Steve Chang, posted the below case in the group (📷 1.58). This implant is an Ankylos implant, discussed often in this book. His post is that he was expecting bone loss after placing Ankylos 6 mm implant, but ratherthe abutment fractured. Now, I hope the readers have some confidence in short implants. If not, let's take a look at a few published papers.

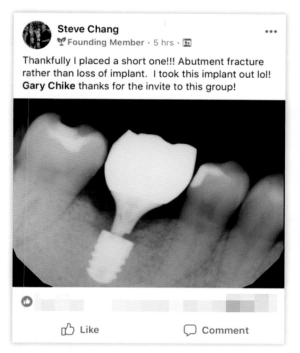

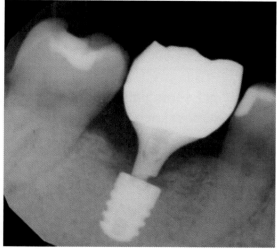

📷 1.58 Dr. Steve Chang's case

Published papers on short implants

> - **Short dental implant (6 mm) versus long dental implants (11-15 mm) in combination with sinus floor elevation procedures: 3-years results from a multicentre, randomized, controlled clinical trial (2018)(journal of oral and maxillofacial research)**
>
>   3 year followup of 6 mm vs. 10 mm+ implants. Success rate & crestal bone loss was measured, with no statistially relevant success rate.

This published paper is a very well designed study that compares implants placed in upper posterior area. 6 mm vs. 11-15 mm, success of implant when simultaneously performed crestal or lateral approach sinus elevation, marginal bone loss, pocket depth, were compared. The followup period was short, but the paper concludes there is no significant difference between the two groups. Thus, I believe that when there is insufficient bone available in upper areas, it is unnecessary to do large sinus elevation just to place long implants. Recently there have many published papers on short implants. But watch out for studies sponsored by Bicon, still thriving like alligators. Let's take a look at just 2 more published papers.

- **Short dental implants: An emerging concept in implant treatment (2014) (Quintessence international)**

  <u>Conclusion</u>

  This is a review paper on short implant success rate. The conclusion is that there is nosignificant difference between short implants vs standard implants, and it actually showsbetter prognosis in resorbed ridge, and that advance in implant surfacetreatment technique has proven effective.

- **Study from Korean Dental Implant paper following up on short implants (7 mm andshorter) placed in lower posterior position (2015)**

  This paper evaluates the following properties of short implants: ISQ, marginal bone loss,and survival rate. It concludes that anatomically, where it is difficult to placea standard size implant, short implants can be a great alternative.

In the previous section in which we discussed about the implant crown-root ratio, we already examined the stability of short implants. There weren't many published papers on short implants, but now there is an abundance. Recently published papers claim that there is no significant difference in success and long term prognosis of short implants vs. standard implants, and that unless it is difficult to achieve initial stability even after going wider in diameter, there is no reason to place longer implants.

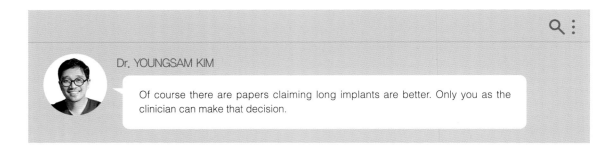

Dr. YOUNGSAM KIM

Of course there are papers claiming long implants are better. Only you as the clinician can make that decision.

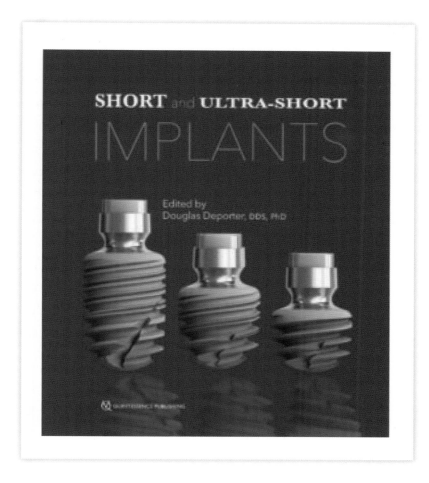

I was reading the monthly version of Quitessence Dental Journal when I found an interesting published paper. In the middle of "Short and Ultra-Short Implants" Endopore implant popped up! And when I finished the whole paper, it was from the developer of Endopore implant! I thought he had retired after selling his company, but... I'm not sure if he started a new company, but the name was Ultra short implants (■ 1.59). It appears that they adopted just the concept of short implant, and gave up on the rough surface and external hex type connection. Because the implants are designed too short, perhaps they couldn't make an internal connection. But maybe because of the previous experience of failure due to external hex type, the new type of implants are half one-body?, and half tissue-level design? Anyway, it's time that we can stop our discussions about the implant length. Even more if the implants are to be splinted. If the implant can be imported in Korea, I would love to try them out, in place of the Endopore implant that I have missed so much...

Below is the updated poster from the world's best implant company: Straumann. They recently introduced a new type of Zirconia implant which catches the eyes, but also something else can be noticed. It's the new 4 mm short implant. To avoid the same problem of internal connection if the implants are designed too short, they made the implant tissue level, with specific abutment & screw to fit the short implant. I've been asking the sales rep for a few years already, but since tissue level implants are becoming less frequent, it's not imported to Korea yet. Even in the US, the implant hasn't passed the FDA yet. Maybe that's why Korea hasn't approved the new short implant yet. In case anybody is interested why Straumann bone level implants can't be made shorter than 8 mm, it's because Straumann internal structure is 6.9 mm. They are having difficulty decreasing the internal structure, so they aren't manufacturing short implants. For their tissue level implants, they have already fabricated 6 mm length as it was used earlier at the Harvard University live surgery case, and the new BLX implants are available in 6 mm only for diameter 5 mm or wider implants.

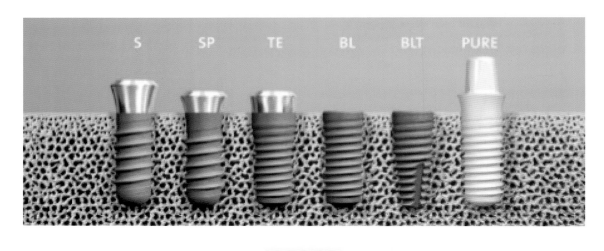

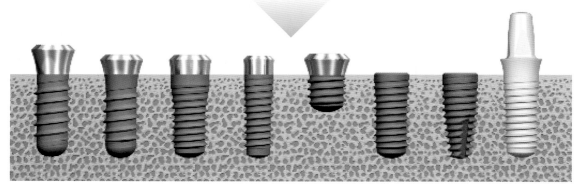

📷 1.60 Changes to the Straumann implant poster

3-2 Choosing Implant Diameter

Mastering dental implants

Diameter of Astra type Implant

Implant generally speaking, there are so many studies that conclude that "Wider implant diameter is more efficient in stress dispersion than an increase of implant length". But more recent studies conclude that, "Implant will integrate to bone and won't break too easily so don't worry too much". The belief that wider implants are always better perhaps began back in the day, back when we used to believe that implants wouldn't be able to function properly, also back when we used to believe that implant crowns have to be designed smaller than regular teeth, and also back when we used to believe that implants shouldn't be placed parallel and placed in a triangular design. I'm not telling you to place thin implants wherever. I'm trying to reiterate that there is no need to try too hard to place wider implants. Let's take a deep dive. Astra implant's internal friction type implant design is used widely from other implant companies, and that's what we are generally used to. Personally I've never placed an Astra implant, but other implant brands that are similar to Astra are 3.5 (mini), then 4.0, 4.5, 5.0 (regular) where the abutment is compatible (📷 2.1).

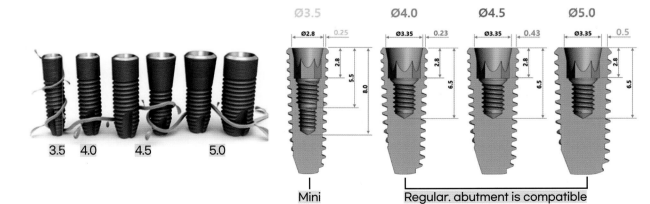

📷 2.1 Astra Implants

📷 2.2 Osstem TS implants (HiOssen ET implants)

Osstem TS is the same in size as Astra implant (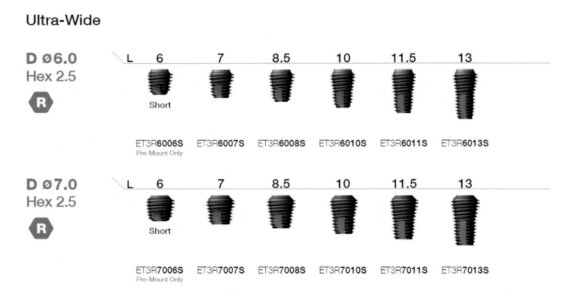 2.2). The image describes the thickness of implant based on the diameter. You can see that for 4.0 regular implant, it actually has thinner implant titanium wall compared to the 3.5 mini. Even though the implant wall thickness is thicker for 3.5 mm diameter than that of 4.0 mm, the stability and durability against lateral forces is more complicated than just the thickness of the wall, and we must also consider the contact surface, etc. Manufacturers claim the same thing, but when we have a thin ridge, we will discuss what is the ideal thing to do.

Ultra-Wide

D Ø6.0 Hex 2.5 R	L	6	7	8.5	10	11.5	13
		Short					
		ET3R6006S Pre-Mount Only	ET3R6007S	ET3R6008S	ET3R6010S	ET3R6011S	ET3R6013S

D Ø7.0 Hex 2.5 R	L	6	7	8.5	10	11.5	13
		Short					
		ET3R7006S Pre-Mount Only	ET3R7007S	ET3R7008S	ET3R7010S	ET3R7011S	ET3R7013S

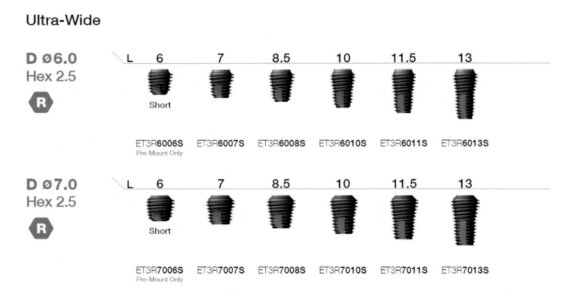 2.3 Osstem wide implants

As seen above in 2.3, Osstem manufactures wide implants in 6.0 and 7.0 diameter. I personally almost never use these. In the past, I have used 6.0 or wider diameter for shorter implants, but as discussed in **Chapter 3-1**, it is no longer necessary. If I were to place such wide implants, it's not for better long term stability but only for initial stability. As forementioned, as long as the implant stays put and doesn't move laterally, it will become osseointegrated. Wide implant can be used when even that initial stability can't be achieved. A good tip when initial stability is low, is to **go one size short and one size wider, rather than go longer.** There is no reason to place a wider implant on purpose and that doesn't correlate to better long term prognosis, but when there is a problem and the implant needs to be removed, there will be bigger trauma, so always keep an eye when placing wider implants. When bone quality is poor, **rather than gaining initial stability through a wider implant, focus more on underdrilling.**

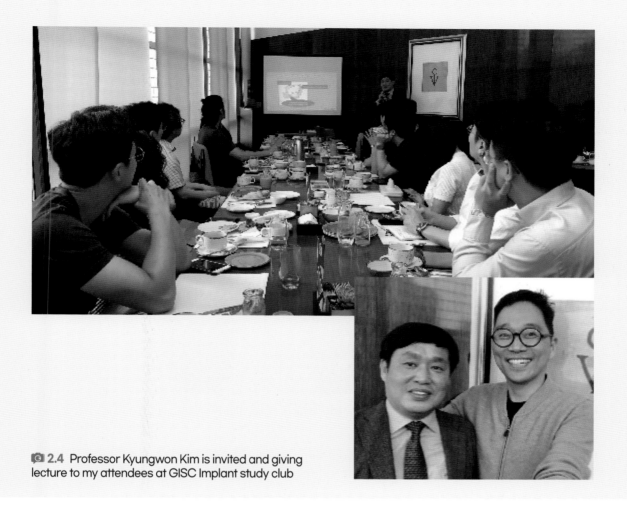

2.4 Professor Kyungwon Kim is invited and giving lecture to my attendees at GISC Implant study club

I was greatly inspired on the diameter of dental implants by another great clinician, professor Kyungwon Kim. Professor Kim is a former professor of oral surgery, he now supervises the research and education at Osstem implant company. He works in implant design, education, as well as private practice, but he says he has only placed the wide implant once. He claims that he rarely finds a need to place an implant wider than 5 mm in diameter. There is a reason that I find this comment very meaningful. Professor Kim is very skilled yet his surgeries are focused on the practical techniques that the students need to learn. He is greatly skilled in all surgeries, but teaches that one should avoid excessive procedures and focus on the practicality, unlike me, who doesn't perform certain procedures because I'm not that great at it... For this reason I think he is a true master. He probably doesn't know that I think so greatly of him because I've just studied his lectures rather than having conversations.

True implant diameter and how it is noted by the manufacturer

OneQ implant from Dentis is another Astra variant (📷 2.5). The position of hex or screw depth is different, but most others are similar to Osstem TS system. One important part to note is the diameters: 4.2, 4.7, 5.2 mm. The surface that meets the abutment is 3.34 mm, 0.01 mm smaller than 3.35 of Osstem. Perhaps it is to prevent implant fracture?

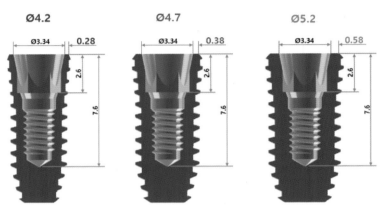

📷 **2.5** My 2nd most frequently used implant system (Dentis OneQ), after Osstem

Let's compare this to a similar size Osstem 4.5 mm implant. The thickness of implant thread can be measured if we subtract the width of internal structure from the manufacturer indicated diameter. For Dentis implants, the number comes out to be 0.3 mm, quite similar to the actual, but for Osstem, the calculated number is 0.145 mm, too big of a difference. How can this be? The reason is, Osstem manufacturer indicates 4.5 mm for convenience, but the actual diameter is slightly wider than 4.5 mm. They did this to make thicker and stronger implant wall and to create a functional thread design. Sometimes, even Osstem numbering system follows that of Dentis. This is because each country has different laws in regards to implants, and often it requires the true dimensions. I now think that it may have been better to increase the threads in the apical portion, and less coronally. I'm not pushing for the microthreads, but rather, make less prominent threads in the coronal portion and increase the diameter of the cortical drills to the full size of implant fixture. Another reason is to have more stable side walls by increasing the titanium thickness, which is beneficial for the long term. Anyway, for these reasons, many implant companies have wider diameter than what theyhave noted.

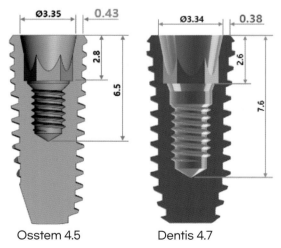

Osstem 4.5   Dentis 4.7

📷 **2.6** Osstem TS vs Dentis OneQ

Wide diameter implants that are unsuccessful

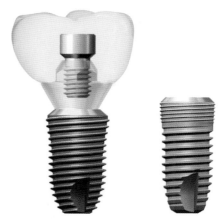

📷 **2.7** Dentium Superline implant and Implantium implant

Thread design is equally important to implant diameter. Asseenin 📷 **2.7** even though two implants have the same diameter, true diameter can differ based on the shape of fixture, as well as thread design and thickness. We have already discussed this point in **Chapter 2-2**, so we will go over just one case now. It's a case I'm really embarrassed to show anyone, but I'm revealing this shameful case to awaken the readers.

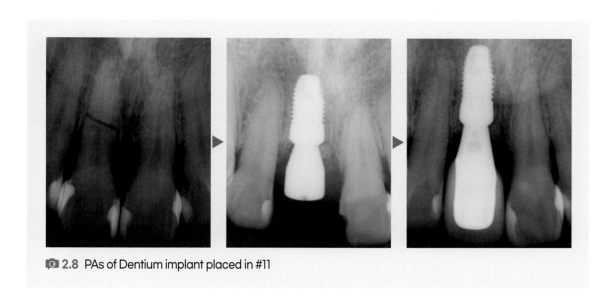

📷 **2.8** PAs of Dentium implant placed in #11

📷 **2.8** It appears pretty good from the PAs. The patient was my distant cousin, who suffered horizontal fracture in tooth #11 (US #8), so I removed the tooth and placed an implant few months later. I was getting my routine equipment ready when the patient specifically asked for Implantium implant. It wasn't one of my go-to implant, and it was actually the first time using it in an anterior implant. Then, I

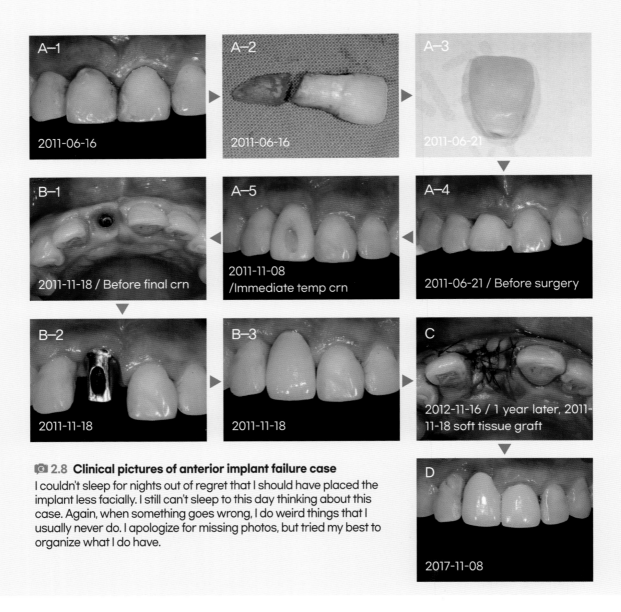

📷 2.8 Clinical pictures of anterior implant failure case

I couldn't sleep for nights out of regret that I should have placed the implant less facially. I still can't sleep to this day thinking about this case. Again, when something goes wrong, I do weird things that I usually never do. I apologize for missing photos, but tried my best to organize what I do have.

let my staff take over to discuss the fees related to the change in procedure.

Generally speaking, I don't like placing implants too palatal, so I try to place it at the incisal line. As I was using my osteotomy drills at the incisal line as usual, it occurred to me that I had to choose the fixture diameter. If it were an other implant brand, I would have placed a 4.0 diameter, but Implantium only offers 3.8 and 4.3 mm. Back then, lots of people believed that we should place a wider implant just like the natural tooth. On top of that, the patient was a young and healthy individual, which led me to place a 4.3 mm diameter implant. It's not my regular implant, and especially it was the first time placing it in the anterior area. Anyway, when one thing goes wrong, everything follows downhill. As I was going up a size, I could feel the drill pushing facially. I felt that it wasn't going to be perfect, but an acceptable result, but when I was placing the actual implant, the microthreads started pushing the fixture facially. I put force on the palate, and then even the facial bone fractured.

I contemplated whether I should go small diameter again, but since I had already fractured the facial plate and 4.3 wasn't even getting sufficient stability, decreasing the diameter to 3.8 mm wasn't going to solve anything. Sweating my pants off, I imagined the final prosthesis in my mind - which seemed possible with angled abutment. Maybe it was just myself trying to avoid the situation...

When I came back to it for the 2nd surgery, it was totally facial. Maybe it was beyond the capability of both myself and my lab tech, but there was no easy solution. The distal papilla, which wasn't great to begin with, started decreasing in addition to the entire gingival contour. During my lectures, I often say that "if you make a vertical incision including the papilla, it means that you will never see the patient again - or vice versa, patient will never return to see you again". But sometimes, this happens. My original plan didn't have vertical incision, but as the implant was pushed facially, I had to put too much force retracting the facial tissue, which led to the tissue being too loose to the point of ripping. This is when I made the tiniest of vertical incision, but this become a nightmare. In all ways. Even my excuses are pathetic. The patient, being a very nice person and a distant cousin of mine, said that it's alright. I gave him a full refund and apologized to him, and promised no-charges on any dental treatments for life.

After about 1 year, I tried some ctg, some soft tissue surgeries.. which made the situation even more. I finally gave up on the case after learning that **for upper anteriors, multiple surgeries will cause scar tissue formation and decreased blood supply, which will make it worse.** Since then, I have decided to live the rest of my life apologizing to the patient.

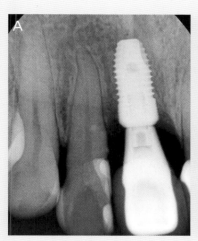
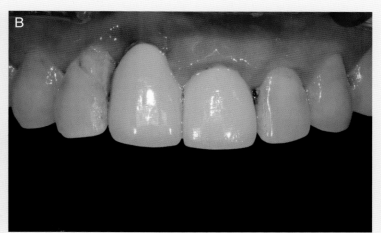

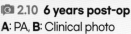 **2.10** *6 years post-op*
A: PA, **B**: Clinical photo

📷 **2.10** is a clinical photo 6 years post-op. Perhaps it is from the microthreads at the cervical part of the fixture, but we can notice some cervical bone loss and inflammation. Patient reported that he has

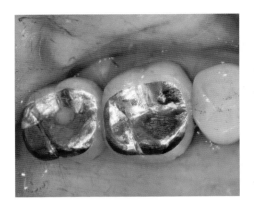
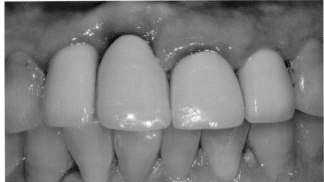
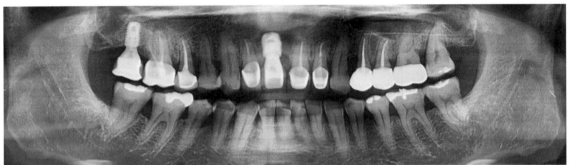

📷 2.11 10 year post-op

some infrequent gingival swelling and was diagnosed with guarded/poor periodontal condition.

In the past 10 years since the implant had been placed, he has visited me with continued trust. During which he received new crowns on upper incisors and upper left premolars, and I also placed implant #17 (📷 2.11). I still hate the papilla. If the soft tissue continues to deteriorate, I am planning on removing the implant and placing a new one palatally. The conclusion is, don't be steadfast in placing a wider diameter implant, but place the right size in the correct angle.

Dentium implant success cases

I don't want to above case to leave a bad impression on Dentis implants as a whole. Dentis implants were actually voted the best quality implants in a survey among dentists few years ago. It's just that I should have understood the characteristics of each implant, but I hadn't done so. For reference, I am sharing a successful case finished with Dentis implants. This patient was an acquaintance of mine, who reached out for help because he couldn't eat due to bad teeth. We had agreed to a payment plan over many years, and finished the full treatment 10 years ago. Because it is quite difficult to find such patients with severe caries in Korea, I took very good care of this patient. I can say that I tried my best, but also due to financial burden, I had to make compromises. It has been over 10 years since the treatment was completed, but the patient still functions very well.

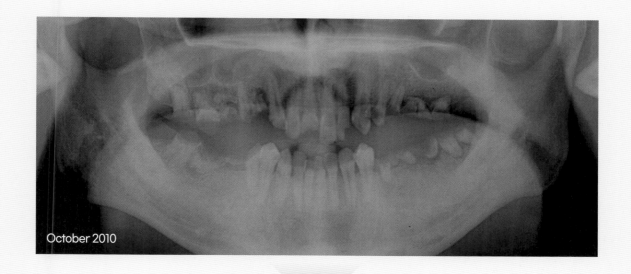

October 2010

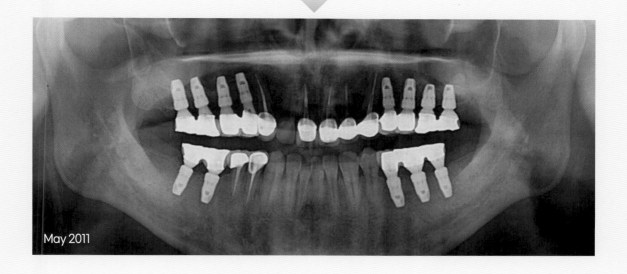

May 2011

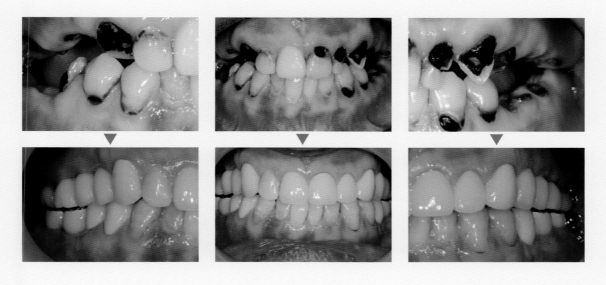

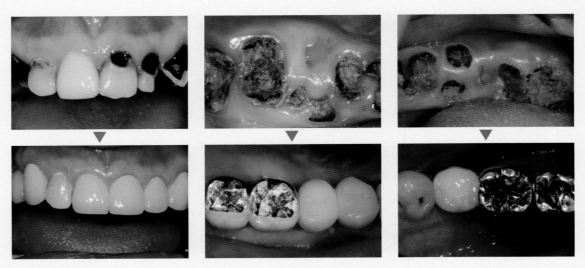

📷 **2.12** Clinical photos

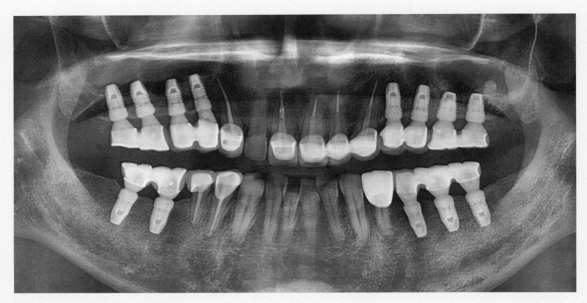

📷 **2.13** June 2021, 10 years post-op

＼ **Note** ／

I have been placing dentium implants for 15 years, but have never ran into tearing problem. Perhaps it's because the crestal threads are thick.

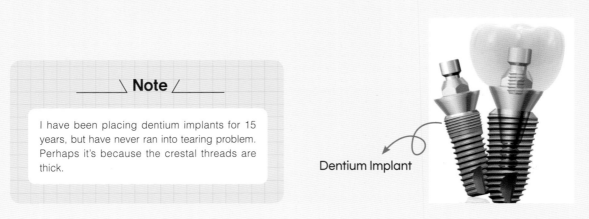

Dentium Implant

Although the different implants may both be noted at 4.0 diameter, but the ones with microthreads at the cervical appear stronger on the xray. As for myself, I have never experienced nor heard of tearing in implants with microthreads like Osstem GS3 for example.

Implant Diameter and Tearing

Implant tearing happens quite often in all types of implants, regardless of the diameter or type. This is especially true for Nobel Biocare implants, which is too thin in the cervical area due to the unique backtaper design. This has led to too many tearing cases.

What are the manufacturer guidelines per each implant company? One specific implant company which sells each fixture at just $10, will exchange implants with tearing at no charge, but not if a 4.0 mm diameter or less was used in posterior areas (4, 5, 6, 7s). Osstem also doesn't recommend single implants of 4.0 mm or thinner diameter to be placed in posterior areas. Then what should one do when the ridge is very thin?

Let's take a brief look at implant tearing (vertical fracture). The biggest problem with internal friction type implant is tearing. If you look at all of the implant cases with tearing, you can see cervical bone loss. Of course, we don't know what happened first. When the fixture has suffered tearing, bone loss will follow. Vice versa, bone loss will lead to implant tearing as well. Then, will there be no implant tearing with no bone loss? We can't be certain, but we know that there is a high correlation between cervical bone loss and implant tearing.

Now let's go back to the question above. What should one do when existing ridge is too thin? Rather than blindly increasing the implant diameter, one must consider if we have sufficient amount of good quality bone in the surrounding. **4.0 mm diameter implant that is surrounded by good quality bone may be better than 4.5 mm diameter with insufficient surrounding bone.** Of course, implant tearing may occur over time through recurring micro-movement from microgaps rather than a single strong force. I believe that micromovements lead to bone loss, and even stress fracture is the cause of implant tearing. This will

Preventing implant tearing Chapter 8-2

- Implant diameter isn't the only problem. You must have sufficient bone surrounding the implant.
- Proper implant Path, Angle, Depth is important (next chapter).
- Most importantly, abutment must be passively placed in the fixture, preventing microgaps and movement. I believe that the continued stress resulting from incorrectly fitting abutment can lead to surrounding bone loss and stress fracture.
- Do not use too much force upon placing the implant. Torque over 60-80NCm may damage the hex, and also destroy the surface treatment.
- Upon crown setting, use only 30-35NCm per manufacturer recommendation (20Ncm for mini implants)

be discussed many times in this book, because it is such an important concept. Now let's discuss my concepts of preventing implant tearing. Implant tearing will be further discussed in **Chapter 8-2**.

Mini implant placed in upper lateral - Case 1

📷 **2.14** and 📷 **2.15** are cases that I placed 3.5 mm mini implant in upper lateral position. 3.5 mm mini implant is best used in these areas because they don't have to withstand too much occlusal load. I generally don't make same day temporary abutment and temporary crown, so I recommend 3 mm

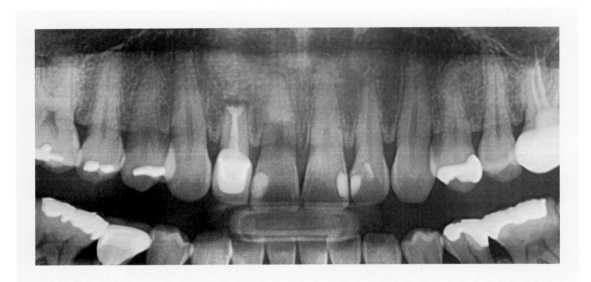

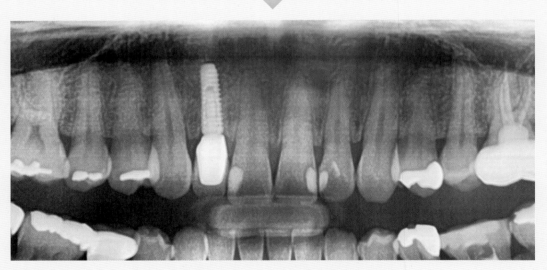

📷 **2.14** Implant placed 12 days after extraction. crown placed 3 months later

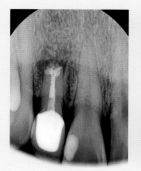
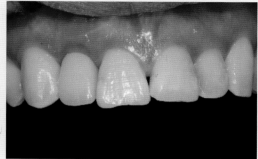

Pre-op

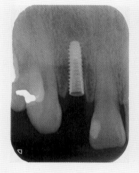

Immediately after implant

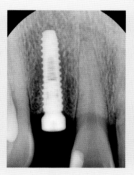

3 mm height HA

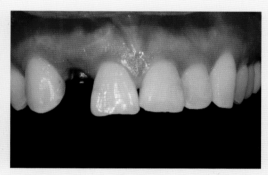

Changed to 5 mm height HA

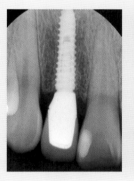
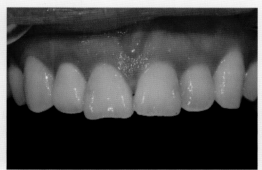

Final crown in place

📷 2.15 General steps in anterior implant

In my clinic, I am no longer involved in the prosthodontic treatments, and the prosth department takes care of it. But generally speaking, if there is nothing in particular, I start off with a 3 mm healing abutment to be just below the gingival zenith, and the prosth takes over. It is generally recommended to change to 5 mm height HA about 1-2 weeks before final impression.

healing abutment height to begin, and change to 5 mm (sometimes 7 mm) 2 weeks before impression for the crown. In this case, I wish I had placed it 1-2 mm deeper.

Mini implant placed in upper lateral - Case 2

📷 **2.16** Straumann BLT 3.3 mm implant was used. I'm presenting this case to show the readers because the diameter is smaller than the 3.5 of Osstem, but Straumann BLT 3.3 is often used as single implant in premolar areas with no problem. I believe that their RockSolid material and small threads in the crestal portion make this possible.

I had placed the immediate implant in a adequate position, but the result by my prosth department

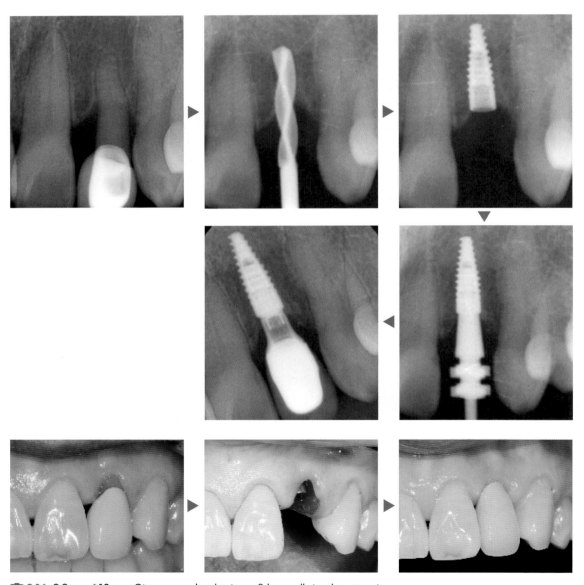

📷 2.16 3.3 mm * 10 mm Straumann implant exo & immediate placement

isn't too satisfying. If they had waited a little longer for adequate gingival healing, we would have been able to achieve more esthetic result.

Mini implant placed in central incisor case

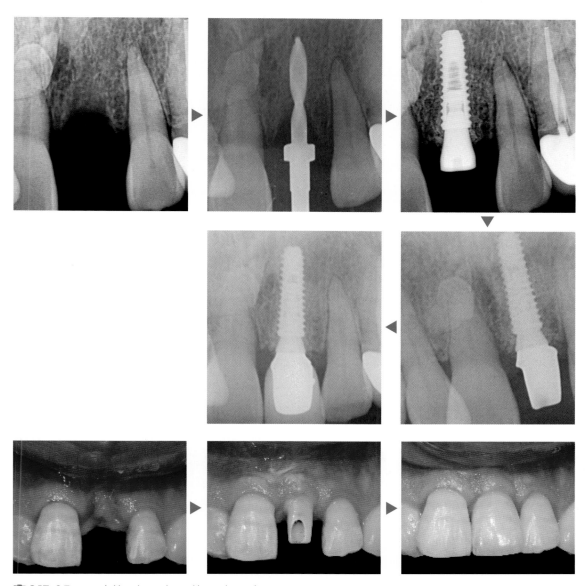

📷 2.17 3.5 mm mini implant placed in male patient

Mini implants can be used in maxillary central incisor position as well (📷 2.17). As mentioned previously, rather than insisting on placing 4.0 (previously, I used to tell to place 4.5 or even 5.0 for central incisors and place such sizes myself), place 3.5 mm in the correct position and angle. If this helps with gaining better quality bone buccolingually, this is what's recommended. In this specific case, because there was very thin bone bucco-lingually, I tried my best to place a 3.5 as centrally as possible, and grafted the facial plate. The implant is positioned slightly facially, but there is no problem esthetically. As I am reviewing the typos for this book in June 2021, the patient came for a recall. He has been using it well for over 5 years so far.

Mini implants used as anterior bridge case

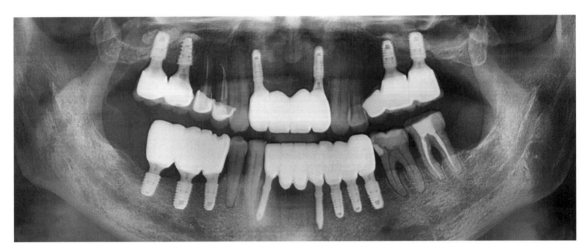

📷 **2.18** mini implants used as anterior bridge case

3.5 mm mini implants were used for a 4 unit bridge for upper incisors. Teeth were removed due to a generalized poor periodontal condition, so I tried to preserve as much remaining bone as possible.

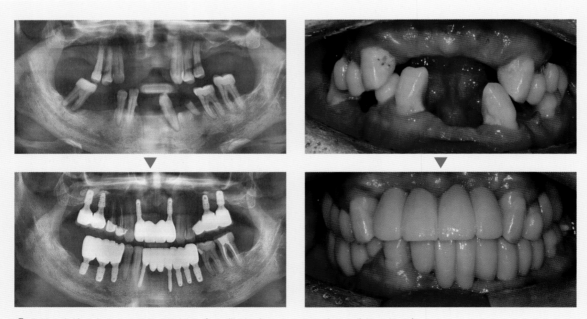

📷 **2.19** mini implants used as bridge (papilla isn't very pretty, but I did my best)

Mini implants were also used in lower left canine and premolar (30s). The surgical plan took into consideration the surrounding bone rather than insisting on wider implants. You can see how much bone loss there was in the below pre-op clinical photo. When I had opened the flap, there was almost no bone, and very thin ridge was remaining. The remaining vertical height was too small, so I had to reduce the occlusion by polishing, and placed the implants. 3.5 mm diameter was used due to very thin ridge.

Mini implant placed in lower premolar case 1

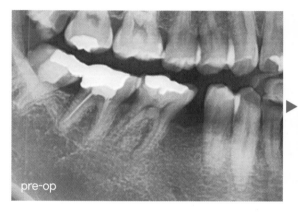
pre-op

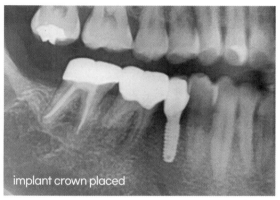
implant crown placed

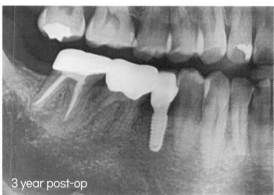
3 year post-op

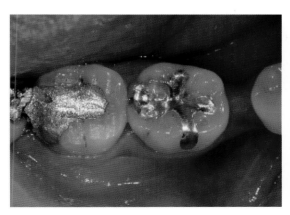

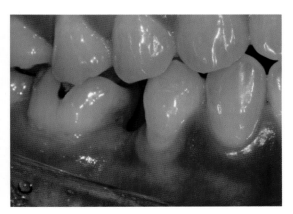

📷 **2.20** 40 year old male patient. the remaining M-D space was so small, I placed a mini implant in premolar area. I wish I had post-op photos.

Mini implant placed in lower premolar case 2

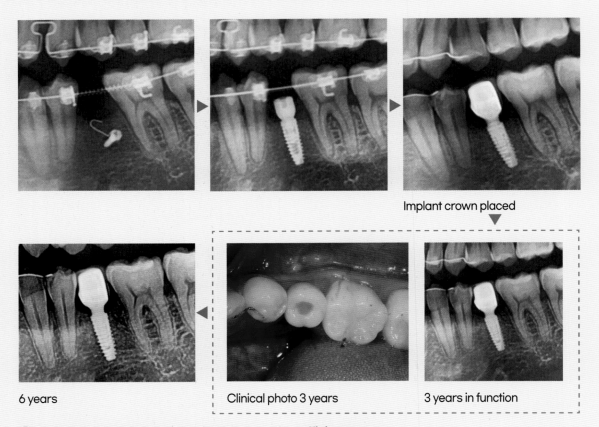

Implant crown placed

6 years | Clinical photo 3 years | 3 years in function

📷 2.21 **Ortho completed prior to implant to make sufficient space**

I decided to place a mini implant for this patient because of the thin bucco-lingual ridge, due to congenitally missing the lower premolar. Looking back at it, I wish I had placed a wider implant a little deeper with simultaneous grafting of the area because it was a young male patient, but I guess I wasn't insisting a wider diameter due to small M-D distance as well. I generally ask my orthodontic department to send over the patient 4-5 months prior to finishing treatment, so that the crown will be ready in about a month before finishing the ortho treatment. The implant has been functioning well 6 years so far and I instructed the patient to return for bite check at least once a year. If I recall correctly, even the 4.0 drill was hitting the neighboring teeth, so I finished with a mini implant.

Mini implant placed in upper premolar case 1

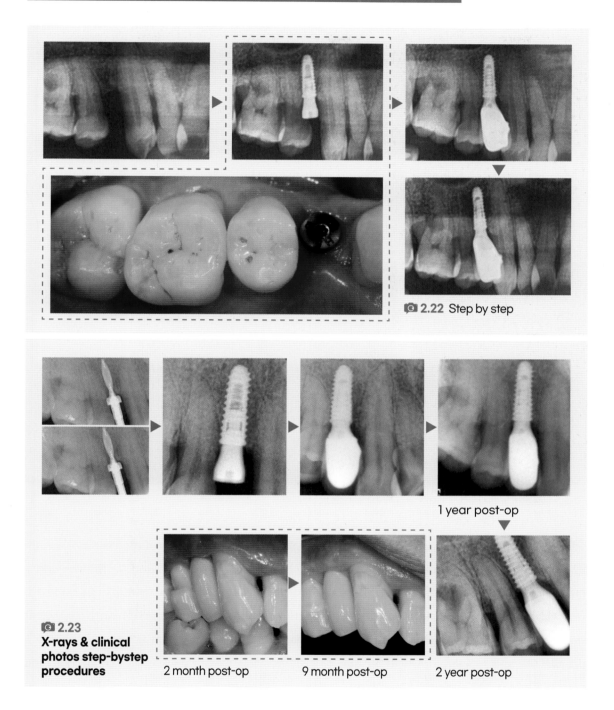

📷 2.22 Step by step

📷 2.23
X-rays & clinical photos step-bystep procedures

1 year post-op

2 month post-op

9 month post-op

2 year post-op

Unfortunately I am missing the pre-op clinical photos, but it is visible that the space is very small and very thin palatal bone (📷 2.22, 2.23). The patient really wanted an implant in this position, so I placed a mini 3.5 mm. Due to thin ridge, I placed the implant where I could find bone so I'm not 100% satisfied with the position, but the result is clinically acceptable. For upper premolars sometimes we have the place the implant slightly buccally angled to consider the emergence profile. If there is severe buccal recession or bone shape is abnormal with defect, it must be taken into consideration. For mini implants, there is higher risk of implant tearing when in combination with bone loss, so the patient was instructed to return to us as soon as possible if he feels the slightest mobility.

Mini implants from other companies (non-Korean)

Straumann BLT 3.3 mm is often found used for premolar areas. I'm sure the dentists have considered everything, but perhaps it is the trust in the strength of Straumann implant's RockSolid material.

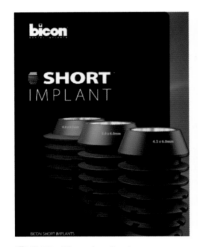 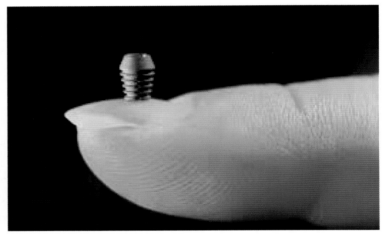

📷 2.24 Bicon implant

This is from Bicon poster, claiming this line of implants will be manufactured soon (📷 2.24). From my research, the smallest implant approved for use by the U.S. FDA is 4.5 mm in diameter and 5 mm in length. But if Bicon is considering this small size, smaller than what's currently FDA approved, why can't other implant companies? The strength of implant and connection with abutment would probably be more important to consider than anything else. Perhaps the reason Bicon can manufacture this type of implant is because it's made of an alloy with no screw for connection, and quite stable once the crown is placed. If this implant is sold in Korea, I'm open to trying this out. 😊

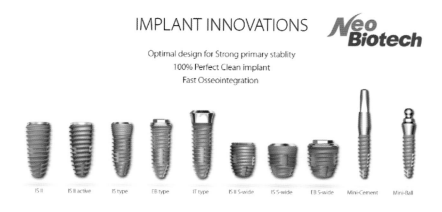

IMPLANT INNOVATIONS **Neo Biotech**

Optimal design for Strong primary stablity
100% Perfect Clean implant
Fast Osseointegration

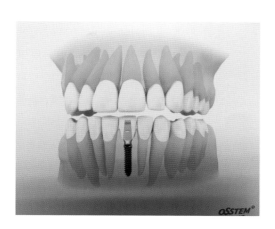

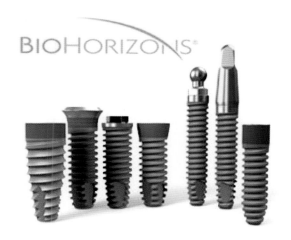

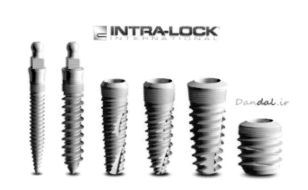

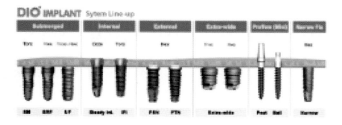

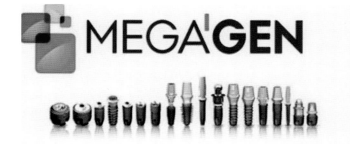

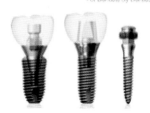

📷 2.25 many different companies manufacture onebody implants

I have been using only **one-body mini implants for mandibular anterior teeth** for quite some time. Onebody mini implants are 3 mm or less in diameter and have the fixture and abutment connected, into a single piece. 2.5 mm diameter is the most frequently used size. Most companies manufacture 3.0 mm as well, but clinicians tend to place 3.5 mm mini, so unless the onebody implant is to be used for lower canine, most often 2.5 mm diameter is used. The onebody implant is mostly alloy (obviously the surface will be RBM) so the implant is very durable, definitely stronger than 3.5 mm mini implant, and **sometimes even stronger than 4.0 mm regular** platform implant. Of course there are more things to consider than just the mechanical strength, so it's not easy to make a direct comparison. Some clinicians tend to avoid onebody implants because the abutment shows above the tissue height, so the implant companies also make 3.0-3.3 mm diameter two body implants as well. To prevent fracture, the material is often alloy titanium with almost no threads. I recommend onebody over two body implants in these areas.

The crown width of lower incisors are about 5-6 mm mesiodistally. The roots are sometimes not even 3-4 mm wide mesiodistally. Very often patients may present with severe crowding and very limited distance from root to root, which makes it physically impossible to place traditional implants. But a 2.5 mm implant makes it possible to place an implant without damaging neighboring teeth. The most stressful surgeries in my implant career are the GBR cases on lower incisors. It can be very stressful because there is a lot of tissue movement and patients tend to play with the area frequently, leading to unsuccessful GBR.

But ever since I started placing onebody implants in lower anterior areas, I was able to avoid doing large GBR in this areas, significantly decreasing the source of my stress. If you are in doubt, please trust me once and give it a try. Most implant companies have started to manufacture these type of onebody mini implants.

There are not many cases I can recall prior to 2014. Only when patients come back for recall and tell me about my other surgeries, I find photos of old cases. In the past 10 years I have only placed onebody (Osstem MS) implants in lower anterior areas.

Onebody mini implant for lower central incisor case

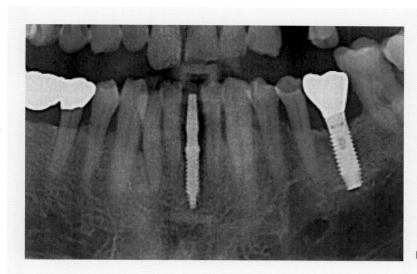

📷 **2.26** 2012 post-op

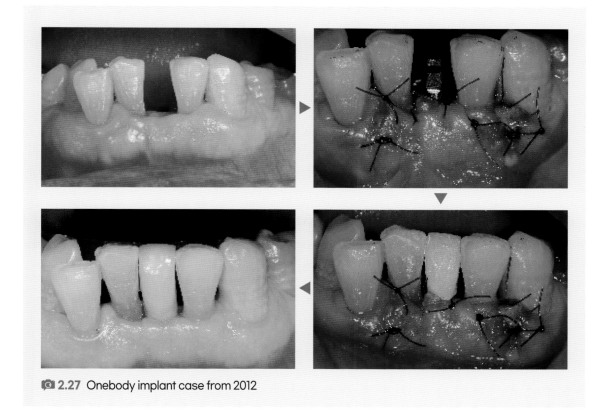

📷 **2.27** Onebody implant case from 2012

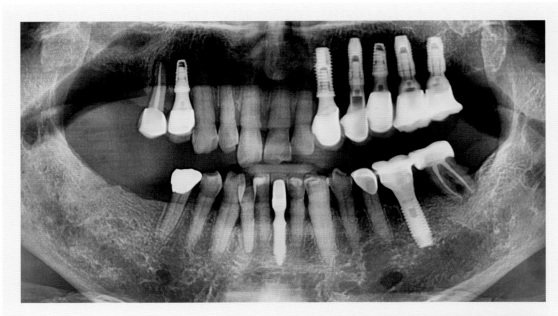

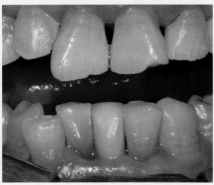

📷 **2.28 After completing implants #4, 23, 25 (May 8, 2019).** #31, 24, 26, 27 had been completed in 2012, #36 completed in 2007

📷 **2.26-2.28** This patient returned to me for a consult regarding another tooth implant, and told me that I had done his implants some years ago, and could find some photos. I don't really like the final crowns, but for an elderly gentleman, he has been functioning well with them. I'm guessing that's why he came back to me for more treatment. I had placed #36 in 2007.

3 things to consider when placing onebody mini implants

1. The surgery is complete after one or two drilling, which makes it difficult if the first angle was incorrect.

This can make it difficult for beginners who aren't as comfortable with implant drilling. Of course, because we are all born with different dexterity, so there is no absolute standard, but as I teach in my live surgery seminars, even most beginners do pretty well with some guidance. However, because it's quite important to understand the qualities of different implants, so it's very important to practice on a model prior to surgery. I always emphasize this in my lectures.

"Onebody mini implants should be placed in one shot - one kill manner"

2. A long abutment is connected to the fixture, so without good initial stability, implant may end up with poor osseointegration.

Initial stability of mini implants if very important, so if bone quality is inadequate, it's best to wait sufficiently prior to implant placement. Generally, I place implants about 6 weeks following extraction, after initial soft tissue healing, but also wait 2 to 3 months if bone quality is poor. During my lectures, I always emphasize, "Think of yourself as a tiger poacher from the 18th century, with one gun and a single bullet". This means that you must have the perfect aim. An imperfect first shot may be costly as it may have been your only chance.

3. It's best to make a temporary crown.

Most people need temporary crowns on the onebody mini implants. Very often the elderly don't need one, but that's an exception. This makes #1 & #2 concepts more important. Basically, it's most important to avoid contact with the opposing teeth and avoid rotational force on the crown at all cost. Onebody mini implants have thin diameter, so it's especially weak against rotational forces. Implant will most likely fail with rotational forces on the implant crown. So, when I had placed 2 of the onebody implants and have the temporary crowns splinted, there has never been a failed case. For single temporary crowns, the temp crowns must be connected to the adjacent tooth. Most of the times the temp crowns are connected by composite to the adjacent tooth.

Single lower canine case

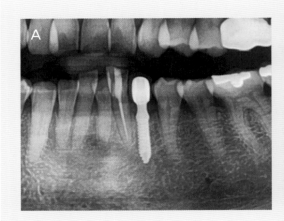 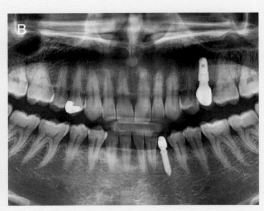

📷 **2.29** Onebody mini implant placed in lower canine area

I use the onebody mini implants in lower canine areas as single crowns too. We generally have 2 options for mini implants: 2.5 and 3.0 mm diameter, and the 3.0 mm is my go-to implant for lower canines, like above 📷 **2.29A**. As for 📷 **2.29B**, a 2.5 mm was used due to congenitally missing lower canine, due to collapsed M-D space. Most of the patients in my country that lose lower incisors is from poor periodontal disease in geriatric population. On the contrary, young females almost never lower anterior teeth, so I have zero cases from young females. We tend to do absolutely everything we can to save such teeth. Because of this, I am able to focus less on esthetics in these areas.

Single implant in lower anterior case

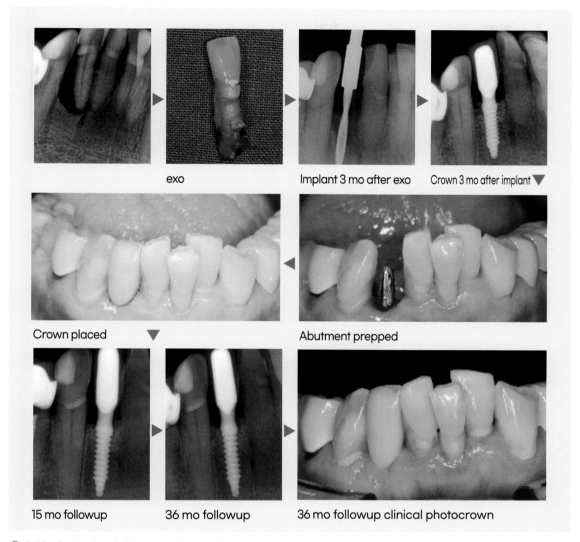

exo   Implant 3 mo after exo   Crown 3 mo after implant ▼

Crown placed ▼   Abutment prepped

15 mo followup   36 mo followup   36 mo followup clinical photocrown

📷 **2.30** Onebody mini implant placed after exo due to perio disease

📷 **2.30** case is a onebody mini implant placed after tooth #43 had to be removed due to perio disease for a 69 year old female patient. I waited 3 months after extraction of #43, and also simultaneously did bone graft using xenograft (Straumann cerabone®).T he final crown isn't very esthetic, I did my best. To accommodate for the different gingival height, manufacturers make various gingival height such as 2, 3, 4 mm. Osstem implants, which I use, have 2.5 mm and 4 mm. I used 4 mm gingival height collar in this case due to generalized poor periodontal condition, which had led to the tooth loss. In case anybody wonders about my grafting policy, I don't place any membrane if an intact periosteum can be achieved from the flap. In this case, I placed the implant in correct position and depth, and placed about 2 mm of non-resorbable bone to cover the exposed threads, and sutured. We will go over my choice of graft materials and membrane in **Part 6**.

Lower anterior 3 unit bridge case

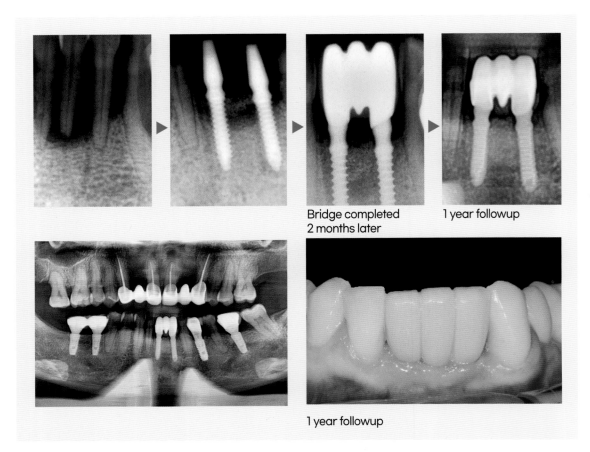

Bridge completed
2 months later

1 year followup

1 year followup

📷 2.31 Anterior bridge after extractions due to severe periodontal disease

📷 2.31 This case was a lower anterior bridge case for a 49 year old patient with some physical disabilities. He was opposed to large grafts and big surgeries. Due to the history of periodontal disease, I waited 6 months after extractions. I did the surgery as I routinely practice, I placed the implants to their ideal position and did about 2 mm xenograft around the exposed implant threads. It is still in good condition to this day.

Onebody mini implant placed for lower 6 anterior teeth

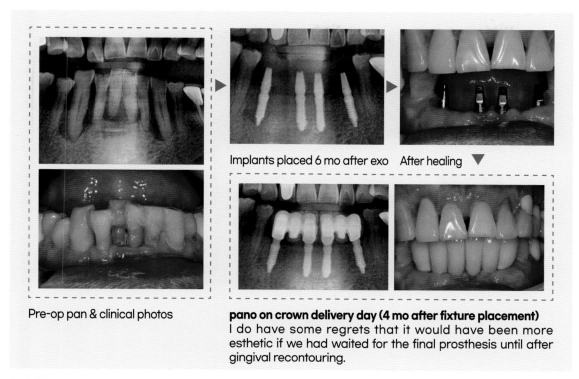

Implants placed 6 mo after exo   After healing ▼

Pre-op pan & clinical photos

pano on crown delivery day (4 mo after fixture placement)
I do have some regrets that it would have been more esthetic if we had waited for the final prosthesis until after gingival recontouring.

📷 2.32

Usually, for lower anterior 6 unit bridge, it's possible to place 2 implants in canine position to make a 6 unit bridge, but it's safer to place one in the middle (📷 **2.32**). As for myself, if finances aren't an issue, I like to place 2 in the central incisor position to make 2 separate 3 unit bridges. As opposed the upper anterior bridge, where esthetic demands, bone quality, and finances are more important, the lower anteriors are somewhat free from such demands. So, we can consider for more stability and function for lower anteriors.

The doc that I met in the U.S., whom I recall to be the quickest and most accurate clinician, places onebody implants in upper laterals as well. I think that he can pull it off being a prosthodontist with such clinical expertise and experience. As for myself, maybe it's my lack of skills, but I don't place onebody implants in upper laterals where high esthetics is demanded, nor recommend for my students. It's possible that I avoid it in upper lateral position because I don't do the prosthesis.

Onebody mini implant for upper premolar case

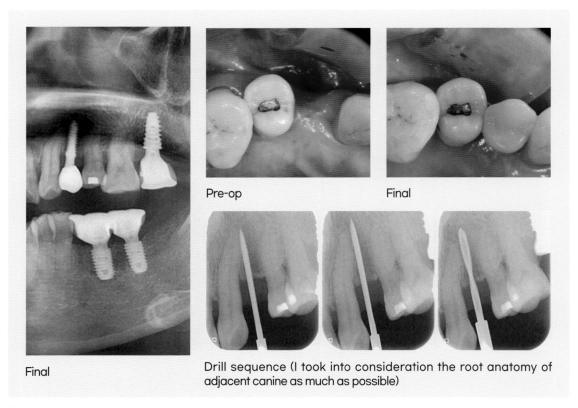

Pre-op　　　Final

Final

Drill sequence (I took into consideration the root anatomy of adjacent canine as much as possible)

📷 2.33 Onebody mini implant used in upper premolar area

📷 2.33 This is the only case that I had placed a onebody mini implant in upper premolar area. Upper 1st premolar had been missing for a very long time, leading to a very tight space. The patient was referred from another doctor. I thoroughly explained to the patient possibility of implant fracture, and agreed to proceed with the surgery. To make the minimal space, #3 distal and 5 mesial spaces were trimmed, then I proceeded to the implant surgery. Because nothing could be done with the distally angled root apex of #3, the surgery wasn't easy, but I made sufficient room facially and placed the implant. I haven't been able to upload any radiographs, but patient is using it well after 3 years, and a strong emphasis must be placed on occlusion check.

We can't skip the discussion of implant fracture or tearing in this chapter. Anyway, onebody can have great clinical success in certain areas. But, just as we avoid placing a 4.0 in lower anterior, we should also avoid placing a onebody implant in posterior or area with heavy occlusal load. It should also be avoided in poor quality bone because of the thin thread design. Obviously such areas are upper posteriors, so there is no need to place onebody implants there. We should check and make sure that even in lower anteriors, there isn't too heavy occlusion. I believe that the best way to prevent implant fracture is to place the implant in correct position and angle.

Short implants & onebody mini implants used for full lower anteriors

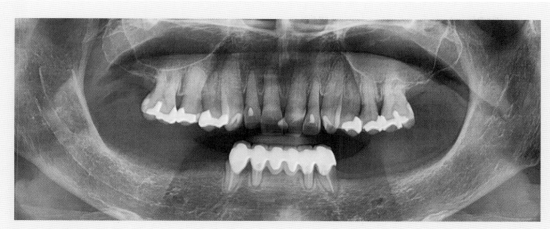

📷 **2.34 Initial pano**
Lower bridge is loose due to root fracture.

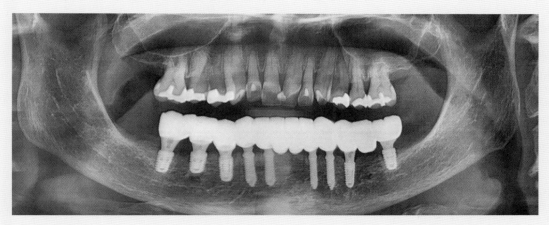

📷 **2.35 Final**
#46, 45 - 4.5*6 mm / 44# - 3.5*8.5 mm / 43-33# - 2.5*11.5 mm / 34# - 3.5*8.5 mm / 36# - 4.5*6 mm

This case was for a 73 year old female patient from Japan. I replaced lower bridge that was used for abutment for lower RPD (📷 **2.34**). Lower bridge was almost fractured and was mobile, so we agreed to remove all remaining teeth and make a full lower denture. Patient was on a form of bisphosphonate, so I couldn't dare recommend immediate implants, and we agreed to wait until after complete healing. The healing was slow, but it did eventually fully heal. The patient was traveling from Japan just for the dental treatments, so it was difficult to come up with a treatment plan.

The patient wanted 2 implants in 3s and 4s, for overdenture, but because the remaining ridge in posterior was very thin and also had very little keratinized gingiva, it wasn't an adequate case for overdenture. So before it was too late, we agreed to have one last attempt at a full mouth rehab with implants.

Usually, I would start off with implants in molar area, re-establish the VDO, then continue on the lower incisors and temporize with temp crowns on lower onebody mini implants, but since the patient didn't have complete trust in implants, patient was insistent on overdenture. So, we agreed to place onebody mini implant for implant supported bridge from 3 to contralateral 3, and place single implants in 4s, for posterior support (I had in mind to somehow convince the patient to convert to full fixed, not overdenture). Then, I placed 4 implants for lower anteriors: #43, 42, 32, 33.

This is when I ran into a major problem. I should have evaluated on CBCT and made a stent, but since I just went straight into surgery, the center of soft tissue wasn't the center of existing ridge, and the patient had unstable occlusion due to being edentulous. On top of that, I started the implant surgery in the 4th quadrant first and moved onto the 3rd, and decided to place #32 and 33 same distance from the midline to 42 and 43, but it ended up too distal compared to the upper teeth. This resulted in all implants in the 3rd quadrant pushed distally.

After finishing the surgery, I asked my prosthodontist to consider #32 as if it were #33, and then splint #33 to the posterior units, but it appears that my requests weren't considered in the final prosthethesis. Anyway, the patient was satisfied that the anterior surgery was simple, and opted to continue to the posterior areas. I placed a short implant in #34 position, and I still wonder how the result would have looked if I could have splinted 33=34==36. Although the implants in the 3rd quad are all pushed distally, the patient was very happy with the result and said that she felt like she was born again, so I consider this a success case by selectively choosing proper implant diameter and length.

_____\ **Note** /_____

Normal implants are two-row thread design with a minimum 0.8 mm pitch, so one turn (360 degrees) places the implant at a minimum 1.6 mm to 2 mm. The Osstem MS implant has 0.6 mm pitch and is a single-row thread design, so one turn would bring the implant only 0.6 mm deeper. A beginner may feel that the implant isn't going in, but actually because it has a sharp apex, the implant still finds way into bone even if the osteotomy site was underdrilled. Hence, it is a good habit to underdrill when placing MS implants (onebody) rather than overdrilling. One more thing to keep in mind is that the tianium is an alloy material, so it is stronger.

I have placed onebody mini implants since 2005. Back then, it wasn't imported in Korea. First, because the implant fixture and abutment was single piece and the abutment end came in various design and shape and because it was advertised that it can easily be used for overdentures, I started placing them even though I had no background knowledge. This is the same time when I first started noticing implant failures, for the first time ever. The ball-type one body implants placed in upper dentition started falling out in just a few months, until every single one failed. In the lower, just a few survived. If I went back in time with my current experience, probably I could have a slightly better chances, but that's what happened back then. So, I stopped using them completely. When Osstem started manufacturing MS implants, I started selectively placing them in lower anteriors, and eventually placed exclusively MS implants in lower anterior areas.

While I was in the U.S., I was invited to a live surgery course hosted by a certain implant company. There I met Dr. Josh Brower, and I was able to learn a lot about mini implants from him. He is actively on social media in his website www.gmdia.dental.

Josh holds many implant seminars sponsored by Sternogold company, and also actively uploads cases in the facebook page: "Mini dental implant masters". He said that I could freely use his cases in my book, but if you are interested, please visit his pages: <Josh Brower's FB> and <Mini dental implant masters>. He also promotes mini implants in a different group as well: "International academy of mini dental implants.

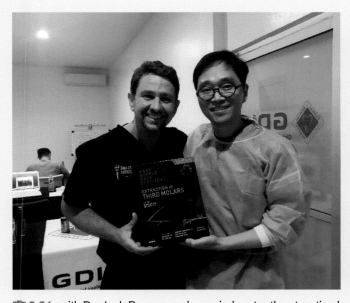
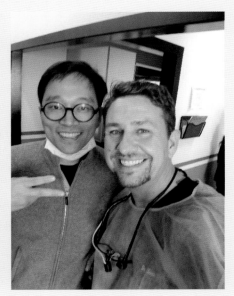

📷 2.36 with Dr. Josh Brower and my wisdom tooth extraction book

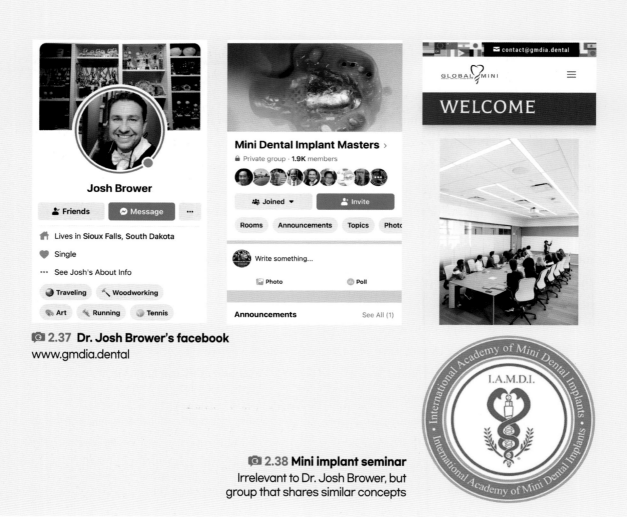

📷 **2.37 Dr. Josh Brower's facebook**
www.gmdia.dental

📷 **2.38 Mini implant seminar**
Irrelevant to Dr. Josh Brower, but
group that shares similar concepts

It seems that mini implants are promoted because of its simplicity in surgery. Even Straumann has started manufacturing onebody mini implants now. From my understanding, Straumann recommends onebody only in overdenture cases, not stand alone crowns.

Anyway, you will run into many different (creative? crazy?) cases using onebody implants. Sometimes, there is sufficient bone width, but some clinician placed 20 implants in the entire edentulous arch for an overdenture support, or placing 2 onebody implants to support a molar. There are very many creative cases. As we can see from Straumann now manufacturing onebody implants, and many different clinicians like Dr. Josh Brower constantly promoting and lecturing onebody implants, there might be a reason for that.. but my thoughts haven't changed yet. As mentioned earlier, it could be that Korenas have such strong occlusion so onebody implants can't work. Unless there is suddenly a huge change, I will still be placing onebody implants in lower anteriors only.

Dr. Youngsam Kim's recommended implant size (Osstem) at a glance

First choice is placing implant in a single in sufficient bone width and length. Second choice is also placing implant in a single but with insufficient bone. For lower posterior, it could be because of proximity to nerve, lower anterior due to prosthetic options. For upper, either due to poor bone quality or concavity, or to achieve high initial stability for immediate temp crown.

Generally, if two units are to be splinted, the diameter could be decreased, and the length can also be decreased unless it is for upper anterior case. For upper anteriors, there is much to consider including potential immediate or early loading, so longer implant may be beneficial. If a pontic & bridge is to be planned, patient's sex, occlusion, occlusal load, and parafunctional habits must be considered..

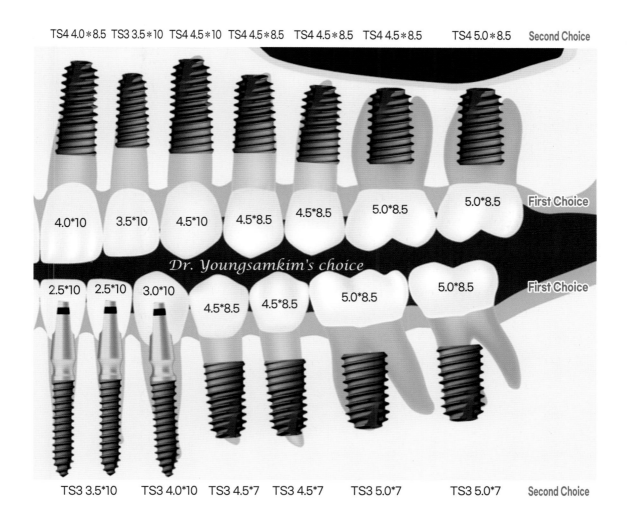

Dr. YOUNGSAM KIM'S

CLINICAL NOTES

EASY SIMPLE SAFE EFFICIENT

MASTERING DENTAL IMPLANTS

The Essential Elements for Success in Dental Implants

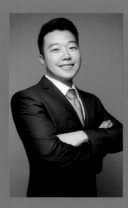

Dr. Jong Wook Hur

I am a general dentist from Australia who graduated from Griffith University School of Dentistry in 2015. I am thrilled to be part of the translating team again after taking part in translation of Dr Kim's wisdom teeth extraction book. I was once a monkey with a pickaxe. Thanks to Dr Kim's guidance, I am evolving into a human-being with a decent implant surgery skill. If you still want more after finishing this book, I recommend you attend his lecture series because what he taught me had a tremendous influence on the development of my career.

4

Ideal Fixture Position, Angulation and Depth (PAD)

What's wrong with having a high standard?

4-1 The Pickaxe

4-2 Fixture Position & Angulation

4-3 The Depth

4-1

The Pickaxe

Mastering dental implants

What is a Pickaxe Implant?

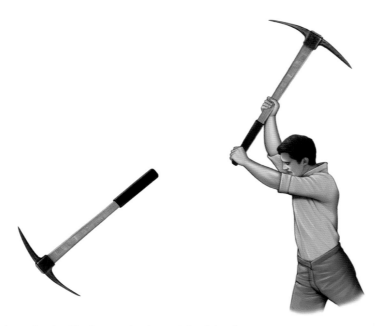

📷 **1.1**   Image I use in my implant lecture series to explain pickaxing.

Many who attended my lecture series tells me that all they can remember is "Monkey" and "Pickaxe". This is because I call mispositioned fixtures "monkey planted" and distally angulated ones in particular "a pickaxe". It's perhaps a most used word in my lecture series.

When dentists who are only used to treating dentition performs an osteotomy, I notice the handpieces tend to tilt backwards causing the apex of the fixture to be pushed mesially. This is a result of a novice implantologist forgetting to assess the edentulous space from multiple view points. The tooth mesial to the edentulous space blocks the operators vision so that the space immediaetly distal to the tooth doesn't get accounted for. This makes the operator thinks that he/she is starting in the

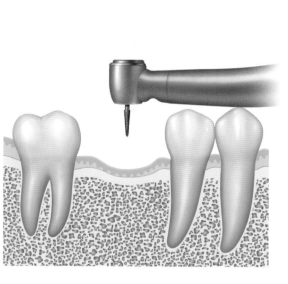
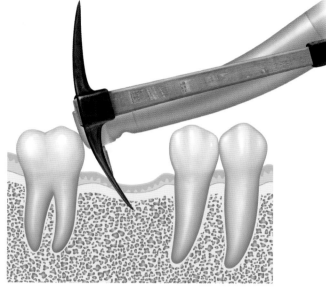
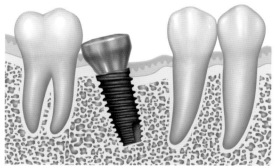

 1.2 How pickaxing happens

middle when they're actually starting further distal then the midpoint. Such confusion then leads to what's shown in 1.2 It is a very commonly observed phenomenon.

When pickaxing reaches its new heights, it finds the distal root of the mesial dentition. Once an operator experiences the heartache from such incident, pickaxing habit is well and truly cured. However, sometimes the operator may go towards the other extreme and starts positioning the implant too far away from the mesial dentition.

I always remind the lecture attendants to focus on developing an eye for excellence by exposing themselves to as many properly placed implants as possible. This needs to happen well before one starts placing implants themselves. Of course this book won't suddenly turn you into an implant master, but I am confident that you will have much higher standard of placement by the end of this book.So let me tell you again. First and foremost step to becoming an excellent implantologist is to develop an eye for properly placed fixtures. Remember that you will be very sad for a while afterwards, because what you've seen and what you've done may be very different. However, as long as you keep working towards your higher standards, one day you will realize that you're there. **You will never improve unless your eyes can tell good from bad.**

Let's look at a few decent pickaxe cases I've discovered while practicing.

Pickaxes from other Dental Practices

We came across the implants shown in images below in our practice. In fact, we encounter them quite often on SNS posts and even in implant company marketing materials. For the purpose of writing this book, I searched our data base for some examples. Obviously, they were no where to be find when I was actually in need of them. With great difficulty, I've managed to find some fairly standard pickaxe cases that I would like to share here. Again, they are incidental findings and NOT placed in my practice.

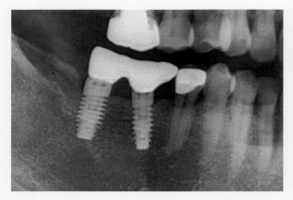 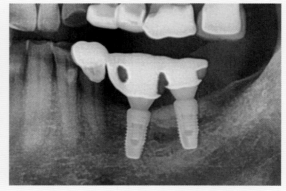

📷 **1.3** Manidbular 6s placed like a pickaxe. They are not severe and happens quite commonly due to the 5s blocking off the operator's vision. I think the operator initiated the osteotomy much more distal then he/she should have.

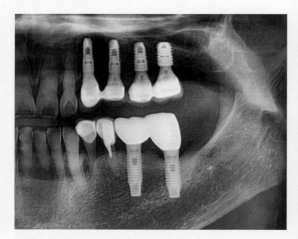 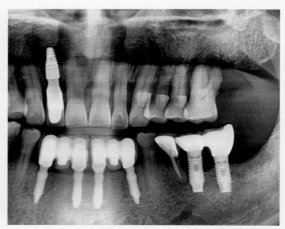

📷 **1.4** 36, 37 placed like a pickaxe. 23-26 were placed by myself.

📷 **1.5** 36, 37 placed like a pickaxe again. 12 Straumann and 33-43 Osstem MS implants were placed by myself. Note the proximity of 36 fixture to the root of the 35.

When the fixture is too far distal from the mesial dentition

As seen from the previous case, pickaxing may often damage distal root surface of the mesial dentition. Such experience drives the operator further away from the root of the mesial tooth, which can lead to the distalising of the entire fixture. While this may not be the only cause of such misplacement, I personally consider pickaxing to be the root of the issue.

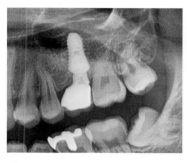 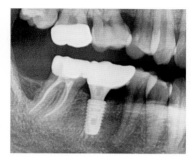 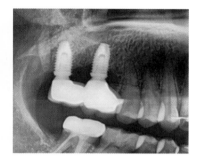

📷 1.6 Fixtures placed much further distally from the ideal position

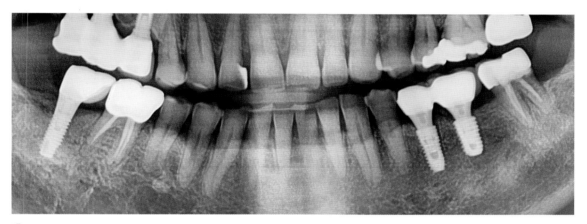

📷 1.7 You can see that #47 was placed too distally. Note the 35-36 which were placed by myself.

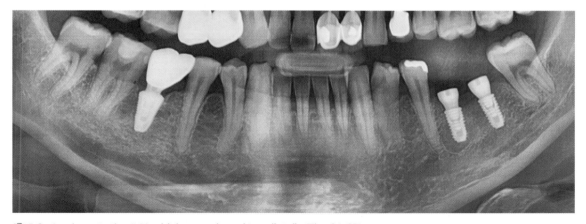

📷 1.8 Again, note the #46 which was placed too distally. The 36-37 were my cases.

7s that are placed a little too far

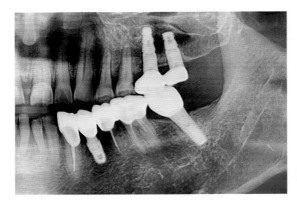

📷 1.9 Surprisingly common #37 which is much further distal. Note the #34 which I have placed.

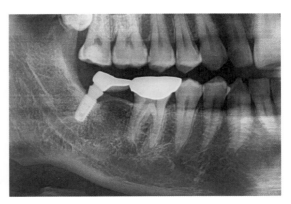

📷 1.10 Is this 47? or 48?

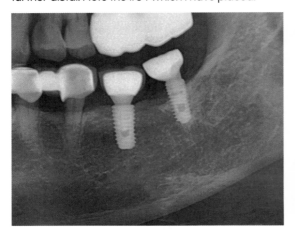

📷 1.11 It looks as though the two were not planted at the same time. Even the 37 crown looks like it's tilting its head in confusion, wondering if it's sitting in the right place.

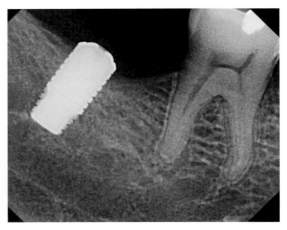

📷 1.12 Image provided by Dr Young Kim, a Facebook friend from the US. He asked what implant system this was as the patient had this placed 10 years ago in Korea. It's a GS2 implant from Osstem but the positioning embarrassed me even though I didn't place the implant.

At this point, I would like to discuss a part of Osseointegrated implant fracture: causes and treatment (Journal of Oral Implantology Aug 2011 Gealh et al.). *In summary, the study states that the "Causes of implant fracture may be divided into 3 categories: (1) defects in the design of the material, (2) nonpassive fit of the prosthetic structure, and (3) biomechanical or physiologic overload." Gealh concluded that "the treatment of implant fractures usually consists of removal of the fractured fragment, installation of another implant, and the manufacture of another prosthesis."* Obviously, it is impossible for the operator to overcome the limitations of a defective implant fixture. Therefore, the only way possible for the operator to reduce the risk of implant fracture is to place the implant at its ideal position, therefore eliminating the biomechanical overload. In **Part 3**, we discussed how to choose an ideal fixture. Which is why we're discussing how to place that "ideal fixture" into an "ideal position" in **Part 4**. We've taken our first step towards learning what the "ideal position" entails; avoid pickaxing at all cost.

Too Far Distal and Too Shallow

Worst possible pickaxed implant fixtures are the ones that are also placed not deep enough (and therefore didn't allow for enough prosthetic space). This creates a cantilever effect which leads to a frequent fracture and/or displacement of the implant retained prosthesis. Subsequently, it increases the risk of the implant fixture fracture and/or peri-implantitis.

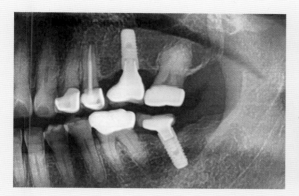
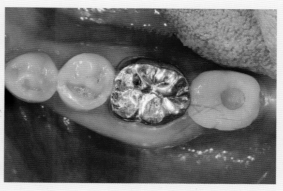

📷 **1.13** We could give the benefit of the doubt for #37 that insufficient prosthetic space was due to the supra-erupted #27. However, #26 placement shows the operator's tendency to place the fixtures too far distally and without sufficient depth.

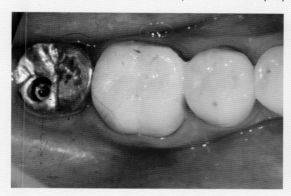
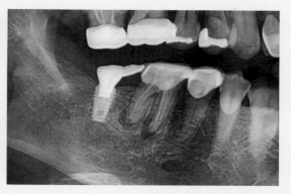

📷 **1.14** Again, placed too far distal and too shallow. Lack of prosthetic space dictated this prosthesis to be a screw-retained crown. I strongly recommend to stay away from screw-retained prosthesis for internal friction type fixture such as this one. The patient's chief complaint was recurring displacement of the composite resin access hole cover. This is most likely due to the lack of resin thickness, which is a result of the lack of the prosthetic space.

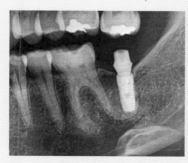
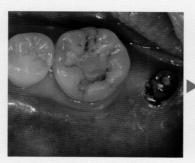
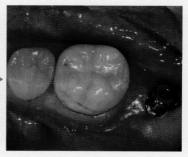

📷 **1.15** The patient visited the practice for the extraction of #48. He specifically requested for us to not touch the #37 implant even during his return visit for the 360 restoration. He said that he is so sick and tired of dealing with the implant crown after recurring implant crown dislodgement, that he doesn't even want to think about it.

Some of my implant lecture attendees sent me photos of their own sightings of pickaxe implant. Let me share a few of those with you.

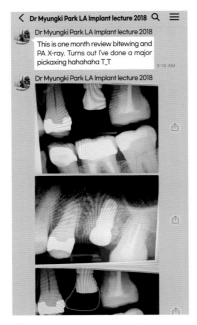
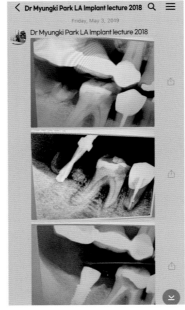
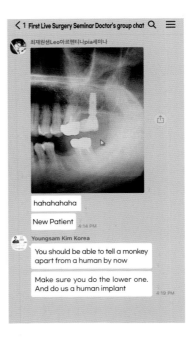

📷 1.16 Pickaxe sighting from overseas

First and second screen capture was sent to me by a dentist in the US who attended my very first US implant lecture. After my lecture he jokingly said that all his past implants were monkeys and pickaxes. It's odd that I've heard people say the same thing time and time again. Third screen capture was taken from a group chat for my first Mexican Live Surgery course attendees. It is still very active even after the 2 years since their course.

The case from the third screen capture was uploaded by one of my most loyal followers. He attended all of my lecture series and returned to Mexico after his first live surgery course for the third time.

It is not a cheap course so I've asked why he kept on coming back and he replied "The US is still the land of opportunity. If you're good at what you do, you can still make good income".

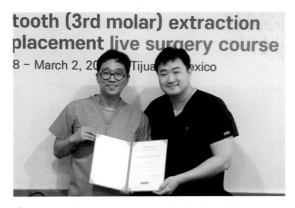

📷 1.17 1st Live Surgery attendee Dr. Leo Choe

Dr Choe lives in Maine, USA and he always invites me over for lobster which is Maine speciality. His father, who is also a dentist in Korea, is a lot older and more experienced than I am. He also attended all my Korean seminars on his son's recommendation.

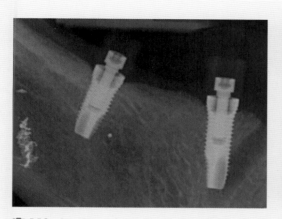
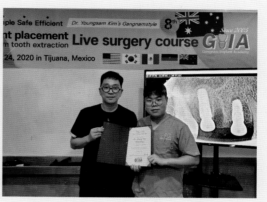

📷 **1.18 An X-ray from Dr Ji-Hyung Kim(left) in Australia. He attended my implant lecture series in 2018 and attended the Mexico Live Surgery course in February 2020, just before the pandemic.**

Dr Kim told me that the implants were placed by a famous oral surgeon in his locality. The surgeon referred the patient to Dr Kim for restoration of the implants. What's interesting is that the surgeon damaged the distal root surface of the #44 during the placement of the #45 and the tooth ended up needing to be extracted. I don't know how the patient was managed but it's surprising nonetheless. Sadly, Dr Kim had to send the patient away to another colleague for the restoration.

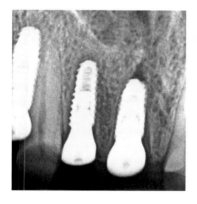
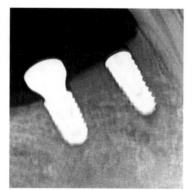
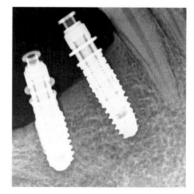

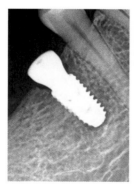
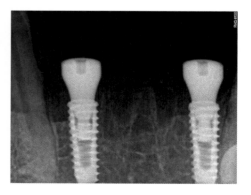

📷 **1.19** Implants placed by Dr Ji-Hyung Kim during the live surgery course. Excellent placement for a novice implantologist

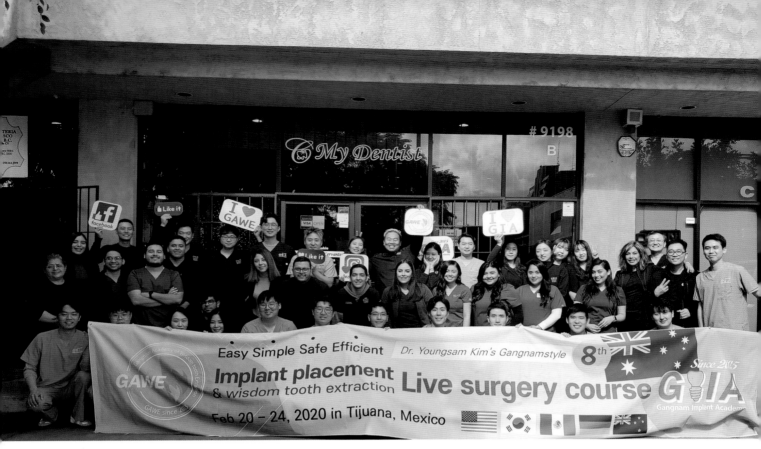

📷 **1.20** A photo from live surgery course immediately before the pandemic in February 2020. The course was planned to resume on Aug 2021. Whilst this book is being finished (May 2021), it has taken just 2 weeks for the August live surgery course to be overbooked with 16 people. Live surgery course always excites me and I look forward to it every single time.

If you're at an early stage of your implantology journey, you might be thinking 'How could Dr Ji-Hyung Kim place all of the implants so well?'. I would say part of it is his talent and part of it is through the help of our excellent teaching faculty. However, above all else, he followed the important principles that I stress upon every live surgery attendees.

Aside from South Korea, most of my live surgery seminars are held in Mexico. Big part of the seminar attendees are dentists from the US, Canada and Australia. Since the pandemic has put a halt on all our operations, I reminisce the past by looking at the photos. Luckily I was able to find 2 photos where the attendees and the faculty members are checking the path of implant insertion together.

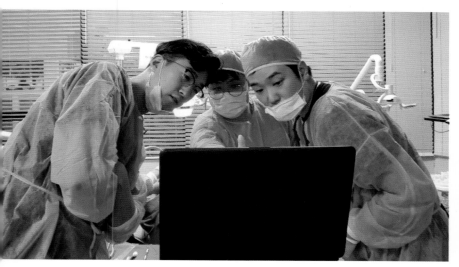

📷 **1.21** Seminar attendees and faculty member checking for implant pathway. From right to left, Dr Chanook David Ahn (U.S.A, Periodontist), Dr Ji-Hyung Kim (Australia) and Dr Young Hoon Pyun (Oral Surgeon, Co-Author of this book and my co-worker in Gangnam Leon Dental)

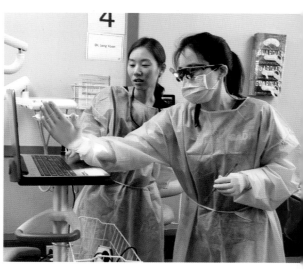

📷 **1.22** Checking the pathway with her hand is the live surgery attendee Dr Jinju Lee from Boston, USA and next to her is Dr Yu-Jeong Jang from Seattle, USA.

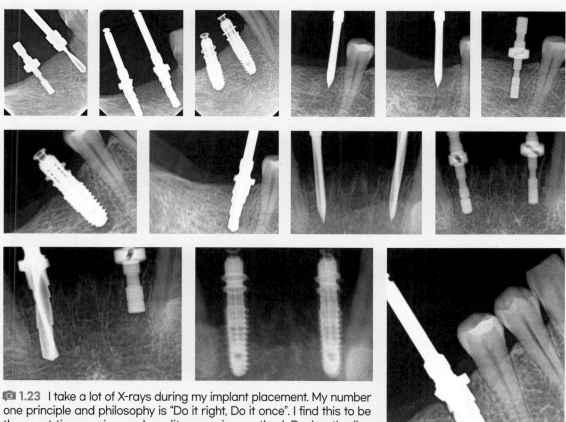

📷 **1.23** I take a lot of X-rays during my implant placement. My number one principle and philosophy is "Do it right, Do it once". I find this to be the most time saving and quality assuring method. During the live surgery seminars, I remove the implant no matter how good it is, if there is no X-ray to show the work. I tell the attendees "If you're that good, don't learn from me" and run these seminars with strict *"Under my roof, my rules. My way or high way"* policy. I am very grateful for the students who follow my ways and they motivate me to do better.

I had a number of associate dentists who worked for me and almost everyone would start off by pickaxing their implant placement. It was as though they didn't know that it was wrong to do so. Perhaps no one had set the standards for them. I personally exo-plant the implant if it isn't to my liking, regardless of who had placed it. As I mentioned earlier, best way to prevent pickaxing is to have an eye for an ideally placed implant. This will change your thinking process and therefore how you do your surgery.

Leon Dental Pickaxe case 1

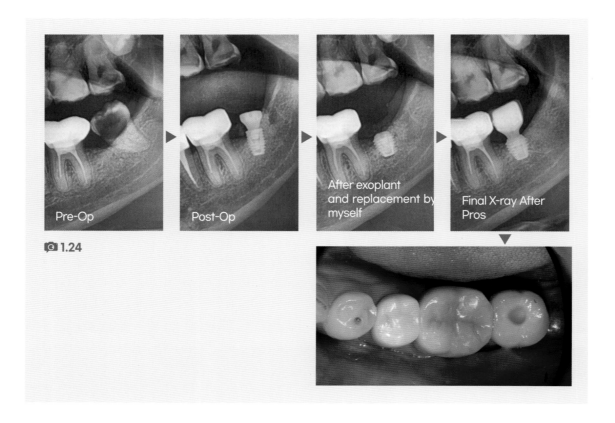

Pre-Op

Post-Op

After exoplant and replacement by myself

Final X-ray After Pros

📷 1.24

Case in 📷 **1.24** was booked in for a dressing appointment with myself as the associate dentist who had placed the implant was on his day off. I had to ask for the patient's permission to remove the implant and immediately replace it. Later my staff had informed me that it was a difficult surgery for the dentist and the patient. It was challenging for myself as well. It is difficult to change the pathway of the implant when the previous osteotomy is not ideal. It is a lot harder than operating on a virgin bone. Previously, I mentioned that **you should consider reducing the length by a size and increasing the** diameter by a size if there is lack of primary stability. I have removed 5×7 mm implant and placed a 6 x6. Although the final X-ray may make the #37 crown seem small, in actual fact the 36 crown was very much over-sized. Note the significant reduction of #36 crown distal surface on the post-operative X-ray compared to the pre-operative one.

Leon Dental Pickaxe case 2

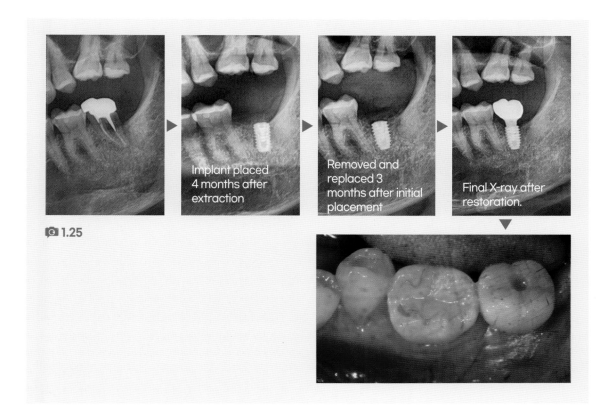

📷 1.25

Implant placed 4 months after extraction

Removed and replaced 3 months after initial placement

Final X-ray after restoration.

📷 **1.25** This patient visited the practice just before the second stage surgery with complaints of discomfort from another region. I've seen the patient as an emergency appointment because the associate dentist who had placed the implant was on leave that day. I've asked where the patient had the implant done only to be stunned by the answer. The X-ray suggested that it was pushed distally into the extraction socket space as the fixture was being inserted. I've convinced the patient for the same day exoplant and immediate replacement surgery. The primary stability was far too inadequate for the healing abutment to be placed. You can also see that the implant was pushed slightly towards where it was originally placed, regardless of how sound my osteotomy was.

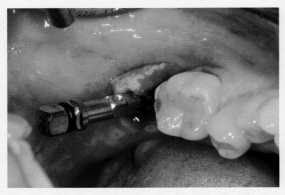

If the occlusion and the location of the adjacent dentition are within normal range, you must always aim to place the implant on the line ex-tending from the central groove of the adjacent teeth.

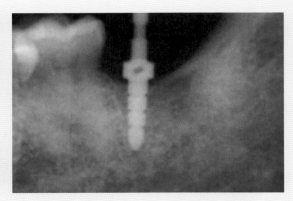

Although the pilot drilling was very challenging due to the socket from the original implant, I still tried to take pathway X-rays on every step. This PA X-ray was taken to check for M-D distance and direction

📷 1.26 What I consider to be an ideal position and how it should apppear on X-rays
I always imagine the crown of the 7 behind the 6 and try to start the osteotomy in the center of occlusion on the imaginary crown.

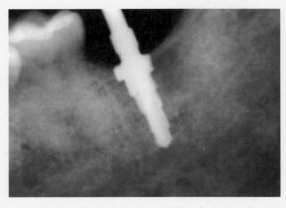

After performing osteotomy with a bur that imme-diately precedes the final bur, I always take an X-ray with the bur in the socket. This is my final confir-mation of location, direction and depth.

I always emphasise the importance of the position, angulation and depth. It's what this chapter is about. 📷 1.26 is how I normally determine the P, A, D. Always place the implant on the extension of the central groove of the tooth immediately mesial to the surgery site and try to place the implant in the center of the imaginary crown. Obtain radiographic confirmation of the P, A, D every step of the procedure.

Leon Dental Pickaxe case 3

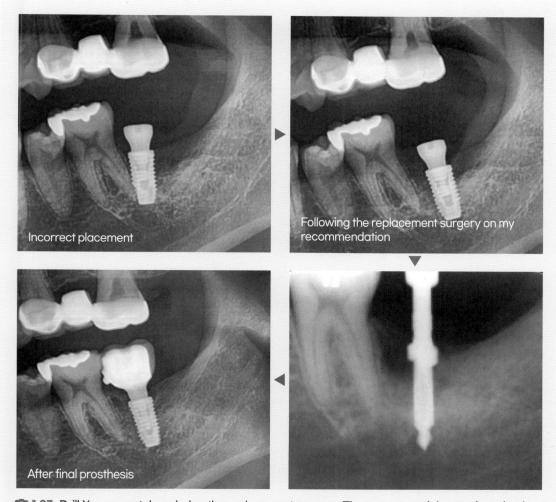

Incorrect placement

Following the replacement surgery on my recommendation

After final prosthesis

📷 **1.27** Drill X-ray was taken during the replacement surgery. They are essential part of any implant surgery in my opinion.

I spotted this case immediately after the initial surgery. The operator happened to be right next to me when I saw the X-ray, so I asked, "Do you want to remove this? or should I?". To which he replied, "I know it looks like the implant has damaged the distal root of the 6, but it actually didn't and the patient is asymptomatic". So I asked him again, "Do you want to? or should I?" and he finally said "I will." I told him that he will be in a lot of trouble if I don't see his work with the X-rays taken in between different drills and only then he took each and every step properly. The final X-ray following the crown insert looks very good (📷 **1.27**). Yes he planted a slightly longer implant but that's forgivable. Pickaxing on the other hand, isn't.

Why did he do a pickaxe in the initial surgery when he was capable of doing what he did on replacement? I think it's because the bar wasn't set high enough. Again, an implantologist must first have an eye for the ideally placed implants.

Leon Dental Pickaxe case 4

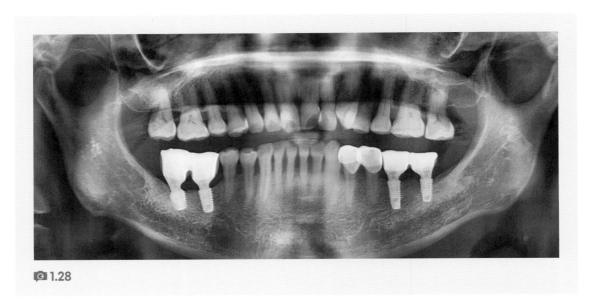

📷 1.28

Quadrant 4 implants gave me heartaches (📷 1.28). The associate dentist who had placed these left the practice a while ago and the patient got referred to me for Q3 implants. Although the sub-par implant placement caught my eyes, thankfully the patient was very satisfied with my work on Q3 and so far had no discomfort from the implants on Q4.

Leon Dental Pickaxe case 5

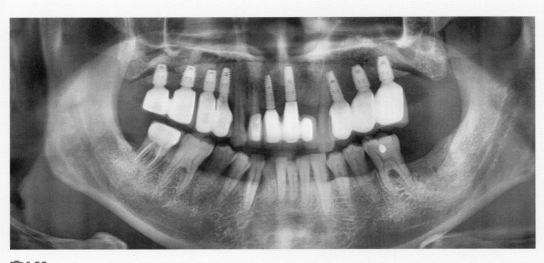

📷 1.29

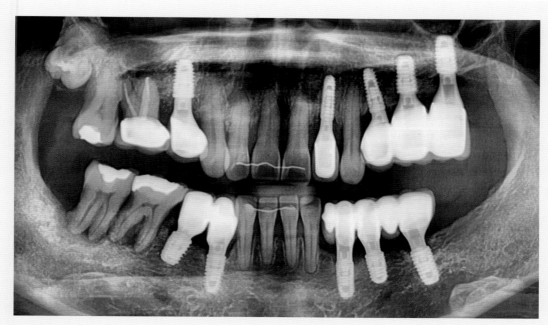

1.30

Was he a mine worker in his previous life? The cases in 📷 **1.29** and 📷 **1.30** were done by the same dentist as 1.28. I've discovered a lot of these pickaxes after he resigned. They were particularly obvious in Q2 implants and this is common amongst novice implantologist. Perhaps this is due to the dentists staying in their usual 9-12'O clock position (relative to the patient) which leads to limited visibility. A lot of the times maxillary 3 and 4 may seem as though they're overlapping. But that's due to the curvature of the arch and often there is space available bucco-palatally. But both of the cases above were blatantly pickaxed.

I've discovered a fair amount of Q2 picaxes in this dentist's cases. Other implants weren't in the best condition either. He was always very confident with his work and I think that may have made me far too complacent with checking his work. I thought the #22 was placed very well. It turned out I had placed it a long time ago.

In recent years, I've been going in and out of Korea a lot for seminars. May be I haven't given enough love to my own practice. My staff members constantly messaged me asking whether an implant should be exoplanted and replaced when associate dentists made mistakes. After meeting the "Surgical Guide Goddess" in the US, I've decided that I can't tolerate the oral surgeons with lots of experience and training to place implants in less than ideal position. So from the end of 2018, I've asked all the associate dentists to place their implants using a surgical guide. Even I started using guides for most cases other than emergency (?) implants. It was more to set the policy of "If I am doing it, you're all doing it". This policy brought a lot of stability and reduced the pressure on me when I was overseas. Currently the staff members have no issues at all with Dr Pyun's work (the co-author of this book and the managing partner of the practice). Therefore the surgical guide policy slowly disappeared unless absolutely necessary. Dr Pyun is an amazing clinician who also studies very hard. I often find myself picking his brain. We study and run seminars together.

Most of the dentists who pickaxed the implants from the cases above had decent oral surgery and exodontia skills. The associate dentist from the 5th case in particular was always very confident and endeavoring. However, his implant placement outcome was unsatisfactory. How could one have decent surgical skills and yet unable to place implant at an ideal position? May be they're incapable, but maybe they've never felt the need to or have never been taught or given serious thought about the importance of ideal placement.

Now let's turn the page and discuss ideal implant placement. Being a good surgeon and being able to place implants at an ideal position are two different things. You need to study it and give it serious thought. Even if you're using the surgical guide, you have to either design it yourself or give approval to the implant company's design. If you don't have an understanding of what is ideal and what isn't, all of that is meaningless. Let's learn how to tell monkeys apart from humans.

4-2
Fixture Position & Angulation

Mastering dental implants

Why we need the SCRP crowns with the access hole in the correct position

I cannot stress the importance of implant position and angulation enough. I guess you could categorize it into good positioning but poor angulatoion and poor positioning but good angulation. But at the end of the day, both position and angulation are equally important and only when both are correct we can say that the implant is placed at an ideal location. Therefore, we need to be able to think in 3D.

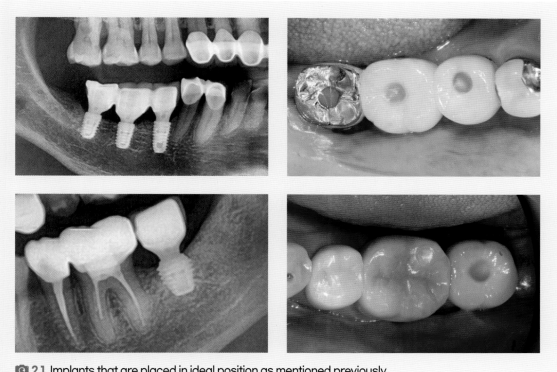

📷 2.1 Implants that are placed in ideal position as mentioned previously

I will briefly go through the theory of what I think is an ideal implant position. What I've learned from practicing at the same location for over 20 years is that, at the end of the day, implant longevity is affected by maintenance. If you've ever removed an existing implant crown before, you will know that removal is harder than placement.

When I first started my journey in implantology, majority of implant crowns were made in gold. They were relatively easy to remove. However, gold price went through the roof and implant prices started dropping and the implant crowns were made out of PFM. More recently, zirconia crowns are very commonly found. Let's say a patient visits your practice with a mobile implant crown and you find out it's a cement retained zirconia crown on a malpositioned implant. You wouldn't know what to do with that. For this reason, I always make my posterior crowns into SCRP crowns. From here on, for the sake of future you, **Just make every posterior implant crowns in SCRP type.**

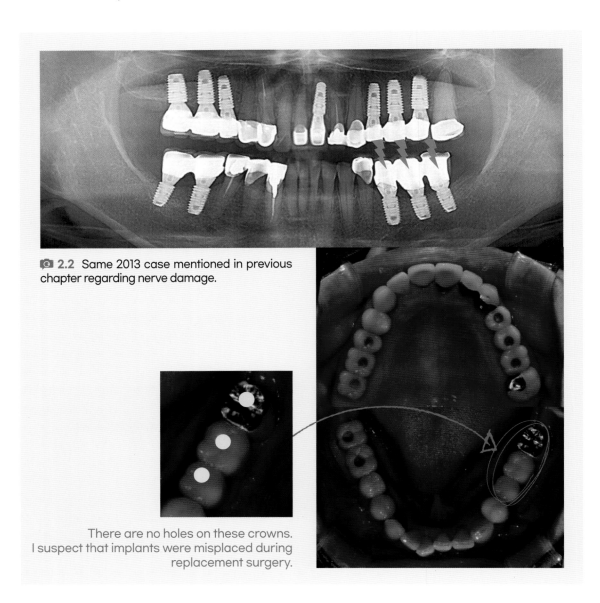

📷 **2.2** Same 2013 case mentioned in previous chapter regarding nerve damage.

There are no holes on these crowns. I suspect that implants were misplaced during replacement surgery.

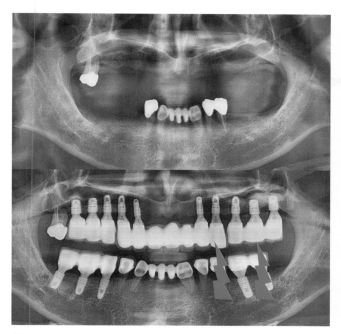

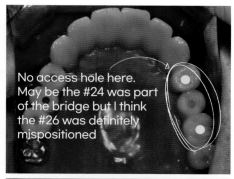

No access hole here. May be the #24 was part of the bridge but I think the #26 was definitely mispositioned

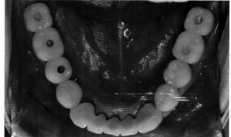

📷 **2.3** A 2015 case

When you place multiple implants in the posterior region or if your implant crowns have to be very long due to severe alveolar resorption, it is extremely difficult to get the access hole position right. Even a minute difference on the alveolar level will completely ruin the access hole position. I recommend using a surgical stent or CAD/CAM guide for cases like these.

Cases from 📷 **2.2** and 📷 **2.3** were done by myself without a guide. You can see I couldn't make access holes for a few of the crowns above. If I was to do it again now, I would probably use a CAD/CAM guide. It helps to position my implants better as well as shortening the surgery duration. Of course I rarely do flapless surgeries. You MUST remember that guided surgery does not equal flapless surgery.

What's really memorable for me is that in 2015 the prosthodontist who restored the implants shared the case with a few of his university colleagues. Their professor asked the prosthodontist whether the implants were placed with a surgical guide. So apparently he replied "No, Dr Youngsam Kim planted these freehand. He's one of the best and quickest among the dentists I've witnessed personally" Now I don't know if this is true or not but it certainly made my day.

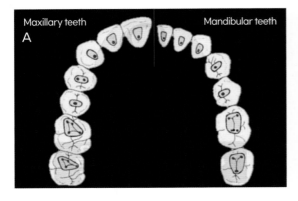

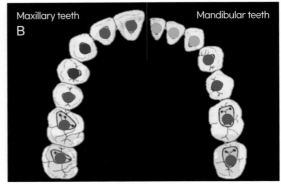

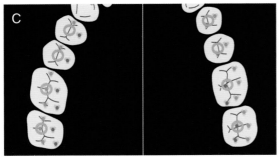

2.4 Implant fixture position (Occlusal access hole position)

A: Access cavity for RCT

B: Occlusal access hole position with reference to RCT access cavity.

C: Occlusal access hole position focused more on the central fossae

So where should we place the SCRP screw access hole? I used to recommend the access hole to be identical to the RCT access cavity to prevent porcelain chipping (📷 **2.4A**). We naturally create an endodontic access cavity to minimise structural damage to preserve tooth integrity. It's also where the roots of the tooth come together and plays a huge part in function.

However, with the advancement of material science over time, we started making the implant crowns out of zirconia. A material that is so hard that we didn't have to worry about fracture anymore. Nowadays, porcelain chipping around the access hole is rarely considered an issue. But if you're used to doing endodontic treatments, you can't go wrong with having the access screw holes where you create endodontic access cavities.

📷 **2.4D** marks points of occlusion, 📷 **2.4E** is location of the screw access. 📷 **2.4F** is the position of screw access hole that I learned when I was studying implantology all those years ago. Back then, we still had a lot of doubts about the implant fixtures and we were taught to place them taking the functionality into account. Longer and thicker the better. However, we now live in an era where SCRP crowns are widely used. If we place the access hole in a region of high occlusal stress, it will lead to excessive wear and/or breakage of covering composite resin. Now that there is no need to question the quality of implant fixtures, it may even be beneficial to place the maxillary implant screw

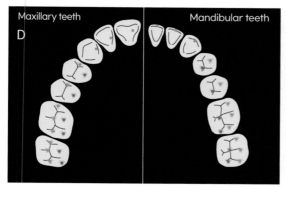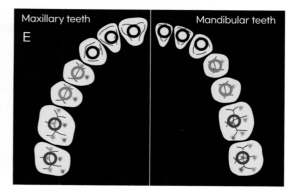

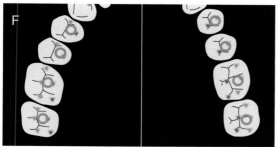

📷 2.4
D: Points of occlusion
E: Access hole position with central fossae as reference
F: Access hole position considering the functionality of the dentition

hole more buccally and mandibular ones more lingually. This will reduce the need for more frequent maintenance appointment caused by wear/fracture and displacement of covering resin. I often tell the following joke to my seminar attendees. "Do your best to position your fixtures in an ideal postion. But if it's tilted a bit towards the functional cusp then say you considered the functionality. If it's tilted a bit towards the non-functional cusp then you tell the patients that you've taken longevity of covering resin into consideration" For me, my screw holes tend to be in the middle if I focus on the arch-form during surgery but if I focus on the opposing dentition, the implants tend to tilt more towards the functional cusp.

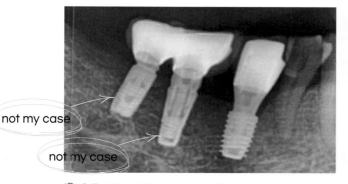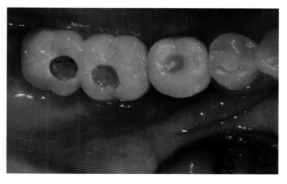

📷 2.5 #46-#47 access cavity are very prone to porcelain chipping and covering resin fracture/wear/displacement.

When we're trying to replace a single dentition, it's relatively simple to position the implant. However, it becomes much more challenging if there is a free end with more than 2 posterior teeth missing. We must consider bucco-lingual angulation as well as the distance between the 2 implants. This is where you can use the opposing dentition as a reference point. So which direction should the center of implant point towards?

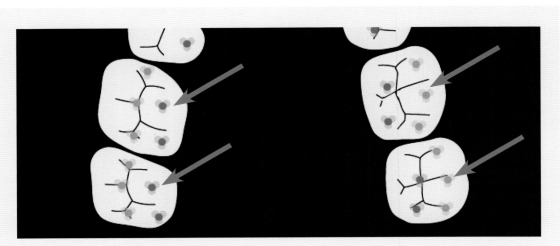

📷 2.6 Blue arrow point towards where the centers of the implants in opposing jaw needs to face towards.
Left: Mandibular (Md) implants to Maxillary (Mx) dentition
Right: Mx implants to Md dentition

As I mentioned earlier, if we set the ideal position of the implants to fall into the center of the crowns, we know that an ideally positioned implants will point towards where the blue arrows are pointing. The implants in mandibular #6 and #7 position will point towards MP cusp of maxillary molars and the implants placed in maxillary #6 and #7 will point towards DB cusps of mandibular molars.

Cases where the opposing dentition were used as a reference

This patient was a mother of a colleague who lives in the USA. There was recurring peri-implantitis due to lack of inter-implant distance and the patient was referred to me by the colleague after the implant crowns were removed.

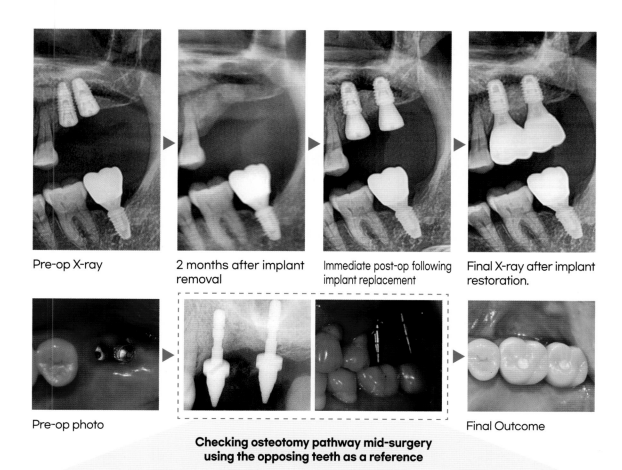

Pre-op X-ray

2 months after implant removal

Immediate post-op following implant replacement

Final X-ray after implant restoration.

Pre-op photo

Final Outcome

Checking osteotomy pathway mid-surgery using the opposing teeth as a reference

In normal occlusion, I measure from the tooth immediately anterior to the implant site whilst staying on the extension of the central groove. If there are more than 2 teeth missing or if the case requires a particularly accurate distancing, I estimate the position, angulation and distance with a guide pin. You can see that the #26 guide pin is pointing towards the #36 DB cusp and the #27 guide pin is pointing towards #37 DB cusp. However, I find myself tilting more towards the center of the opposing dentition when I use this method. I think I subconsciously think about the importance of the functional load bearing. This results in my access holes for the first molar to be positioned more palatally and the second molar to be more mesiopalatally.

📷 **2.7** Using guide pins to estimate fixture position and angulation

You can see that the existing implants were placed too shallow and too buccally. They're also too close together. I made re-entry at 2 months mark after the implants were removed. To make sure I don't make the same mistake as the previous operator, I used the guide pins to check for pathway and sufficient inter-implant distance. Then I used the opposing dentition to decide B-P angulation. In addition, I've performed a sinus elevation using my most commonly used crestal sinus lift procedure which is also my favorite.

This is a very useful approach when the arch is missing from the premolar onwards. But ironically, I noticed the tendency for the implants to point more towards the center of the opposing dentition rather than the functional cusps. Even when I double check with the opposing reference teeth. When

the implant is pointing towards the center of the opposing dentition, the screw hole tends to end up
closer towards the implant crown functional cusp tip. Perhaps I put more weight on the functional load
bearing deep down in my mind.

Ideal implant positioning: It's a trend!

So why does implant position really matter?

When your implant positioning is bad

- ☑ You're embarrassed in front of your staff
- ☑ Taking Impression is difficult and there's bigger room for error
- ☑ You feel bad for your lab technician
- ☑ Your restorative componentaries
- ☑ You have less restorative options
- ☑ Your lab fee will go up
- ☑ It can be less aeshtetic
- ☑ So you're embarrassed in front of your patients
- ☑ Increased foodpacking
- ☑ Occlusal force distribution is less efficient
- ☑ It will lead to frequent abutment and screw loosening and/or fracture
- ☑ Increased risk of peri-implantitis
- ☑ Patient goes to another practice and tells them who had done this. Ruins your reputation and cause embarrassment

I am sure that not everyone would agree with me. There has always been debates about similar issues and the market tends to decide who to follow. 15 years ago majority of the seminars were focused on large GBR surgeries to fit long and thick implants. Just 10 years ago I felt uncomfortable going into a surgery without bone cutting and fixation instruments for block bone graft, such as a trephine bur or a piezoelectric unit. I rarely use any of them these days. Since about 10 years ago, the importance of correct implant positioning over length and thickness of the fixture was highlighted in the field. A lot of companies came up with tools to help operators place implants in the right position. In fact, you can say almost all the companies developed one of these tools (📷 2.8).

Recently, I can see that the supplementary tools (📷 2.8) to help the operators position their implants are losing popularity. I think it's because the CAD/CAM surgical guides began to dominate the market very quickly (📷 2.9).

Flapless surgeries are gaining popularity along with the surgical guides. But as I said, we must not think that guided implant=flapless surgery. As soon as you consider the two to be the same, the implants will move out of its ideal position to look for bone. As you know, I take implant positioning very seriously and I rarely do flapless surgeries. When you're performing implant placement surgeries, your sole focus must be on correct positioning of the fixture. Nothing is more important than that.

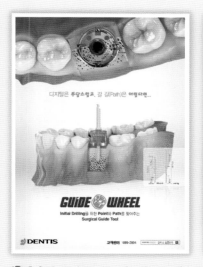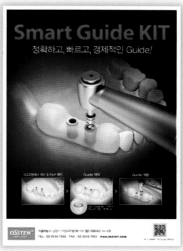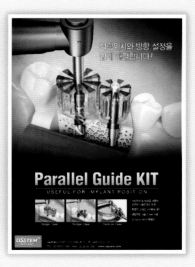

📷 2.8 Supplmentary implant guide tools

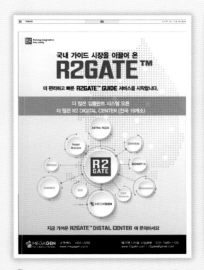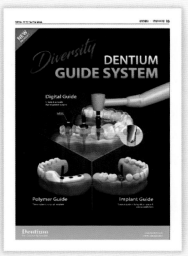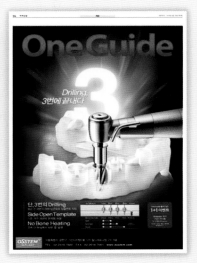

📷 2.9 Advertisement for CAD/CAM surgical guides

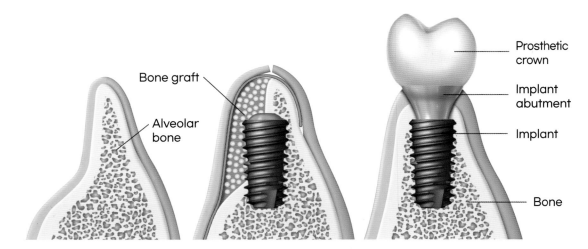

📷 **2.10** Implant fixture placed in an ideal position followed by GBR

What do you do when there is insufficient bone or an inclined plane where you want to place a fixture? As a dentist, you would've given a lot of thought on this matter already and will continue to be your biggest challenge. What I described below is only my way of approaching this issue, not an absolute answer to the problem.

Anyhow, when you find an inclined bone plane, how should we position the implant? Especially for lower molar teeth, unless the extraction was done due to a severe lingual root abscess, most of the time you will fine the buccal bone to be lower than the lingual plate. So do we lean against the lingual bone? Or do we tilt the implant buccally to the fixture is lower towards the buccal plate? I say ignore all of the above and just place the fixture where it should be. you actually need to plan your surgery considering how the implant may get pushed towards the buccal plate where there is less bone (📷 **2.10**).

Clinically, minor cervical exposure of the implants on the buccal surface are quite commonly observed. A lot of researches suggests that it is very rare for such exposures to lead to implant failure and that success rate of implant doesn't show a significant difference. Of course this doesn't mean that this is a desirable clinical outcome. All I am suggesting is that having the implants in the correct position can be better than changing the position of the fixture for the sake of submerging it in the bone.

I've also heard time and time again that implants where most its' threads are exposed, even the ones with the apices sitting outside the bone have decent survival rate. So let me stress this one more time. Don't place implants away from its ideal location just for the sake of submerging them in the bone.

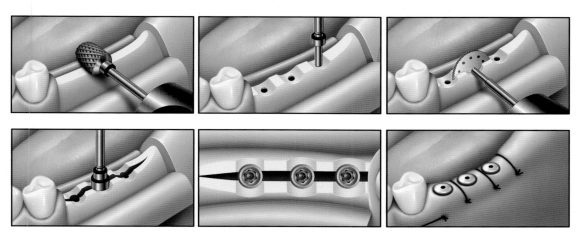

📷 2.11 Illustration of how to use the ridge splitting kit

I no longer perform ridge splitting for one reason; it's difficult to place fixtures in the ideal position. I don't do blockbone graft anymore either. I simply don't think that they're worth the risk of post operative bleeding,pain and swelling. In my opinion, there are other ways of dealing with the lack of bone issue and the above mentioned complex grafting techniques just make ideal implant placement more challenging.

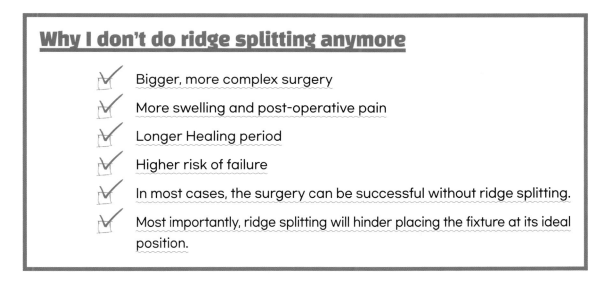

Why I don't do ridge splitting anymore

☑ Bigger, more complex surgery

☑ More swelling and post-operative pain

☑ Longer Healing period

☑ Higher risk of failure

☑ In most cases, the surgery can be successful without ridge splitting.

☑ Most importantly, ridge splitting will hinder placing the fixture at its ideal position.

How do we place implants in a lingually inclined bone caused by buccal plate resortpion?

This is a big question for us dentitsts. Everyone might have different approach to the question but I prefer to place mine as shown in 📷 2.12A. Place where the implants should be and perform GBR as required. Of course the GBR technique must vary depending on the size of exposure and the anatomy of the region. However, if the GBR needs to be large enough that you're considering a ridge split or a blockbone techniuqe, I recommend using a titanium mesh which can be connected to the fixture itself.

A

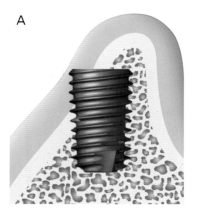

Fixture placed in its ideal position

📷 2.12

B

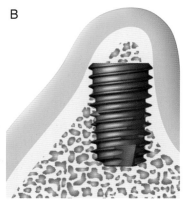

Implant placed lingually to avoid exposure of the buccal threads

C

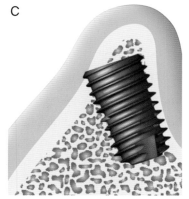

Implant tilted buccally to avoid exposure of the threads

The titanium mesh you see in 📷 2.13 below is the one I highly recommend. Traditionally the titanium meshes or ti-reinforced non resorbable membranes were fixed using bone tack screws. It's a bigger and more technique sensitive procedure in itself and carries a higher risk of failure. However, the meshes that connects directly to the implants as shown below are a lot easier to use and therefore carries

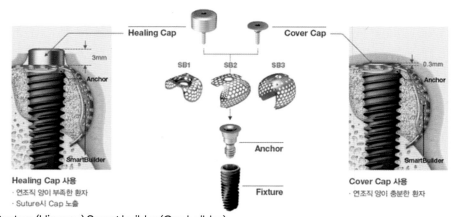

Healing Cap 사용
· 연조직 양이 부족한 환자
· Suture시 Cap 노출

Cover Cap 사용
· 연조직 양이 충분한 환자

📷 2.13 Osstem (Hiossen) Smart builder (Oss builder)

less risk of failure. This can be a very useful tool to keep in your inventory if you're just starting out.

A case where the Ti-Mesh was used

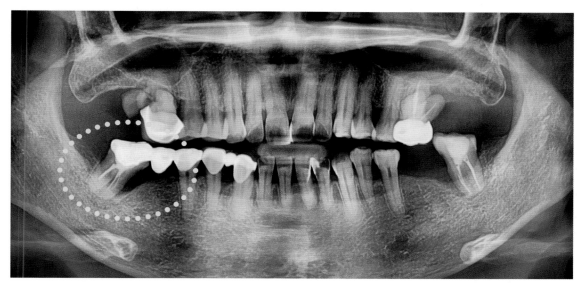

📷 2.14 Pre-operative OPG

Again, a colleague's mother who visited our practice for periodontal management. (A lot of dentists comes to me for their implants or wisdom teeth removal. Some send their parents or in-laws to my practice. Personally I find the recognition from my colleagues to be more rewarding than anything and I do my best treating them) Let's take a look at Q4. Most people would think that I've used the TI-Mesh on #47 position. Truth is, the #47 location had plenty of bone width and I just used a standard resolvable collagen membrane. The #46 position is where I actually used the TI-Mesh. It has been a long time since the #46 was lost and therefore I was left with a very narrow ridge. So I placed the#46 fixture at the ideal position and performed GBR using the Ti-Mesh shown in 📷 2.13

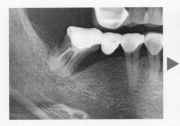 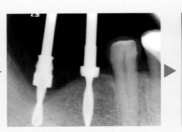

6 months after extraction

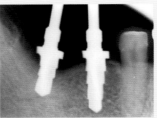

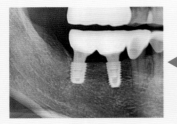

14 months after final restoration. 20 months after fixture placement

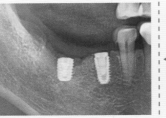

3 months after first stage sugery. Before and after the second stage surgery

You can see the Ti-mesh on the X-ray

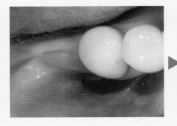

Note the lack of buccal bone where the pontic used to be.

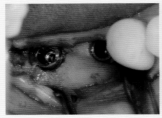 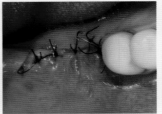

#47 horizontal and vertical thread exposure, #46 horizontal buccal thread expsorue. GBR with Ti-Mesh and sutured.

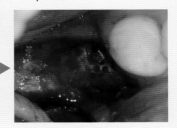

3 months after fixture placement. Re-entry to remove the ti-mesh

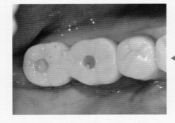 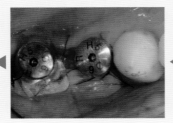

Louis Button (Dentis) was used to help with the formation of vestiuble and to preserve attached gingiva.

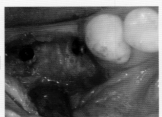

You can see that the graft material had ossified successfully

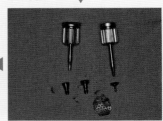

Removed screw and the ti-mesh

On the CBCT

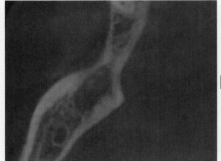

Pre-op Mandibular horizontal section

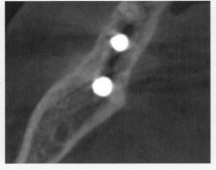

Horizontal section 6 months after restoration

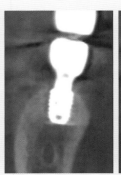 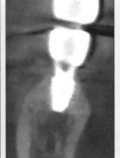

Coronal section showing plenty of bone surrounding the implants

📷 **2.15 Osstem (Hiossen) Ossbuilder case**

38 y.o female patient. She had the #12 implant placed 10 years ago. On the X-ray it's hard to fault the placement. Good depth and stable bone level even though it was an external hex type fixture.

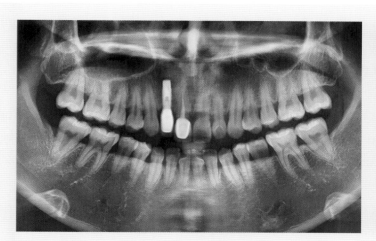

The fixture seems to have been placed at a decent position

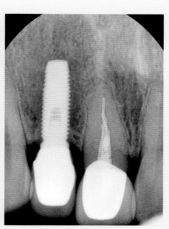

PA X-ray of the implant

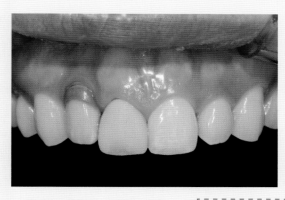

Frontal view, 10 years after placement.

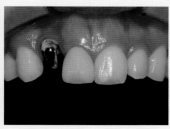

Patient visited the practice as she lost the implant crown

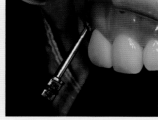

Placed the screw driver to re-tighten the abutment screw. It shows just how buccally tilted this implant was.

📷 **2.16 An anterior fixture placement direction failure case**

However, when you look at the clinical presentation, you can see just how wrong this was. How could one do this to a female patient in her early 20s? Yes the implant placement protocol was less defined back then, but if you saw your implant tilting this far buccally, you should've removed it and replaced it instead of dealing with it using pink porcelain (I guess it's easy for me to say this in hindsight). The patient told me that she lost confidence in her smile since then. Maybe the tooth was better off replaced with a bridge. The issue here wasn't just the aesthetics. When an implant is tilted this far buccally, it increases the frequency of crown displacement and/or screw loosening. I have had to retighten and recement the implant crown for this patient.

In my experience, the direction of the implant in the anterior region may vary depending on the position of the fixture, thickness and shape of the soft tissue etc. Even if your implant isn't necessarily pointing towards the singulum, at the very least the access hole shouldn't fall beyond the incisal line.

I would like to briefly touch on cases where you try your very best to place the fixture in the ideal position and the direction changes as the fixture is placed (Refer to the case from **Chapter 3-2**). This can happen in a few different scenarios; immediate implant cases, when you're lacking a boney wall and when you have soft buccal wall and hard palatal (lingual) wall.

"The fixture is thicker than the drill". It's a statement I always stress onto the live surgery course attendees. I think it's also the most overlooked statement during implant surgery. The modern implant fixture threads comes in variety of shapes and also in general, a lot larger. Thread size averages 0.3-0.5 mm and the fixture can be up to 0.6-1.0 mm larger than the equivalent drill. So if the bone hardness is relatively uniform around your osteotomy site as shown in 📷 **2.17A**, the fixture will go in as you've drilled. However, if you're missing a wall or if the bone quality is poorer on one side, you may notice the implant to bend and move towards that side after placement. You can imagine that 1 mm displacement at the fixture level will become 2-3 mm difference at the occlusal plane level.

📷 **2.17C** shows exact same issue as 📷 **2.17B**. When we're replacing a single rooted dentition, we need to place the implant along the lingual wall. You will notice that in most cases the implant will want to move buccally. To solve this issue, you need to make sure that the palatal wall has same density and strength as the buccal wall. Or you just drill along the palatal/lingual wall with the bur identical to the implant diameter and just obtain primary stability from the apex (Refer to the Ankylose technique mentioned previously).

A

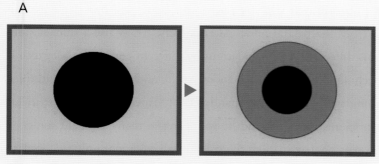

The fixture will follow the osteotomy pathway without any deviation when there is uniform bone density around the osteotomy site.

B

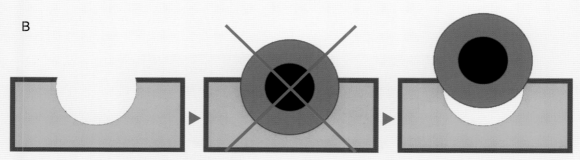

If there is an open plane after osteotomy, the implant will deviate towards it. This is very common in maxillary anteriors and lower posteriors where there is severe buccal bone resorption.

C

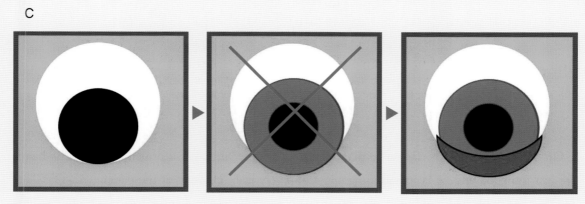

I've drawn the diagram above for immediate implants. If you prep your ostetotomy where the black circle is on the far left the fixture will never remain in that position. It will be pushed towards the socket. To avoid this, you need to drill with the bur diameter equivalent to the fixture diameter as shown in the far left marked with red. I call this the ankylose technique. You can apply this technique in every implant case and not just maxillary anterior immediate implants. Always remember that best place to obtain your primary stability is the apex where the bone density is the lowest.

📷 2.17

I usually finish my osteotomy with a drill that is 2 size shorter in length and one size bigger in diameter to help reduce resistance from the palatal bone. Alternatively, I may use a thicker side-cutting bur also. You will come across different recommendations by different companes. Megagen is pushing for the "Root Membrane technique" (Also known as Socket Shield) and they recommend thick diamond bur. Some recommend using straight low-speed handpiece. I visited a periodontist in LA once to observe his upper anterior implant placement and he was using so many different tools (2.18). It was amazing to witness him passionately shaping the palatal wall using not only the implant motor but 2 high speed handpieces AND a piezo unit. He was basically shaping the palatal wall into that of the fixture itself. I felt like I've learned a lot about how to place the upper anterior implants well.

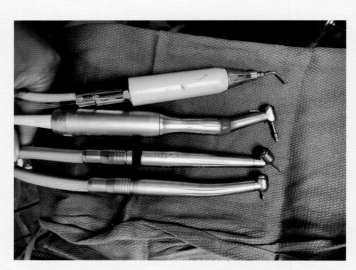

2.18 Upper anterior palatal wall shaping tools used by the LA periodontist. (I may add that he's quite handsome as well)

On the other hand, the fastest implant surgeon I've met in LA is a prosthodontist. His hands are just too good and he keeps his armamentarium very lean. He stays at the patient's 12 O' Clock position and applies a lot of bodily pressure from above to make sure that the fixture is leaning against the palatal wall. I think he strives for better primary stability because he predominantly uses Hiossen (Osstem) implants with sharp threads and also because his inner prosthodontist deeply cares about his temporary crowns.

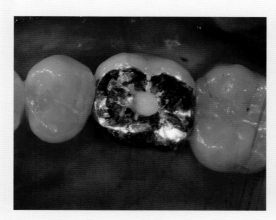 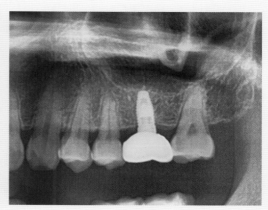

📷 **2.19** Fixture in correct position.

Patient visited our practice with complaints of mobile implant crown (📷 **2.19**). I've asked him to go back to the practice where the implant was placed but the patient had refused. He said he had spent a significant amount of money on the dentist's account as he/she said that this was "the best implant in the world", but the crown kept coming off and he was sick and tired of dealing with it.

If we only look at the positioning of the fixture, it is pretty well placed in the middle (may be ever so slightly pickaxed). The issue actually lied in the depth of the implant. The fixture turned out to be Nobel Biocare Replace Trilobe. It's an internal fit type fixture (*not internal friction) but the implant was not placed deep enough that the crown was exposed to huge cantilevered stress. If only the fixture was a little bit further in, this whole situation may have been avoided. Moreover, all the non-friction type implants are exposed to higher risk of vertical fracture (or tearing). In this case I am a little worried about the fixture fracture which may happen from the 1-2 mm thats sitting above the alveolar crest. In the next sub-chapter, we will discuss more about the depth of the fixture.

4-3
The Depth

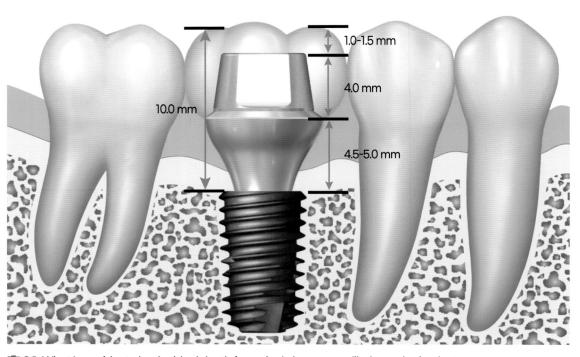

Ideal Lower Molar Implant Depth

1.0-1.5 mm

4.0 mm

10.0 mm

4.5-5.0 mm

📷 **3.1** What I consider to be the ideal depth for a single lower mandibular molar implant

This sub-chapter may be summarized into the following sentence: "Minimum requirement for what I consider to be the ideal depth for a single lower mandibular molar implant." On average, the thickness of abutment gingiva from crest of the bone to the proximal contact point is 4.5-5 mm. If there is a significant height difference between the buccal and the proximal bone, then the abutment gingiva might be a bit thinner on the buccal side (3-4 mm). I am talking about bare minimum here.

You need at least 4 mm of abutment height for crown retention but try to stay under the 6 mm mark. This you can shorten if you're making a bridge and the fixture can't go any deeper.

I gave 1.0-1.5 mm of occlusal thickness. To be honest my main focus is surgery and I've never had to give too much consideration about this. However, majority of technicians told me that 1.5 mm is the thickness they're most comfortable with. The occlusal thickenss can be easily managed in the crown fabrication stage at the laboratory. So unless the implant was placed very shallow, you don't have to worry about this too much.

For bone level fixtures, ideal depth needs to account for early marginal bone loss and passive fitting of the abutment. This is usually around 1 mm below the bone level. Even when you're performing GBR, you want the top of the implant to be approximately 1 mm below the graft material.

Submerge the implant a little deeper in following situations; there is less than 10 mm crown height, thin gingival biotype and/or when you need to match the depth of adjacent implants. Even when there is a plenty of prosthetic space from the opposing dentition, when the gingival biotype is thin, I tend to over graft when doing GBR. I build the graft 2-3 mm above the implant so that I can get sufficient gingival height.

Why they suggested 0.5 mm subcrestal implants in the past

When I was first learning about implants, there weren't any considerations about distance from opposing teeth or gingival height. You just open up a flap, osteotomy and place fixture 0.5-1 mm below the bone level. The reason is even funnier. They used to teach that bone just dies when it has even a whiff of air. Science behind implantology has come a long way since then. A lot of studies have proved that the bone doesn't die with the whiff of air. Now we consider the distance from the opposing dentition and the gingival height before anything else when deciding how deep the fixture should be. If we do go far subcrestal for some reason then it's usually to prevent bone-loss from pathological conditions such as peri-implantitis and to stabilise the implant.

Reason behind 4 mm abutment preparation (core) height

In page 193 of the <Contemporary Fixed Prosthodontics> written by The Journal Of Prosthetic Dentistry Chief Editor Stephen F. Resentiel, a single crown is best retained with at least 3 mm core height and less than or equal to 10° of preparation taper. Molars require longer core height as they're wider teeth.

When I was first learning implant we were taught to always make a cast-metal crown when there was less than 5 mm space from the opposing dentition. You would need 1 mm of crown thickness which would've meant that the core height (abutment preparation height) was not tall enough to provide retention for a cement retained crown. However, this isn't how I do it anymore. If there is less than 5 mm crown space from the opposing dentition, remove the implant and place a shorter implant deeper. I wanted to get this point across in this chapter.

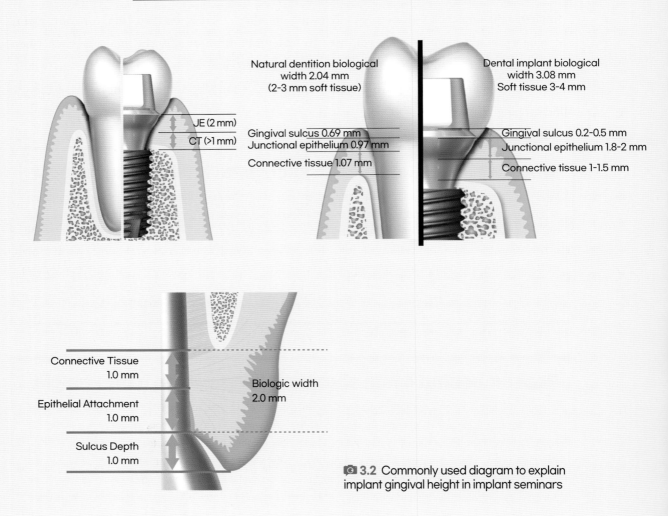

Tooth		Implant
Periodontal ligament	**Connection**	Osseointegration
Periodontal mechanoreceptor	**Proprioception**	Osseoperception
25–100	**Axial mobility**	3–5
Shock absorbing	**Load bearing**	Stress concentration at crestal bone

Natural dentition biological
width 2.04 mm
(2-3 mm soft tissue)

JE (2 mm)
CT (>1 mm)

Gingival sulcus 0.69 mm
Junctional epithelium 0.97 mm

Connective tissue 1.07 mm

Dental implant biological
width 3.08 mm
Soft tissue 3-4 mm

Gingival sulcus 0.2-0.5 mm
Junctional epithelium 1.8-2 mm

Connective tissue 1-1.5 mm

Connective Tissue
1.0 mm

Epithelial Attachment
1.0 mm

Sulcus Depth
1.0 mm

Biologic width
2.0 mm

📷 3.2 Commonly used diagram to explain implant gingival height in implant seminars

You must've seen the diagrams used in 📷 3.2 before. Either in Seminars or online. Yes the implant is different to natrual dentition. However, I don't think this illustration encompasses all the variations that are results of different implant systems, protocols and operators. It's too summarised to analyse the more dated studies.

📇 3.1 Studies regarding the biologic width around natural teeth or dental implants

	Natural teeth		Dental Implants		
			Non-submerged	Submerged	
	1961 Gargiulo et al. 57 30 human skulls	*1994* Vacek et al. 58 10 human skulls	*1997* Cochran et al.53	*1991* Berglundh et al.71	*1996* Abrahamsson et al.71
Sulcus depth (SD)	0.69 mm	1.34 mm	0.16 mm	2.14 mm	2.14 mm
Junctional epithelium (JE)	0.97 mm	1.14 mm	1.88 mm		
Connective tissue attachment (CT)	1.07 mm	0.77 mm	1.05 mm	1.66 mm	1.28 mm
Biologic width	2.04 mm (JE + CT)	1.91 mm (JE + CT)	3.08 mm (SD + JE + CT)	3.80 mm (SD + JE + CT)	3.42 mm (SD + JE + CT)

Reference: Dr. Mohammed A. Alshehri. The maintenance of crestal bone around dental implants. 2011.

Let's take a look at the more recent literature review (📇 3.1). The table compares a few different data on biological width. This literature review was done somewhat recently (2011) but the cited data were all from a long time ago. So we can't trust everything on there regarding implants. I agree that the biological width is roughly 1-2 mm wider than the natural teeth but a lot has changed since the data were collected in the 90s. Implant body shape, abutment shape, surface treatment to name a few. In addition, our understanding of implant length and width, as well as crown and crown margin types have all had significant advancement in that time. You can always refer back to these older studies but why don't we discuss more conventional ideas? The trend lies with bone level internal friction implants and we need to revisit some core principles.

What is Biologic Width?

You must've heard of the term "biological width" over and over again in periodontics or prosthodontics lectures. Basically it's a minimum tissue thickness which protects our body. I often compare it to the DMZ (De-Militerised Zone) in my lectures. There is a total of 4 kms of DMZ between South and North Korea. 2 km each from the border. It's a minimum amount of cushion zone required for the civilians to live safely. I say bone (Civilians) is safe underneath this cushion zone. If another war breaks out and the military demarcation line (MDL) needs to be re-defined then we will still need the cushion zone from the new MDL line. If, for example, the MDL moves 5 km south, we would have 2 km of DMZ and civilians will live at least 7 km from the MDL. In other words, if you're trying to protect the civilians, you need to see how far up the civilians are and form a MDL at least 2 km above where the civilians are. That's how you decide depth of your implant in surgery.

A new definition of biological width was suggested at the 2017 World Periodontology Workshop Co-Hosted by American Academy of Periodontology and European Federation of Periodontology. In summary, the biological width is defined as the thickness of the "Supracrestal Tissue attachment" which consists of the junctional epithelium and the connective tissue that sits above the alveolar crest. I think the reasoning behind this decision was because the term "biological width" wasn't very scientific and the term opened it up to individual differences. There is also the difference in natural teeth and dental implants. However, I think the term "biological width" have stuck quite well with people. No one around me uses "Supracrestal Tissue attachment" yet.

Studies about fixture depth

> ## Minimum abutment height to eliminate bone loss: Influence of implant neck design and platform switching.
>
> The International Journal of Oral and Maxillofacial Implants. 2018.

This study suggests that shorter abutment height leads to greater marginal bone loss. It had also found that the abutment height had a greater influence in the marginal bone loss in the platform switched, internal friction type implants compared to the non-platform switched internal fit type implants.

> ## Prosthetic avutment height is a key factor in peri-implant marginal bone loss.
>
> Journal of Dental Research. 2014.

This study compared the marginal bone loss of the same internal conical connection type implant when the abutments were either longer or shorter than 2 mm. They found that marginal bone loss was significantly greater in the cases with abutments shorter than 2 mm. They also found that the abutment length had a greater influence on the marginal bone loss compared to the presence of graft material, smoking and pre-existing periodontitis.

> ## Influence of abutment height and implant depth position on interproximal peri-implant bone in sites with thin mucosa: A 1-year randomized clinical trial.
>
> Journal of clinical oral implant research. 2017.

This study aimed to assess the influence of abutment height on the interproximal peri-implant bone height. Interproximal bone between implants are where the marginal bone loss is most common and they compared the high abutment group (3 mm) with the low abutment group (1 mm) in an area with thin mucosa. This study conclude that high abutment group showed significantly less inter-implant bone loss. In a 12 months follow up, the high abutment group showed only 0.12±0.33 mm inter-implant bone loss as opposed to the low abutment height group which showed 0.95±0.88 mm of inter-implant bone loss.

Dimensions of the healthy gingiva and peri-implant mucosa.

Clinical oral implants research. 2015.

This study measured biological width/supra crestal tissue attachment thickenss through measuring transmucosal sounding. Transmucosal sounding measures the probing depth at which the bone contact is felt by the patients under local anaesthetics.

Measurements were taken from facial, mesial, palatal and distal. On average, biological width in natural teeth was 3.2±5 mm and in implant it was 4.4±0.8 mm. For implants, average measurements for each aspect are as follows; Facial 3.7 mm, mesial 4.48 mm, Palaltal 4.06 mm and distal 5.08 mm.

As mentioned previously, implant biological width is larger than that of the natural teeth. On average, interproximal BWs were larger than that of buccal or palatal. Therefore, according to this data, an ideal depth of the implant fixture is 4.5-5 mm below the interproximal papilla and (if there is a significant difference between interproximal and buccal wall height) 3.5-4 mm below the buccal gingiva. However, we must learn to take this data with a grain of salt because I have also noticed a lot of loopholes. However, I think this study is meaningful in a sense that they were able to quantify the average gingival height in different surfaces of the implant.

We must not focus on the average

I think failure rate is much more significant than success rate in implant therapy. So we must look at the extremities of the bell curve instead of focusing on the average. I have a habit of multiplying the S.D by 2 when I read any journal articles. For example, from the journal above, average gingival height around implants was 4.4 mm and standard deviation was 0.8 mm. So I double the standard deviation and add it to the average (6.0 mm).

In general, the distribution of the probabilities in a normal distribution curve is as shown in the graph below. (Left) If we then input the data from the study above, you can see that there is 2.3% probability of gingival height being greater than 6.0 mm. Obviously we can never account for all the outliers in our clinical practice but it is not a bad habit to double the standard deviation value before adding or substracting from the mean. Particularly if the standard deviation is quite large.

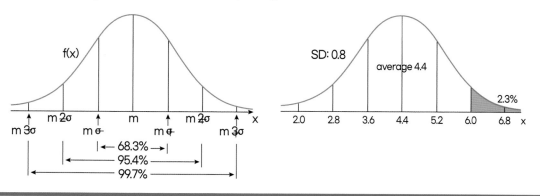

How to avoid cantilever on the abutment

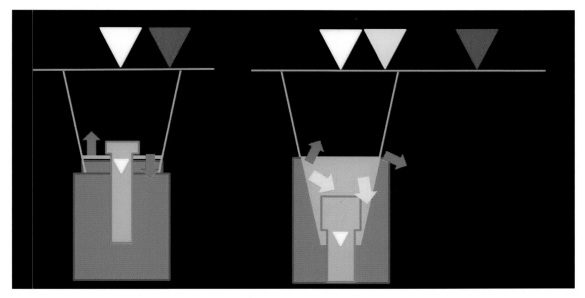

📷 **3.3** Simplified schematics of how I think the masticatory force is transferred into the abutment in an external hex type implant and an internal friction type implant. It's a lot more complicated in real life.

I think cantilvering (when one side of the abutment moves away from the fixture) is just about the worst thing that can happen to an abutment (and implant). For external hexa types, you get cantilevering as soon as the direction of the force moves away from the centre of the screw. If the force is applied from beyond the size of the abutment, you can get huge cantilevering force on the abutment. However, for internal friction types, if the force is within the extension of the internal angle, it can still get dispersed without any cantilevering. The force needs to be applied from much further outside the extension of the internal angle in order for cantilevering to occur. So how can we reduce this? We just place the implants deeper. If the fixture is deeper, even if the force is applied from a point that is fairly far away from the center of the crown, it would still be within the extension of internal angle.

Some may question "what about the crown-root ratio when you place the implant too deep?" But I've already mentioned previously that crown-root ratio works differently in implant supported crown compared to natural teeth. A larger crown-root ratio actually allows for the stress to be distributed more evenly across the body of the implant.

Let's take a look at this diagram (📷 **3.4**) of a mandibular first molar occlusal surface. The main areas where the

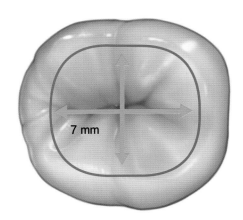

📷 **3.4** The occlusal force applied to the area inside the blue line will be redirected to the fixture as an excursive force.

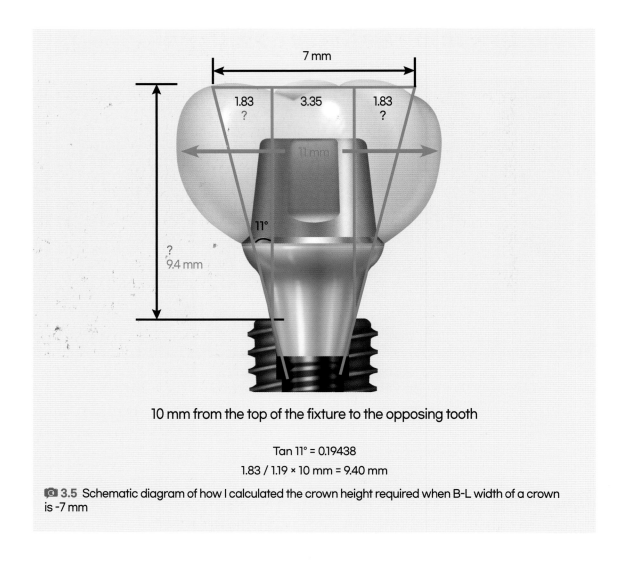

7 mm

1.83
?

3.35

1.83
?

11 mm

11°

?
9.4 mm

10 mm from the top of the fixture to the opposing tooth

Tan 11° = 0.19438
1.83 / 1.19 × 10 mm = 9.40 mm

📷 **3.5** Schematic diagram of how I calculated the crown height required when B-L width of a crown is -7 mm

occlusal forces are applied and directed towards the fixture are more towards the center of the occlusal surface. On average, the diameter of the area was about 7 mm buccolingually according to my measurements. So let's put that into a cross-sectional diagram to calculate the height of the crown required.

Minimum desired crown height turned out to be -9.4 mm. So I concluded that at roughly 10 mm crown height, the cantilevering force on the abutment is greatly reduced. It also increases the Crown-root ratio which helps dissipate the occlusal stress onto the fixtures rather than being so focused on the crestal bone. In other words, deeper fixture means longer crown which is mechanically advantageous.

Case study : Implants that were planted too shallow

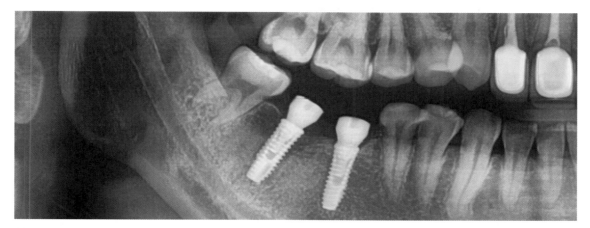

📷 **3.6** Implants placed in one of the "Dumping Dental Practices". Size estimated to be 4.5 x 12-13 mm

Chief complaint of this patient was actually the #48 but I couldn't help but ask where the implants were placed. Turns out they were placed in one of the "dumping dental practices". I mean, I know they advertise for cheaper treatments, but this sort of placement makes even their pricing seem expensive.

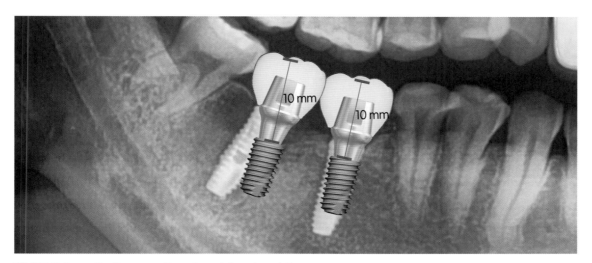

📷 **3.7** Schematic diagram of how I would've placed them

If I was to place implants for this patient, I would've place them with 10 mm crown height in mind (📷 **3.7**). If you were to splint the crowns, you could get away with a shallower placement. However, since this patient is quite young, a deeper placement would've been beneficial in having a better long term prognosis. If the #48 was planned to be extracted, the #47 implant could've been placed a bit more distally. If the #48 was in the way of placement it could've been extracted during the placement surgery. I mean yes I was grateful that the patient was referred to our surgery for the wisdom tooth removal but if the implants were placed where they are already, why extract the #48?

When IAN canal is too close from the occlusal plane

Let's take a look at this #47 case below. We were taught to leave 2 mm above the IAN canal when deciding implant length in the region. This was a consideration for the thickness of the IAN canal. These days CBCT is widely available to most dentists and they all have the habit of taking a CBCT for a peace of mind. I am from the OPG generation and I rarely look at the CBCT scan. I just never felt the need to. The CBCT scans I take these days are to collect images for the seminars.

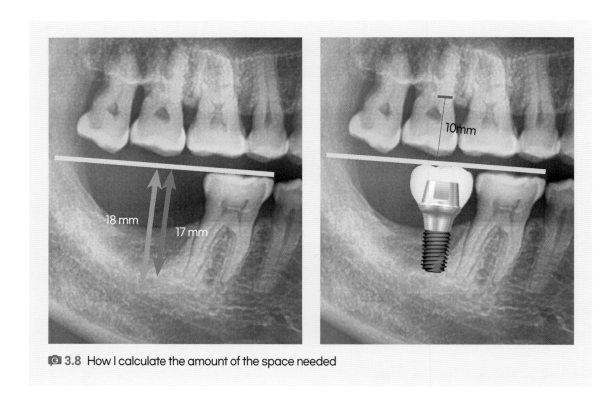

📷 3.8 How I calculate the amount of the space needed

When we look at the OPG image above, the orange line (18 mm) is measured from the occlusal plane to an imaginary point which is 2 mm above the IAN canal. However, I tend to use a slightly longer drill for my osteotomy and the drills themselves are -1.5 mm longer than the fixtures. Therefore, I take another -1.5 mm off from the orange line (Blue). Safety above all else. If you have to decide whether you need to drill down further, you can always take a PA with the bur in the socket.

We rarely get a perfectly flat and even bone surface and not many osteotomies goes exactly according to the plan. Anyway, you can see that the blue line is about 17 mm long, which means we need to place a 7 mm implant so that we can ensure we have 10 mm distance from the occlusal plane to the top of the fixture.

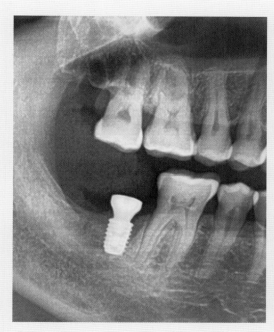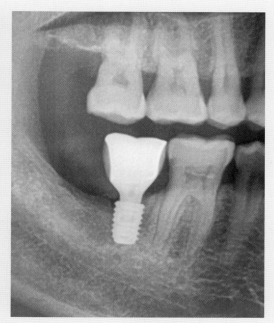

📷 **3.9** OPG taken after placement and following final prosthesis

You can see how the case actually turned out in 📷 **3.9**. Because I do lots of third molar extractions, I come across just as many lower 7s implant. Some of the cases I've witnessed that were done in other practices were too focused on the bone height and the implant length that they ended up with insufficient prosthetic space. Don't forget that the distance from the occlusal plane to the implant is much more important than the length of the implant.

\ Note /

Textbook second molars are about 20 mm long. But when I do endodontic treatments, I find that the Koreans tend to have a slightly shorter roots. Statistically, even the average Korean teeth size is 1-2 mm smaller and since the apical foramen are mostly sitting further superior to the actual apex, we can estimate that Korean average 2nd molar length are closer to 15-16 mm.

Considerations for fixture depth in implant supported bridge

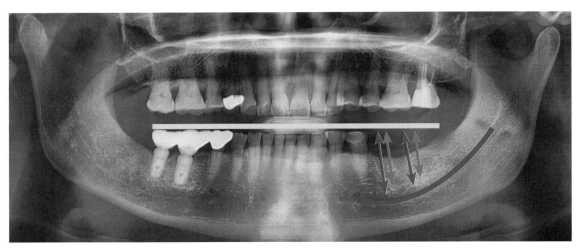

📷 **3.10** Schematic diagram of how to calculate fixture depth in a bridge case

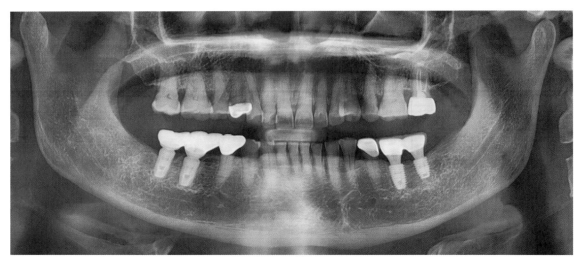

📷 **3.11** After final restoration

I was planning to splint the crowns after placing 2 implants in #36, 37 position. I placed a 8.5 mm length fixture for #36 and 7 mm for #37. After the placement, I've measured how much distance I had from the top of the fixture to the occlusal plane and I had roughly 9 mm for #36 and 8 mm for #37. So in this case, where should we get the other 1-2 mm? I left the "abutment neck" (4 mm) alone and obtained my crown thickness by reducing the height of the "abutment core". I think in this particular case, the core height was 2-4 mm instead of 5 mm.

To be honest, I thought the #37 was placed a little bit too far mesial. So I did consider not sharing this case on the book. But I couldn't resist sharing this case because there is a prime example of what

NOT to do in the 4th quadrant. I think this case is growing on me because I used it in all the lecture series.

Deeper the Better?

We've discussed that shallow implants are disadvantageous for maintaining the biological width and reducing cantilevering force on the abutments.

So, is deeper better? There are studies which suggests that they are. People who support this idea such as myself, are very supportive of the shorter implants. Sometimes the fixtures need to be shorter to ensure sufficient abutment and crown height. Most of the time, I aim for 4 mm gingival height and 5 mm HAs but some short implant enthusiasts aim for 6 mm gingival height and 7 mm HAs. I've seen up to 8, 9 mm HAs in some cases. Their argument is that the deeper placement stabilises the crestal bone level. I am also in agreement with shorter implants placed deeper.

So what issues could you encounter when the implants are placed too deep? Well firstly, if you're doing 2 stage placements, it will be very difficult for you to look for the cover screw. It's also more challenging to achieve passive fitting of HA, impression coping and the abutments. Obviously, deeper the implant is, more obstacles there are. When I place implants I tend to remove all the surrounding structures (hard and soft) that may be of hindrance to the passive fitting of the HA. Deeper the fixture, more hard and soft tissue structures to consider there are. This introduces inaccuracies when we connect the final restorations to the fixture.

You will commonly hear about the importance of "re-tightening" in these deeper implant cases. Personally, I rarely do any re-tightening and yet I rarely get screw loosening. This is because I remove anything that may get in the way during the surgical phase and stress the importance of the "sudden stop" in any abutment screw tightening. Everyone had felt the sensation of the healing abutment gradually tightening. Most of the time people push the soft tissue aside by just tightening a bit more. I just unscrew it entirely and remove anything thats in the way of the abutment. If it's bone, I trim it away, if it's gingiva I either cut it or hold the flap out properly and put the HA back on. It's much easier to do in the surgical phase because it will cause you a massive headache when you encounter this issue in prosthetic phase.

So what do we do? Right from the surgical phase, I use a HA that is either identical or larger than the final abutment size. Then you put the HA on while getting the feel for a passive fit and the "sudden stop". When there's metal to metal contact, there can't be such thing as a gradual tightening. It needs to have a gentle spin followed by an abrupt stop. Radiographical evidence isn't accurate either. Even if it appears to be snug on the X-ray, there may still be microgap in there. Our body runs away from stress by default so any gingiva you applied pressure on will be resorbed away in a few days. This leads to abutment loosening. You don't want to be a slave of re-tightening. Make sure you get it right from the beginning. Yes. Just like me.

Just because this is an important point, let me stress this once again. On principle, I agree that a fixture needs to be placed deep enough. Therefore, I recommend that you clear the pathway of abutment insertion at the surgical stage to allow passive fitting of the healing abutment. Always remember that the HA size needs to be equivalent or larger than that of the final abutment and you as an operator need to feel the "sudden stop" when the HA is fitted.

Case 1. Fixtures that were placed too deep

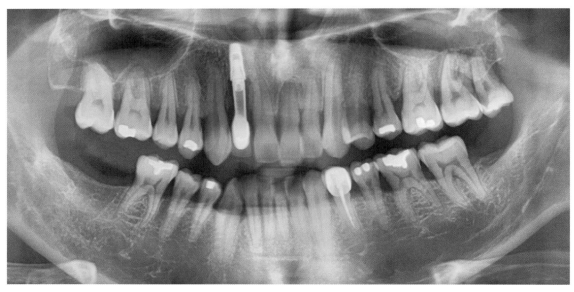

📷 3.12 **Longest abutment I've seen**
This is way too long. In other words, the fixture is way too deep. Surprisingly, aesthetics was decent, I am still wondering how they did the second surgery and the final restoration.

If deeper is better then 📷 **3.12** just about hits the mark. But you can imagine just how challenging servicing this implant will be. I think screw loosening and abutment/screw fracture may be more common due to the length of this abutment. I also question which screw driver they would've needed to tighten the screw. They must've asked for the super-long driver that are only used by the dental technicians.

I used this case in my lecture during 2017 Osstem World Symposium and I had the honor of donating this OPG to my mentor Yongsuk Cho so he could use it in his lecture.

Case 2. Fixtures that were placed too deep

This patient visited our practice for Q4 implants and I was taken by surprise with the length of #17 abutment. I don't know whether to call this implant bone level or sinus level but everybody makes a mistake. Although I think in this case, it would've been better to admit to your mistake, retrieve the implant and re-enter in a few months. When you rush your surgery, you end up forcing your fixture where the bone is. Remember that you shouldn't let that happen. You have to place your implant where you think the bone will form, not where the bone is. I've added how I managed the Q4 implant treatment below for your interest.

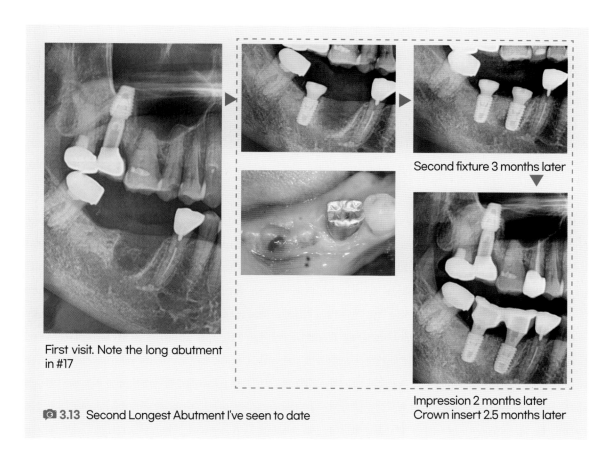

First visit. Note the long abutment in #17

Second fixture 3 months later

Impression 2 months later
Crown insert 2.5 months later

📷 3.13 Second Longest Abutment I've seen to date

It had been quite a while since the extraction of #36 but as you can see in the photo above, shape of the gingiva was unusual. During surgery, I noticed a root fragment underneath. Most roots don't cause any inflammation even when they're left behind but I think this particular fragment had pre-existing infection. Socket was filled with granulated scar tissue instead of bone so I only placed the #47 implant, thoroughly curretted the #46 socket after the root fragment removal and closed it. 3 months later there was no sign of inflammation but still didn't have much bone left in the area. I placed the fixture, grafted without membrane and fitted a healing abutment. As I've mentioned previously, implant will osseointegrate as long as there's no excursive force applied to it. I had to hold this implant in place with hand but still could restore it 2 months later.

Case 3. Fixtures that were placed too deep

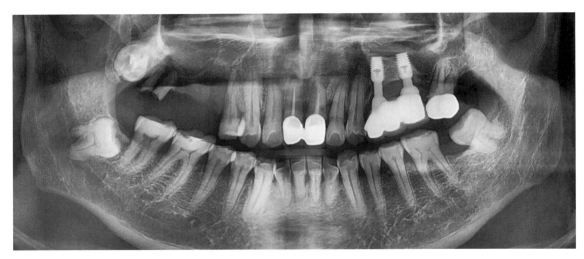

📷 **3.14** Fixtures in 24, 26 region are placed very deep (OPG supplied by Dr JunYong Kim, Allbareun Dental Clinic, Cheongju, South Korea)

Dr Jun Yong Kim is one of my students from the 2nd Korean Live Surgery courses (The fixtures were NOT placed by Dr Kim). All my students are fully aware of the importance of the abutment length and he forwarded this OPG so I could use it in my lecture series. The fixtures looked like Bicon implants (or similar). The Bicon type implants with cold welding can get away with shorter abutments when compared to the internal friction type, so it's a shame how deep these fixtures were placed. They could've been at least 2-3 mm shallower. As I said, if you have doubts about your fixture placement, best time to fix it is during your surgery. I always stress this upon my students who attend the live surgery course and if there is anything wrong with their PAD (position, angulation and depth) I ask them to remove the fixture and try again. This is how training implantology should be. As I always say in the live surgery courses, "Placing implant is the easiest part, you get that wrong it will follow you around forever with failed prosthesis. Don't do that to yourself. Just get used to doing the easy part twice"

Case Study of insufficient HA tightening 1

Passive fit is what I consider to be one of the most important part of my implant teaching and it all begins with using an appropriate HA that gives you a "sudden stop" sensation. I haven't seen anyone emphasizing this as much as I do yet. I've seen cases where the HA isn't fully tightened more times than I can count. Considering how some of the cases where the HA appears to be fully seated on the X-ray isn't actually fully seated, if it's not even fully seated on the X-ray, it means its just not in. If it's not fitted well on the radiographs, you just need to remove the HA, clear all the tissues that stops the HA from fitting and seat the HA again.

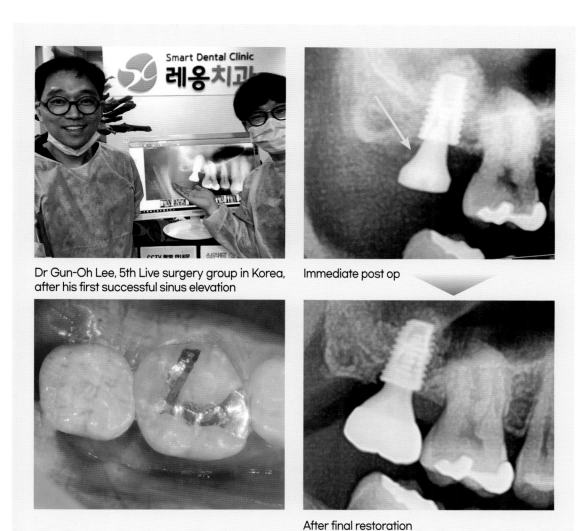

Dr Gun-Oh Lee, 5th Live surgery group in Korea, after his first successful sinus elevation

Immediate post op

After final restoration

📷 **3.15** Photo taken to celebrate my live surgery course student's first successful sinus lift

Regardless of how much I emphasize certain things, some students just don't follow. I always ask whether they've felt the sudden stop. I ask them to get used to the sensation while practicing on the model first. Even then, simulation model and real patients are completely different. You won't be able to learn without doing it yourself.

Dr Gun-Oh Lee from **3.15** is a Kanagawa dental school (Japan) graduate who also passed the Korean licensing exam. The patient was his cousin who is also a medical doctor. After his successful first sinus elevation and celebratory photoshoot, I've noticed that the HA wasn't seated fully. I always tell my students that people don't make mistakes because they're dumber than you. They're all smart and decent operators, but they didn't fully focus to do their best. That's how mistakes happen.

PAD of final prosthesis isn't bad, but I think it could've been submerged 1-2 mm more. When you perform sinus elevations, you need to familiarize yourself with what size and shape of dome you can create with the amount of graft material you used. It will vary depending on the anatomy of the sinus floor and morphology of the elevated sinus membrane. This is hard to describe in words and only way for you to learn is by experience. Dr Lee brought a lot of his friends and families to his live surgery course and left behind trail of fantastic implant cases. If I ever write a sequel of this book, I would like to share a few of his amazing maxillary anterior cases with you.

Dr. YOUNGSAM KIM

I think 2 mm thickness of bone surrounding the fixture is just right in the sinus. In fact, any more than that reduces the quality of the bone formed and is worse off for the implant. So if you're trying to simply stop the sinus membrane from touching the fixture and putting a lid on top of the fixture, (I call this a helmet) I tend to use 0.2 cc (-0.1 g)

If the implant is 3-4 mm into the sinus like the case shown in **3.15**, I would use about 0.5 cc (0.25 g). I would put 2/3 of the graft material in and then take an X-ray with a bur inside the socket first. For this particular case, I've asked Dr Lee to put the entire 0.25 g but I think maybe about half had made it in. The HA wasn't able to be fully seated because when he performed the papillary saving incision, he left too much of 16 distal papilla due to lack of vision. The remaining papilla was resisting the seating of the HA. So we ended up excising the small portion of papilla to achieve passive HA seating.

Graft material used in this case was the Ovis Bone(β-TCP 80% + HA 20%) by Dentis. They sponsor my live surgery course in Korea. I used Ovis bone because it was the only graft material produced by the company at the time, but it's very radio opaque and that makes it an excellent material for sinus elevation training. However, the β-TCP will resorb over time and you may notice the area to be more radiolucent compared to immediate post operative X-ray. New bone will form as the β-TCP gets resorbed. Somtimes the white particles become whiter over time. Time will tell in this case though. Mostly I use xenograft for my sinus elevations (A-Oss from Osstem and Cera Bone from Straumann).

Case Study of insufficient HA tightening 2

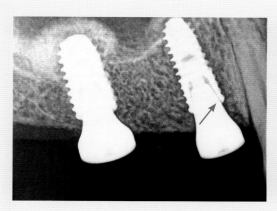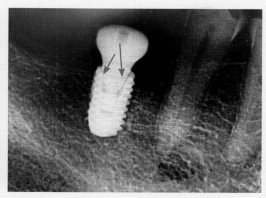

📷 3.16 Cases from my first Mexico Live Surgery course. You can clearly see a gap where the red arrow is pointing.

Incomplete seating of HA is a common observation even in my Mexico Live Surgery courses. Even when I ask my students whether they felt the "sudden stop", they can't really give me a clear answer. If you didn't feel the sudden stop, it means the HA isn't fitted passively. If you force it down when you're only feeling gradual tightening, the force will be used either to push the gingiva away or to damage the fixture. NEVER force the abutment connection.

First you must find out whether it's bone or gingiva thats in your way. Usually throughout the surgery or at the end of the surgery, X-ray will show whether it's the bone. Of course the 2 will give out different feel to you but it will be difficult for an inexperienced clinician to differentiate. If it is the gingiva than you can excise the excessive gum away. The only time you can take a conservative approach is when the lingual keratinized gingiva is on your way. They're weak and it doesn't affect the seating much and they can also be forced away a little bit as well. If its a thick interproximal gingiva, you must get rid of it to achieve a passive fit.

Removing proximal bone for passive seating of bigger healing abutment

If you made the incision properly, most of the time HA will catch the proximal bone (Mesial in most cases). If you're a seasoned surgeon, you would be able to remove that part with just any bur. I just use whatever is available. However, if you're inexperienced, your handpiece grip is unstable and you will find the burs to be bouncy. Losing control can lead to bigger problems such as damaging adjacent gingiva. Few of the companies came up with solutions to deal with this issue.

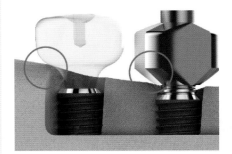
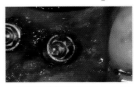
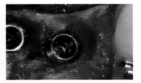

BoneShaper

Easy alveoloarplasty available with proper emergence profile secured when subcrestal implant placement needed

Prevents abutment screw loosening and fracturing

📷 **3.17** Tools to help you shape the bone so you can achieve passive seating of HA (Sold by Medipia Kr)

The bone shaper was first made by an implant company called Acrodent but I think it's sold elsewhere now. As shown in 📷 **3.17**, the the bur is in contact with the implant while the bone around it is being shaped. I thought it might damage or overheat the fixture but the company states otherwise. I've purchased a lot of this and given out to my live surgery course attendees as a gift.

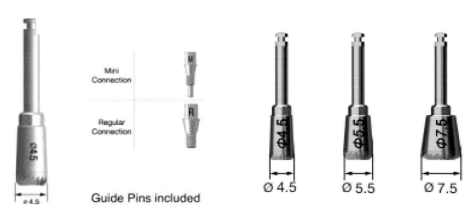

📷 **3.18** Osstem Bone Profiler

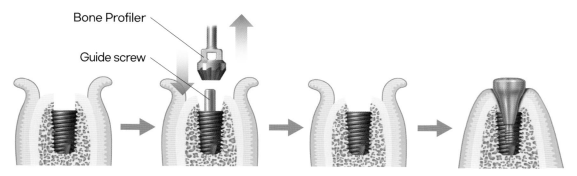

Bone Profiler

Guide screw

📷 **3.19** Osstem Bone Profiler Schematic diagram

📷 **3.18** is Bone Profiler from Osstem. They connect a guide pin with the fixture and remove bone around it to prevent fixture damage. I've heard good reviews about it. Dentis is also selling similar products in a kit and so are a lot of other implant companies. The market seems to be more focused on passive fit of the abutment. Whatever you do, you can't have healing abutment not seating fully.

Dentis Bone Profiler kit

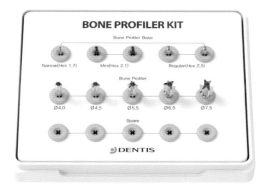

I purchased this Dentis Bone Profiler recently. I haven't had to use it too many times yet but I absolutely love this product. I would recommend it to everyone. It comes in a kit so the staff finds them easier to manage.

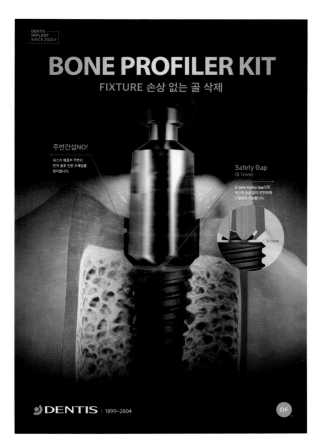

"How do I know if the implant is placed in the right position and depth?" It's a question many people have thought about already. I was one of them and I tried to come up with a tool to help answer this question a long time ago.

📷 3.20 is my invention from 2009 which I named the "YS-Pin". I had to ask a technician to make this for me. I've made molar and premolar YS-Pins to the 90% size of their respective textbook average so I can account for cases where there is less M-D space. I've used them a few times but soon I got tired of them. It was a little side hobby of mine but I think the fixture part could've been a little shorter in hindsight. I've asked around a few different companies but none of them showed enough interest to commercialize this groundbreaking invention. I thought you could just make this out of

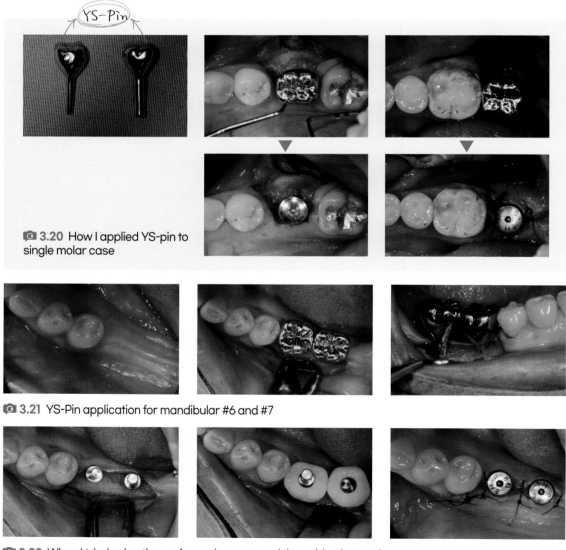

📷 3.20 How I applied YS-pin to single molar case

📷 3.21 YS-Pin application for mandibular #6 and #7

📷 3.22 When I tried using the preformed crowns and the guide pin together autoclavable radioopaque plastic to make it work.

YS-Pin was able to tell you if you had the right position from the top and also if you had the right depth by looking at it from the side. I've made the crown part 8 mm high to account for bridge cases. However, this would've required too many different pins, one for each tooth in the mouth. So I tried using a guide pin and a preformed crown to mimic the same effect but not one company was interested in commercializing this idea either. So in the end I just gave up.

5 mm length healing abutment with sufficient width that I use instead of the YS-Pins

You can't really change the position of your fixture towards the end of the surgery. However, the depth of your fixture is something you decide towards the very end of the surgery. As I've become more aware of the importance of gingival height and the distance from occlusal plane, I've started using 5 mm length HA exclusively.

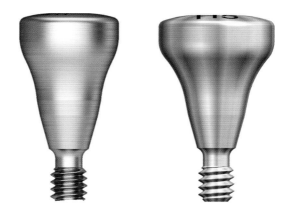

📷 **3.23** I use Osstem HA Ø5.0 x H5 for premolars and Ø6.0x H5 for molars.

A lot of people wonder why my seminars are so popular but I think there can only be one reason. If you do as I say, it works. I wasn't born with some sort of ingenious talent. I work very hard to overcome my challenges. I wasn't born with an eye for beauty and aesthetics but I got given a little bit of OCD. I always take the same road, eat the same food, wear the same clothes. Naturally, I repeat same protocol persistently. That's why I only ever use 5 mm height HAs. 5 mm diameter for premolars and 6 mm for molars. I complete my surgeries in single stage 98% of the time unless I use a membrane and yet I always end up using the 5 mm HAs. Sure it may be a little different for anterior teeth depending on how I plan to temporize them. Osstem came up with this HA a few years ago and it instantly became my favorite due to their C-shaped curvature. Even when I place a fixture from another company, I still use this HA. The C-shaped concavity meant that I would be getting dense gingiva around that area much like the HA from Ankylos company. It also meant that less soft or hard tissue would be able to disturb its passive seating. The HA made my surgeries very convenient.

How do we get the healing abutment depth right?

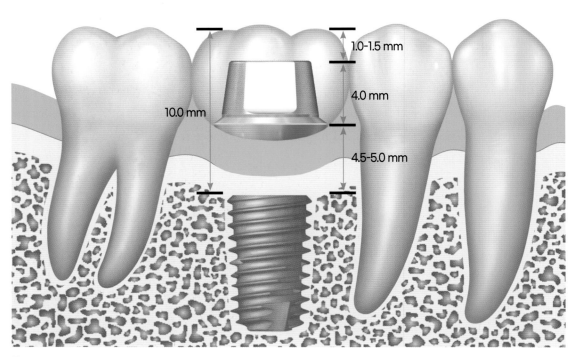

📷 3.24 Ideal implant depth

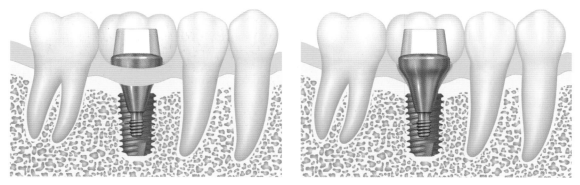

📷 3.25 When you connect a healing abutment that is identical in size and shape as the final abutment. HA shouldn't come up above the gingiva more than what is shown above..

Place your fixture, connect the HA. If the top of the HA is level with the height of the proximal gingiva (papilla) and you can see 1-1.5 mm of the HA above the buccal gingiva for mandible and 1 mm for maxilla, you got the depth right. This is a bare minimum depth. If you can see any more than that, you need to go deeper with your fixture. However, this isn't everything. You must remember that we need 10 mm from occlusal plane to top of the fixture. So make sure you have at least 5 mm space above the 5 mm HA. If you have less than that, even if you have to use a shorter implant, bury your fixture deeper. I use the HA diameter to estimate the amount of crown space available. A dentist I know uses his mirror handle because he says its 5 mm diameter. It's a good habit to come up with your own way of doing things.

I already had a habit of placing my fixtures a bit deeper than some of the other practitioners I've seen. However, after observing my implant patients for a long time, I've decided to place them even deeper. I now place my fixtures about 1 mm deeper than when I first started to ensure long term stability of implants even in challenging cases.

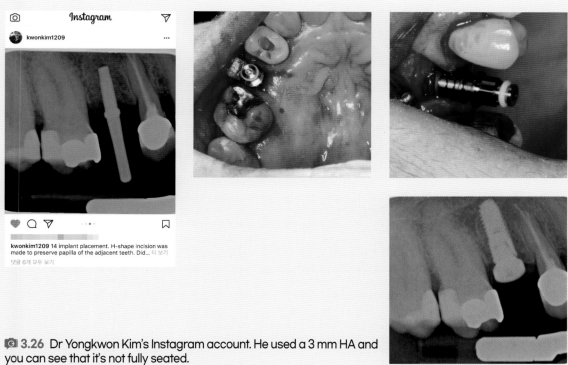

📷 **3.26** Dr Yongkwon Kim's Instagram account. He used a 3 mm HA and you can see that it's not fully seated.

Few years ago, I became friends with Dr Kwon Kim (Toronto, Canada) commenting on one of his Instagram post. Initially, I was only letting him know that the healing abutment wasn't fully seated. As the conversation carried out, we found out that him and I shared the same Kim lineage. I happened to be his distant grandfather of sort (Translator note** Dr Kim stresses that he's only a grandfather by lineage, not by age, or looks). Since then, I've shared my philosophy on longer HA, passive fit and gingival height. Even for the case above, I suggested that he could've gone down a size in length to fit a 5 mm abutment. You can see the implant mount in 📷 **3.26**. Looking at the mount height in the photo where the fixture isn't fully inserted, I think the final implant depth is actually close to ideal.

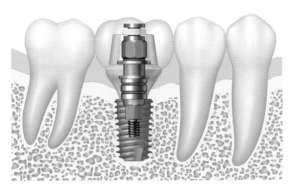
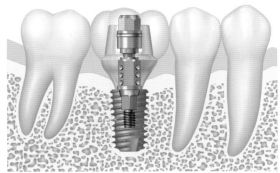

📷 3.27 Superimposed the mounts onto my ideal implant depth diagram

🔍 ⋮

Dr. YOUNGSAM KIM

Most dentists around the globe use mounts to gauge the fixture depth. Every company is slightly different but most of them offer pre-mounted implants. On average, the mounts are about 8-10 mm long so that the operators can measure the distance from the opposing dentition. If mounts were any longer than that, it would make it more challenging to gauge the depth and it can also affect the fixture stability as opposing dentition may apply too much force onto it while you're checking. Most mount systems have length marks on them to help you measure gingival height. For example, Osstem mounts are 9 mm length in total with 2 wings at 3 mm and 5 mm mark. Strauuman mounts are 10 mm in length and they also have similar length measures on them. It is important that you're fully aware of the dimensions of the mounts you use. At this point you may wonder why I don't use mounted implants. Firstly, not many Korean companies offer mounted implants. They also cost more and I don't really feel the need to use the mounted implants for a moment of convenience. Removing mount is an additional step in the surgery and it can cause issues of their own. Please refer to the general characteristics of mounts in "**Chapter 1-1 History and Latest Trends in Implants**" for more information. As I said, I just use 5 mm HA to gauge my fixture depth.

The shape of healing abutment I use

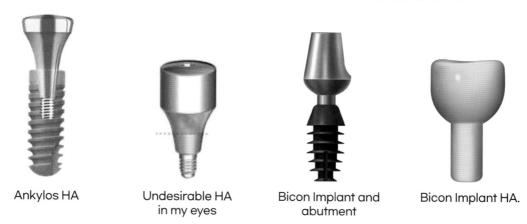

| Ankylos HA | Undesirable HA in my eyes | Bicon Implant and abutment | Bicon Implant HA. |

📷 **3.28** Healing abutments

I think the very first healing abutment with S-shaped concavity was developed by Ankylos. Their internal friction angle was 5.7° so I guess they had no choice but to have the abutment come up straight before spreading outwards. Seeing as Bicon implant with the internal angle of 1.5° made a HA that looks like a lollipop on a stick, the S-curve design by Ankylos was truly groundbreaking.

I often say that I don't understand why HA would need a parallel flat surface on the side. No restorative component above the fixture itself contain anything that is parallel to each other. So why did they design the HA like that?

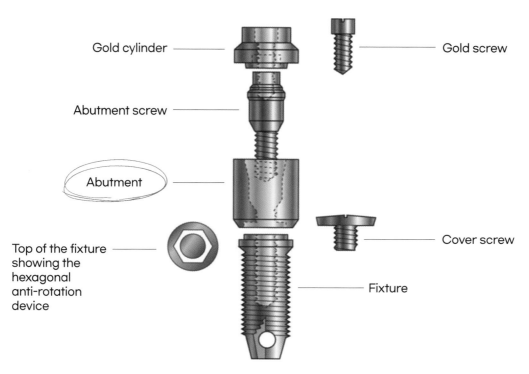

Gold cylinder ⸻
Gold screw
Abutment screw ⸻
Abutment ⸻
Top of the fixture showing the hexagonal anti-rotation device ⸻
Cover screw
⸻ Fixture

📷 **3.29** Schematic diagram of early stage Brånemark Implant

It probably all started with Brånemark implants. Strauuman was pushing tissue level so they didn't really put that much effort into healing abutments. But Brånemark implants started as 2 stage surgeries as we know it today (Bone level placement, second surgery, screw retained prosthesis). So back in the days, they made so called "standard abutments" parallel from the top of the fixture to the gum level. It was basically a gold cylinder connected to a crown. However, now the abutments have the S shaped curves like natural teeth so we don't really need a portion that's parallel and cylindrical. Modern healing abutments would have a small parallel cylinder in top 1-1.5 mm and below that are mostly curved concavity or straight cone shaped at the very least. The 1-1.5 mm exists so that the HA can still appear flat despite the height difference between buccal and proximal gingiva. Now we rarely get healing abutments that look like the head of a sperm whale.

📷 **3.30** compares older Osstem HA versus newer ones. It was a huge design improvement and also made the surgeries easier. The concavity really helped reduce the bone getting in the way of passive HA seating.

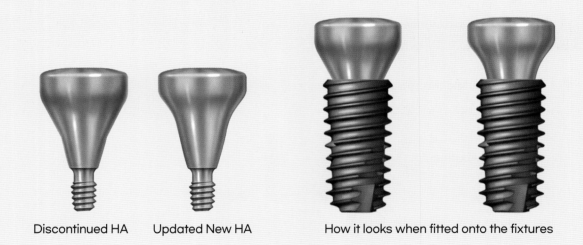

Discontinued HA   Updated New HA   How it looks when fitted onto the fixtures

📷 3.30 **My favourite Osstem Healing Abutment**

Case study : Healing abutment used in live surgery

I get all my live surgery students to use 5 mm height HA. Alway claiming "Under my roof, my rules". The Korean live surgery course is actually sponsored by Dentis, but I still use Osstem healing abutments. That's how important the 5 mm HA with the concavity is. It's such a big part of my implant surgery. Even in the OPG below, the #46 implant is from Dentis, but the HA is Osstem. The #36 was done by another student from the previous course. You can see that the final abutment used is the same size and shape as the healing abutment (📷 3.31).

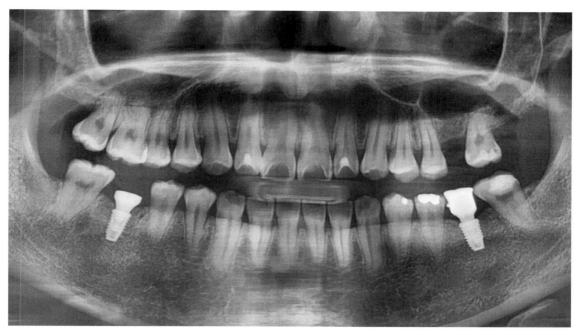

📷 **3.31 OPG taken immediately after the #46 placement at my live surgery course from a few years ago.** You can see that the HA is seated passively without any interference from surrounding tissues thanks to its concavity. In hindsight I think the fixture could've been placed a little deeper (by about 1 mm) but at the time of the surgery I thought this was already plenty deep.

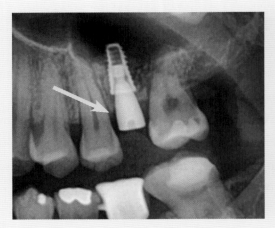

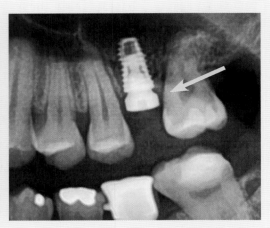

Fixture was placed too deep and 7 mm HA was used.

fixture was placed too shallow and 3 mm HA was used.

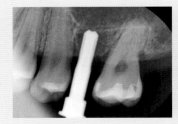

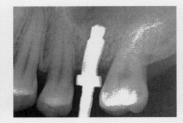

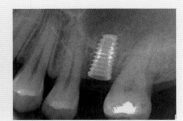

Osstem CAS Kit was used

PA X-ray with the drill and the graft material in the sinus

PA X-ray to check implant depth. You can see that there isn't enough graft material in the sinus.

📷 **3.32** How 26 implant was placed

#26 was placed immediately after the #46. M-D space was very narrow for a molar tooth (📷 **3.32**). Due to the patient's financial circumstances, we decided to only place the fixture during the live surgery. It was a simple sinus elevation case and it ended up with a student who was also very close to me. I've instructed him to use the 5 mm HA and allow about 0-1 mm of HA visibility from buccal side after seating. I was running 2 live surgery chairs on my own at the time so I would often give these instructions and move on to the other room. Then, the operator made 2 mistakes. Firstly, I've asked him to put every single granule of the graft material into the sinus and he didn't. Sometimes I wish people would just listen to me without me having to use swear words. He thought what he had used was enough and just left it there despite my very specific instruction of "use every single particulate". Needless to say, he had to take a long and threatening (for him) lecture from me regarding sinus volume after this incident.

Second mistake was him using 7 mm HA because he thought the fixture was placed to deep. He unwound the fixture and all of a sudden we had no primary stability. If I was to do this case, even without the primary stability, I would've just used a wider healing abutment to fit snugly into the cortical bone and gingiva to obtain stability and closed it up. As I've mentioned earlier, even the fixtures you hand torque will integrate as long as you don't expose it to any lateral excursive movement. Anyway, I removed the fixture that day and we got the patient back in the month after. Again, if it was a case from my practice, I would've left it for another 6-8 weeks. However, because this patient came in through the live surgery seminar, we decided to make a re-entry the next month.

Same operator, same protocol, I had left him to attend to the student in the next room. When I returned I noticed that he had placed the fixture a little bit shallower and used the 3 mm HA. I was going to do it again but the patient was already ready to leave. I changed the HA to 5 mm couple weeks before the impression was taken for gingival remodeling. Honestly, people won't listen to my instructions unless I get angry and throw around a few curse words. Now I sometimes just act angry to get a point across.

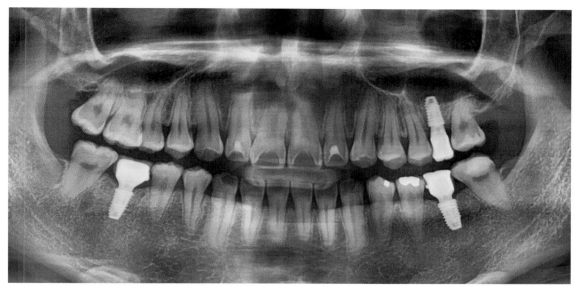

📷 **3.33 Final OPG taken after All 3 cases were finished**
3 implants, 3 different dentists. All of them were their first ever implant in a live patient but they still look very good. Again, if I was to do it now, I would probably place it about 1 mm deeper.

The final OPG after the cases were finished (📷 **3.33**). #26 sinus still bothers me because it's not even 1/3 of what I asked him to use (For your information, I recommend xenograft for sinus lifts). Due to lack of space, the shape of the bone around the fixture isn't bad but I think it could've gone in by another 1 mm or so. If only he used the 5 mm HA on his first attempt as I've suggested. Regardless, for someone's first ever implant placement, they've all turned out well. My students who attended these seminars often told me that the fixtures they've placed during live surgery under my guidance were still their best placement. It's not because I do anything special, I just ask them to follow my principles that I've set. One of which is the "5 mm HA rule". We need at least 3 mm space (5 mm

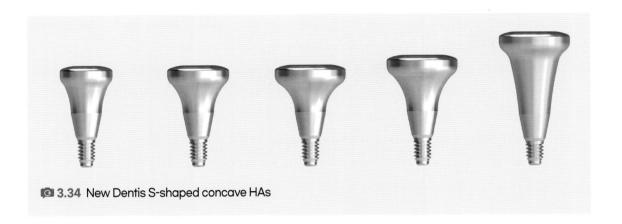

📷 **3.34** New Dentis S-shaped concave HAs

recommended) between the 5 mm HA and the occlusal plane. Not just for ideal prosthesis but also to stop any mastication stress being applied to the HA. Novice operators are often satisfied with the HA simply not touching the opposing tooth. However, occlusion is never that simple. We also don't know and have no control of what the patient is eating. This is why I recommend at least 3 mm gap above the HA.

Dentis finally came up with the HAs as shown in 📷 **3.34** after all these years of my protest. Larger concavity, shorter parallel cylinder component. Smaller 4.8 and 5.8 diameter as well. For myself, smallest I would use for premolars and molars are 5.0 and 6.0 respectively so I use the 5.8 and 6.8 from Dentis. So far it's been very good. Dr Ji-Sun Kim from Sunshine Dental Clinic in Seoul (Also a co-author of this book) changed both her healing abutment and final abutment to this design and she has been very satisfied with it.

Healing abutment as a reference for immediate implants

My placement principles remain the same for immediate placements. The healing abutment placed at the end is a great judge of the depth. For immediate implants, I tend to try and get the top of the HA to be equigingival. Usually the gingiva shrinks by about 1 mm as it heals and it ends up looking similar to what you would get after the placement surgery on an edentulous ridge. 📷 **3.35** shows a case I've done on a female colleague who came for an observation at my practice and asked for a same day immediate implant. Sure I was short on time and the surgery was rushed but I regret not placing it deeper. Even by just 1 mm.

Few months later, she sent me a follow up X-ray and photos (📷 **3.36**) She said she's happy with the implant and location of the access hole, but I wasn't. During placement, I thought my initial plan was a little too deep, so I got the HA flush with the gingival height as if I was placing on an already edntulous space. Later I found that there was lack of bone in the distal side. I think the pre-existing inflammation on the distal root had prevented the healing process. 3 years later she sent me a follow

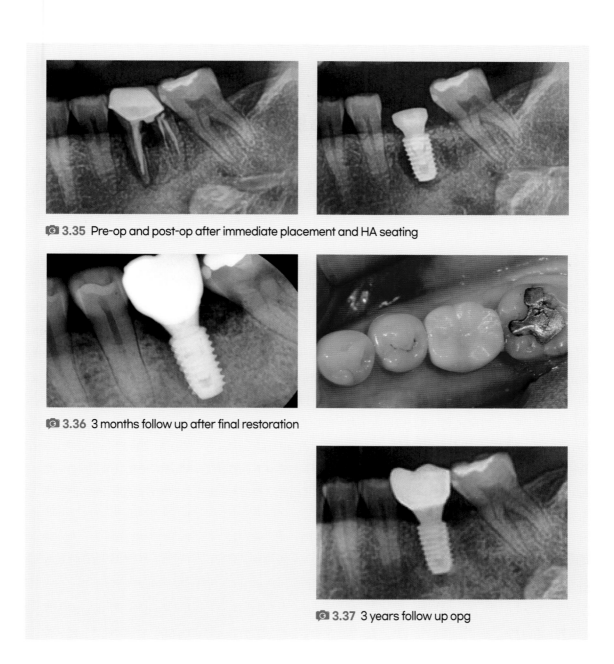

📷 **3.35** Pre-op and post-op after immediate placement and HA seating

📷 **3.36** 3 months follow up after final restoration

📷 **3.37** 3 years follow up opg

up OPG (📷 **3.37**). The image quality is poor but you can still see a decent bone level. Still gives me heartache to not have placed this fixture deeper by another 1 mm. I was known to place my fixtures too deep amongst my colleagues back then and I think may be I was too conscious of that reputation. Nowadays I just place the immediate implants slightly deeper than my usual placement by about 1 mm to take healing gingival shrinkage into consideration.

Case study : Inadequate placement depth

📷 **3.38** is a case of my associate dentist. I've only found out about this case after the final restorations were placed. If I had known about this earlier, I would've removed the fixtures sooner. If I notice the fixtures to be placed wrong, no matter how long ago it was, I just remove them and place them again.

I asked him why he used 3 mm HA in place of the 5 mm. He told me that he thought the opposing dentition is supraerupted and the 5 mm HA would engage the opposing dentition. If you encounter similar issues, you just need to decide how much you will reduce from the opposing dentition at the prosthetic phase and place the fixture accordingly. In this particular case, he had plenty of good bone all around and he just needed to place the fixture deeper. You can see that the final crown shape is very unusual. I've asked him why he used the 6 mm implant in 47 and he said it's because he couldn't get the primary stability. If I was to handle this case, I would've removed both and replaced fixtures at a different location. Thankfully(?) because the whole PAD were less than ideal, even if I had replaced the fixtures, I would've still been able to achieve a decent primary stability for both. For your information, the #26 was placed by myself. You can see my placement principles in the X-rays. The only regret I have with this case is not removing mesial surface of the 27 prior to fabricating the #26 crown.

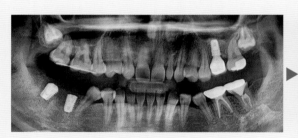

Immediate post-op after #46, 47

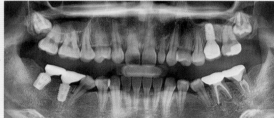

Two Pickaxes after final restorations

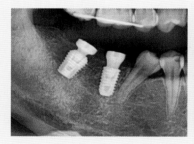

Immediately after the second stage surgery and HA seating

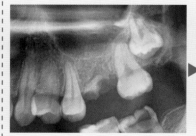
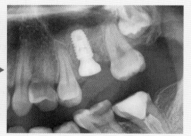

Before and After of my #26 placement

📷 3.38

Case Study 2 : Adequate depth control

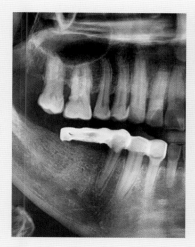 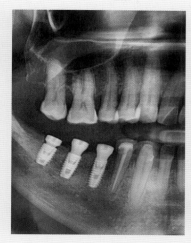 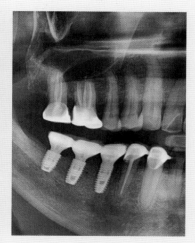

📷 **3.39** My placement when there is insufficient prosthetic space between the fixture and the opposing dentition

📷 **3.39** is a case similar to 📷 **3.38** that I have done a while ago. I was visiting China a lot to do implant surgeries 10 years ago and the patient was a father of the nurse who used to translate for me. She claims that she hasn't seen anyone who is better than I am in the whole of china, how could I not look after her? Look at the ridiculous cantilever on the pre-op X-ray. Crowns were so bent that they were digging into the gingiva. 17 was supraerupted enough to touch the opposing gingiva, causing pain and swelling of the area. First, I've asked the prosthodontics department what their treatment plan was. They've advised me that to reduce the height of the crown by at least 3 mm, they were going to perform root canal treatments and crowns. It would've been easier to get reference for fixture placement if we had reduced the 16 and 17 first, but in most cases, the placement surgeries get done first to account for the healing time. The 5 mm HA was contacting the overerupted 17, so I had to use the 3 mm HA. As I've mentioned before, the HA needs to be absolutely clear of the opposing dentition. I've changed the HA to 5 mm after the RCT once the crown preparations were completed. I didn't take any clinical photos then but I remember it to have at least 2-3 mm clearance from the opposing dentition. 7-8 mm prosthetic space is enough for implant retained bridges and we had plenty of room to successfully place the final prosthesis. As I've mentioned earlier in the chapter, you can see that the prosthesis were made to the occlusal height, not by reducing the gingival portion of the abutment but by reducing the core height part of the abutment.

Fixture depth in guided surgery

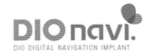

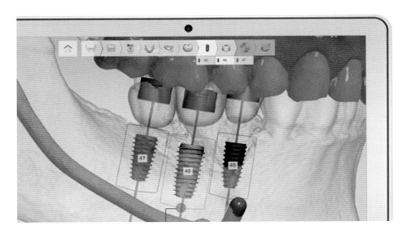

📷 **3.40** DioNavi Advertisement

📷 **3.40** is an advertisement image of DioNavi company who pioneered in digitally guided surgery in South Korea. People think that surgical guides are only about the fixture pathway, but I think height setting is also very important. According to my placement principles, the #47 plan design sparks a question mark. I am only talking about the image itself, not what it could've been in real life. In guided surgeries, you must never design your fixtures shallow. This is especially the case in mandibular D1 bone cases. You can encounter "Stuckers" where you can neither retrieve nor wind it down deeper. Of course if if happens, you must remove it at all costs to replace the fixture properly. Anyway, because the fixtures are larger than the drills, I've seen so many guided surgery cases where the fixtures in lower posterior regions have just stopped going in. If the flap was raised during the surgery, you would've been able to visually confirm, remove fixture, prepare your osteotomy again and then place your fixtures. But for those who just does flapless surgeries, they have no choice but to stop there. If the abutment is short on the design phase, it will cascade to bigger problems in practice.

Comparing the depth of fixtures placed in another practice to mine

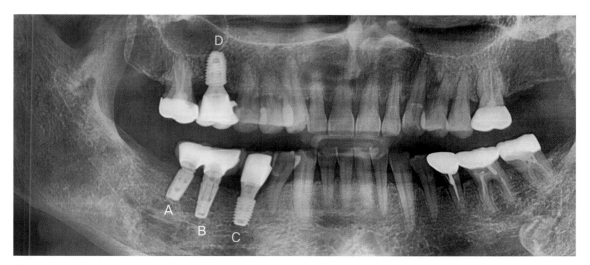

📷 **3.41** A, B from another dental clinic VS B, C placed by myself

I've used Shinhung Luna Implant for this patient as she was the mother of a Shinhung company employee. I used to place a lot of them. Even in this book, you would be able to point out a few of those. My own mother has a few Shinhung Luna Implants in her. You can differentiate them on the X-rays. I mainly place Osstem TS implants nowadays, 20-30% Dentis fixtures and Strauuman if the patients want imported implants.

If you've read this far, you should be able to tell that the #45 is a better placed implant than the #46 or #47. D appears as though there is no bone on the distal but there is more than enough seen on a PA X-ray.

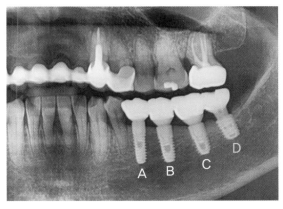

📷 **3.42** A, B and C from other practices and D placed at our practice

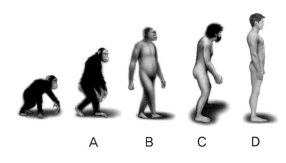

Out of all 4 shown in 📷 3.42, the #37 is the only fixture that was placed at my practice. A,B and C are splinted together and #37 is a lone standing single crown. You should know by now that 6 mm implant for the most posterior mandibular tooth is no longer an issue. This was placed by Dr Young Hoon Pyun who is also the co-author of this book. You can see his principles align with mine by looking at the distance from the top of the fixture to the occlusal plane which is longer than the length of the fixture. A-B-C-D almost feels like looking at the evolution of human species.

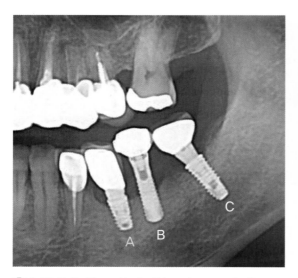

📷 3.43 B, C : Placed in the "dumping practice"

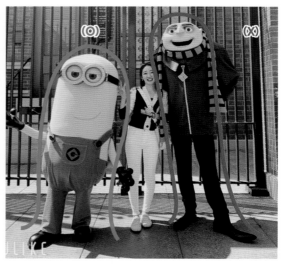

📷 3.44 Saehee Lee is one of our Dental Hygienist at Leon Dental. The photo was taken at Universal Studio in LA.

📷 3.43 Photo credit to a colleague in Busan. All 3 were done at the same practice which is notoriously known for their overtreatment (Another dumping practice). They have high dentist turnover and it shows on the work that just lacks consistency. They're all wrong but A is probably better out of the three.

I use the 📷 3.44 on my lecture series. If you compare the characters to fixtures, the minion on the left is closer to ideal. The fixture must never look like the tall guy on the right.

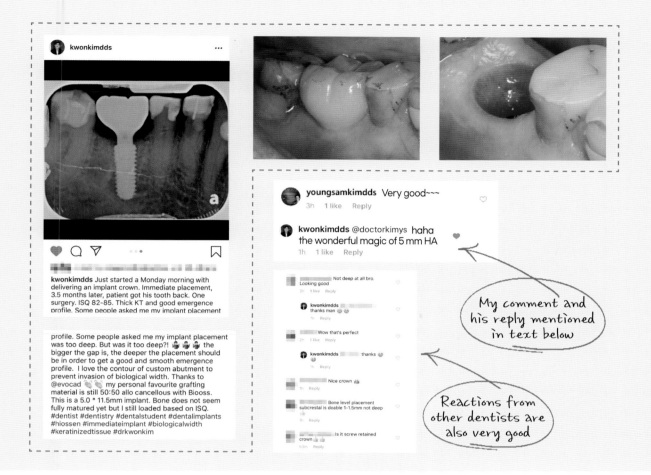

📷 3.45 Dr Kwon Kim's Instagram

I've left a complimenting comment on Dr Kwon Kim's (Toronto, Canada) Instagram. He replied saying "The magic of 5 mm HA" which is what I told him in our discussion over the phone. The fixture looks a little too long but it's because he placed it before attending my implant lecture series. When he invited me over to Canada to deliver a lecture series, he complained that all the fixtures seem so small compared to the larger framed Caucasian population. Particularly so for immediate implant cases. So I told him "Yes I understand, but you must consider how much worse Korean diet is for the longevity of implants when compared to the westernized diet, so if it works for Koreans, it will work for Canadians"

Dr Kwon Kim now attends my live surgery seminars as a faculty. He was already an excellent clinician before we've met so he's of a tremendous help to me.

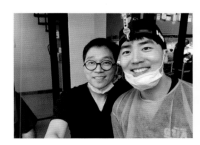
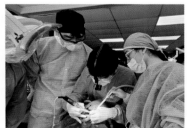
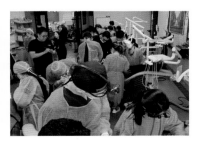

Advertisement posters need to change for the basic principles of fixture depth to change

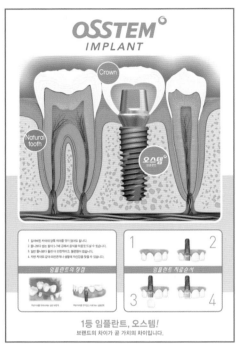

📷 **3.46** Osstem implant poster

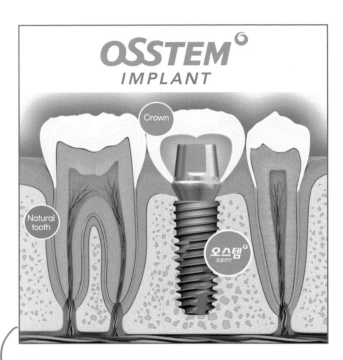

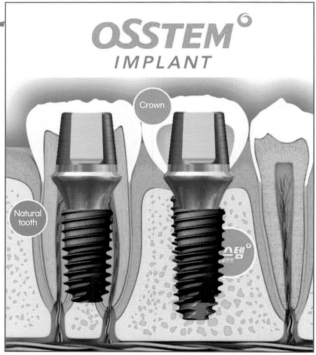

📷 **3.47 What I think the poster should look like**
5.0 x 8.5 mm fixture, 5 mm abutment gingival height and 5 mm crown

This is an advertisement material for Osstem implants which is the brand I use the most (📷 **3.46**). When I am looking at this poster, I just want to re-draw this. I know it's only a schematic diagram for the patients but novice dentists can see it and get the wrong idea from it. Just as an estimate, it looks like a 4.5×11.5 mm fixture with 2 mm Abutment gingival height and 7 mm crown height.

This poster needs to change like the 📷 **3. 47**. 5×8.5 mm considering it's a mandibular first molar AND placed about 2 mm deeper. As a big Osstem fan and user, I really hope they consider this change seriously.

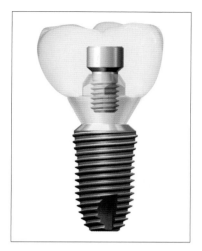

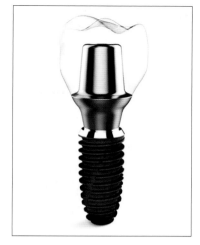

Dentium Poster

Acrodent (Korean implant company) Poster

 3.48 Fairly realistic Implant Schematic image

You can see the abutment length had increased in the Dentium Poster (**3.48**). Although I don't know why the crown is screw-retained out of the blue (May be it's an abutment poster, not an implant poster). Next to it is an implant made by the company which made the Bone Proshaper from earlier in the chapter. You can see that they take the passive abutment fit very seriously from the long abutment neck. If any implant company is reading this, please consider the contemporary trends and science on your posters. It will help the dentists develop an eye for well placed implants. It will help them tell monkeys apart from humans as I always say in my lecture series.

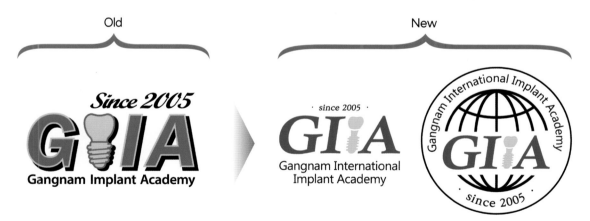

3.49 It's a new logo I made while I was adding the word "international" into it. I even made the abutment longer in our new logo when compared to the old one.

Dr. YOUNGSAM KIM'S

CLINICAL NOTES

EASY SIMPLE SAFE EFFICIENT

MASTERING DENTAL IMPLANTS

The Essential Elements for Success in Dental Implants

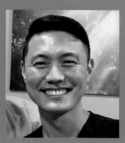

Dr. Joung Lee

Dr. Joung Lee earned his Bachelor's of Science degree in biochemistry from Georgia Tech with the highest honor. He completed his Doctor of Dental Medicine at Nova Southeastern University School of Dental Medicine in Florida with oral surgery honor and won the award from Academy of General Dentistry. Following his move to San Antonio, Texas, he has been working as a general dentist.

Implants and Soft Tissue

Soft tissue can deform hard tissue

5-1 Attached Gingiva and Vestibule

5-1

Attached Gingiva and Vestibule

Mastering dental implants

What Is The Key to Implant Maintenance?

What else should we consider if an implant is placed in the right position, angulation, and depth as discussed in the previous chapter? Soft tissue! You probably won't recognize the importance of soft tissue until delivering implant crowns unless there is exposure of implant threads or grafting materials in the mean time. Many dentists tend to start paying attention to soft tissue when they have patients with some discomfort after implant crowns or observe bone loss around implants radiographically.

One of the greatest strengths of my implant experience is the fact that I have been consistently practicing implant dentistry for 20 years at the same place. In addition, most of my implant patients are very compliant to recall visits since many of them are my friends and acquaintances. So, I was able to monitor and follow up many of my implant cases for an extended period of time. Compared to my colleagues, I did not have problems like mechanical fracture of implant fixtures, and that's probably because of my constant effort to place implants in the right position, angulation and depth.

However, I have been constantly observing some soft tissue problems though. People who received implant treatments from me 20 years ago in their late teens, 40s and 60s are now in their 30s, 60s and 80s respectively. Based on the observations of my implant cases for the past 20 years, it seems that **natural teeth are getting older as patients are getting older, but implants merely change over time except for some porcelain fractures of crowns.** On the other hand, soft tissue around implants is changing with (or even faster than) the surrounding tissue as soft tissue around natural teeth changes.

In this chapter, I will be discussing how to manage soft tissue following the ESSE concept, so anyone can easily apply it to their daily practice. Once, I took a lecture in periodontics, and it was about keratinized gingiva and vestibule around implant. They said "Keratinized gingiva is not that important. Actually, **stable marginal gingiva from deep vestibule is more important.**" They also reported good prognosis with vestibuloplasty without free gingival graft and mentioned that flap surgery is recommended to prevent peri-implantitis if pocket depth is greater than 5 mm. Their conclusion was that the key to implant maintenance is to have stable marginal gingiva without any fluctuation.

Overall, I agree with them, but there are a few questions: "They said it's not good to have 5 mm pocket depths, but what about people who want to place implants deeper (more subcrestal) so have 6 to 7 mm pockets all the time?" Those people who place implants deeper use this analogy: "even though hurricanes produce extreme waves on the sea surface, the deep sea is calm" I think both groups are right. I have never heard about any problems with having deep periodontal pockets around implants, but actually good things about them though. Anyway, I accepted both opinions and concluded that it would be better if **we place implants deeper and have deep vestibule for stable marginal gingiva.**

Recently, I have read some researches saying that having a few threads exposed out of the bone does not affect the prognosis of implants much and the attached gingiva is not mandatory for implant success. And I figured that these researches are frequently referenced in seminars that are sponsored by companies that emphasize on guided implant surgeries. So, they are basically trying to promote their products and to eliminate doubts in guided surgery. Speaking of which, many people teach flapless surgery as one of the advantages of guided implant surgery, but you don't want to correlate the terms "flapless" and "guided" too closely. Actually, it has to be the other way around; **you need to consider guided surgery when flapless surgery is the only option for some reason.** For instance, I do flapless guided surgeries only for medically compromised patients in order to minimize complications.

Anyway, I like keratinized gingiva. I studied and took exams about the difference between attached and keratinized gingiva in dental school, but clinically I merely see any difference between them. There are some people who are very strict about this matter and say that the two terms have to be used separately. However, in my opinion, your skill will not be improved if you focus too much on theoretical things rather than trying your best to place implants correctly. Only students need to know about the difference between the two. If you are a dental student and reading this book now, I strongly recommend you stop reading and start studying about the difference between them because you might not be able to pass the boards by reading this book. In this book, I will use both terms interchangeably. ☺

I often hear many dentists saying that 2 mm of keratinized gingiva is enough, but I disagree with that. Actually, the more, the better. When they say that statement, they only think about the width of keratinized gingiva around implants. However, it is important to have more keratinized gingiva towards the vestibule since it's better to have moveable soft tissue as far away from implants as possible.

When I was in dental school in the 90s, I occasionally saw vestibuloplasty cases from oral surgery clinic for denture patients since implant dentistry was not common back then. They often used stents made of self-cure composite resin in order to avoid apically repositioned vestibule from moving coronally. Even nowadays free gingival graft is done by securing mucosa at the apical part of vestibule

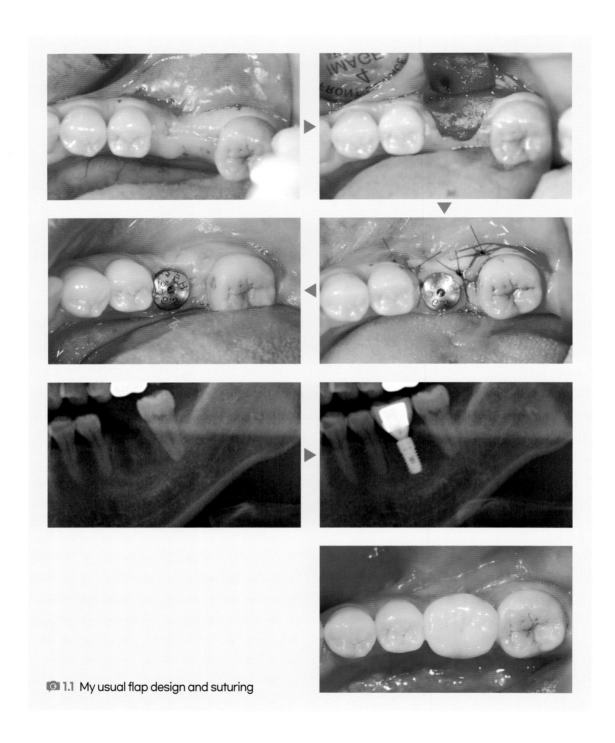

📷 **1.1** My usual flap design and suturing

followed by applying some materials like COE-PAK to maintain apically repositioned vestibule in place. That's because having non-moving and stable vestibule is the key to success.

This is my usual flap design and suturing technique for implant surgeries. Papilla-sparing flap is apically repositioned and sutured so that the keratinized gingiva can be positioned buccally and the depth of vestibule can be leveled with adjacent sites. Here, the keratinized gingiva is acting like COE-

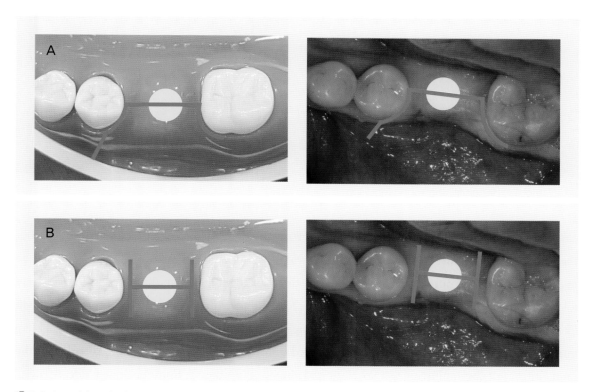

📷 1.2 **A**: Incision design that I used as a beginner, **B**: H shaped incision design to spare papillae

PAK that keeps the vestibule at the apical position. The case in 1.1 is an old case from 2008 and has been used for all of my implant lectures to show how I consistently use the same technique for a long time. I still use this technique for most of my implant cases.

📷 **1.2A** was the most common incision design when I first learned implant dentistry. The design includes a vertical incision at the distal line-angle of a tooth in front of an implant site. When bone grafting was needed, I used to make the vertical incision at the mesial line-angle of one tooth or two teeth in front of the implant site. Recently, many young dentists told me that implant seminars are now teaching an H shaped incision design mainly (📷 **1.2B**). That's probably because it usually causes more swelling, post-op pain and delayed healing if papillae are incised. I assume that the shift of incision design has started ever since implant surgeries started to be considered as minor surgeries.

When you perform many implant surgeries, you come to realize that there is no need to use wide and extensive incision designs. I felt the same way, so from some point on, I ended up not including papillae if possible and making as minimal incisions as possible. Actually, this is something we need to learn and think about when starting implant dentistry, but after a certain period of time, we tend not to care about the incision design anymore.

However, when using the H-shaped incision design, two problems can occur. The first is that an assistant must retract the lingual flap during surgery. Otherwise, it will continue to block the site

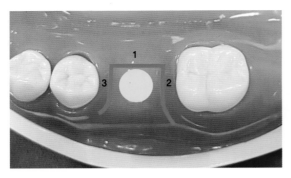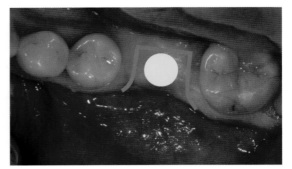

📷 **1.3** Incision design for the Youngsam Flap

and can cause some difficulty when drilling. Anyway, let's say that the surgery is over somehow, but then how can you suture up the flap around a healing abutment? Normally, the buccal flap can be re-positioned apically, but in fact, we can't do much about the lingual flap. It will seem to have been folded under the healing abutment. Over time, the folded lingual flap will be slowly absorbed and look like that it was cut in that form from the beginning. If you don't want this to happen, the lingual flap must be cut before suturing. Then, there is no need to leave the gingiva over the lingual aspect of the implant from the beginning unless the keratinized gingiva is insufficient from the lingual side.

So, after deciding the ideal implant position, I first make a horizontal incision at the straight line that touches the lingual aspect of the implant. And then vertical incisions are made about 1.5 mm away from papillae to preserve them as much as possible. Most of my implant surgeries are done using this flap design as in 📷 **1.3**, and many students were surprised to see this design. I guess there was no one teaching this way, so I named it "Young Sam Flap". In my live surgery courses, sometimes we need to use other flap designs for specific cases, so the term "Young Sam Flap" is used to distinguish it from them. For my students, I always use relatively expensive implant models that have gingival portion. This is because practicing implant placement without the gingiva is meaningless. Implants have to be positioned on the gingiva, so I think the gingiva is more important than the bone when deciding the ideal implant position .

Once a flap is raised based on this design, initial drilling can be done buccolingually at a distance of about 2 mm (a radius under the premise that a 5 mm diameter implant is placed) from the horizontal incision line. This is also very helpful in positioning implants. When drilling like that, the osteotomy gets bigger gradually and the lingual side of the implant comes into contact with the lingual gingiva finally.

However, when teaching beginners, I see many of them make incisions like 📷 **1.4**. As explained in the previous chapter, this happens because the mesial aspect of an edentulous site is not easily visible, so wider mesial papilla is left than the distal one. If the incision is made like this, from then on, you will have to start drilling from a slightly mesial position, not from the middle position where the incision was made. Anyway, the principle is to make incisions as large as possible without including papillae. So, without cutting any keratinized gingiva, the flap is apically re-positioned and stablized by sutures.

If suturing is not easy because of too much keratinized gingiva, or if final prosthesis has to be delivered without having sufficient recovery time for the gingiva, I usually cut the gingiva around healing abutments slightly. I once taught my students to cut the gingiva in the healing abutment space in circular or triangular shape, but surprisingly, it was difficult for them to control blades, and they cut too much. Since then, I tend to tell them to just suture the gingiva rather than cut it.

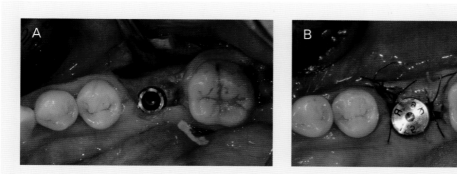

📷 1.4 Usual incision design and suturing for beginners following my method

This is my case, done the way beginners do (📷 1.4). I still use this picture every time I give a lecture. Even today, when I'm in a hurry, it happens a lot like this. When I do implant surgeries, I do not think of them as simple incisions and suturing, but I consider them as FGG and vestibuloplasty in all cases. But, is vestibuloplasty really necessary in all cases though?

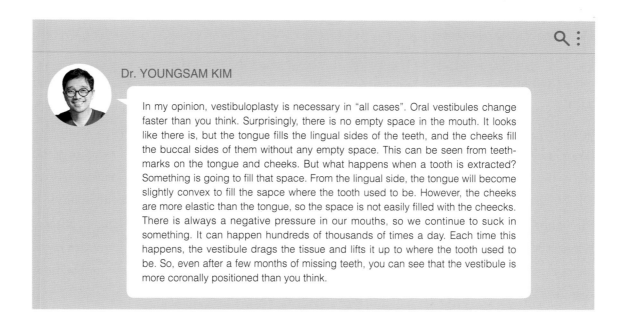

Dr. YOUNGSAM KIM

In my opinion, vestibuloplasty is necessary in "all cases". Oral vestibules change faster than you think. Surprisingly, there is no empty space in the mouth. It looks like there is, but the tongue fills the lingual sides of the teeth, and the cheeks fill the buccal sides of them without any empty space. This can be seen from teeth-marks on the tongue and cheeks. But what happens when a tooth is extracted? Something is going to fill that space. From the lingual side, the tongue will become slightly convex to fill the sapce where the tooth used to be. However, the cheeks are more elastic than the tongue, so the space is not easily filled with the cheeks. There is always a negative pressure in our mouths, so we continue to suck in something. It can happen hundreds of thousands of times a day. Each time this happens, the vestibule drags the tissue and lifts it up to where the tooth used to be. So, even after a few months of missing teeth, you can see that the vestibule is more coronally positioned than you think.

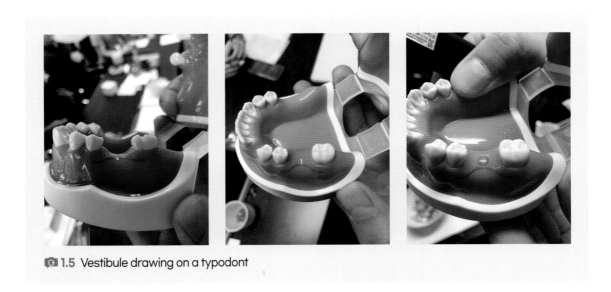

📷 1.5 Vestibule drawing on a typodont

Even when practicing on typodonts, I always ask my students to draw the shape of virtual vestibules on the typodonts before practicing incisions.

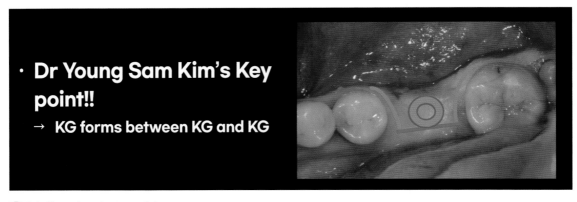

📷 1.6 One of my lecture slides

If a band of keratinized gingiva is narrow, I tend to make incisions as large as possible and spread the buccal and lingual aspects of the band of keratinized gingiva as far apart as possible. This is because, by secondary intention, spacing between two keratinized gingiva will always result in a keratinized gingiva. During my lectures, there are several things that I simply say to memorize, and one of them is that "A brand new keratinized gingiva will form between two keratinized gingiva".

Looking at the literature on the next page, it is mentioned that in the case of epithelium, it is affected by the underlying connective tissue to form keratinized or non-keratinized gingiva. If there is a gap between two keratinized gingiva, granulation tissue is formed from the connective tissue under the two keratinized gingiva. Since both are connective tissues that promote the formation of keratinized gingiva, of course, keratinized gingiva will be formed as a result.

J.Periodontal Res. 10:1-11

The role of gingival connective tissue in determining epithelial differentiation

T.KARRING, N.P.LANG AND HARALD LOE

Department of Periodontology, Royal Dental College, Aarhus, Denmark

Note: Whether keratinized or non-keratinized gingiva is formed depends on the underlying con-nective tissue. If there is a space between soft tissue, granulation tissue is formed from connective tissue that is surrounding the space, and then keratinized or non-keratinized tissue is formed thereon (For a space between two keratinized gingiva, both granulation tissue is formed from con-nective tissue that promotes the formation of keratinized gingiva).

However, incision designs vary greatly from case to case (📷 1.7). If everything is perfect, a small flap that just fits the implant site can be raised. For other cases, I may need to extend incisions more apically, mesiodistally or lingually as much as needed. When it is thought that bone grafting is necessary even before raising a flap or it is expected that an implant needs to be buried with a cover screw and membrane, the incision design can be quite extensive.

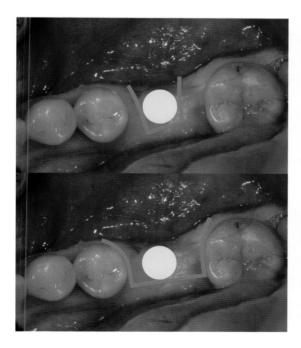
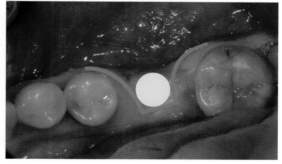
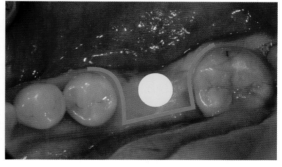

📷 1.7 Even with the same implant location, the incision design may be different depending on the gingiva and the shape and amount of bone.

Youngsam Flap case 1

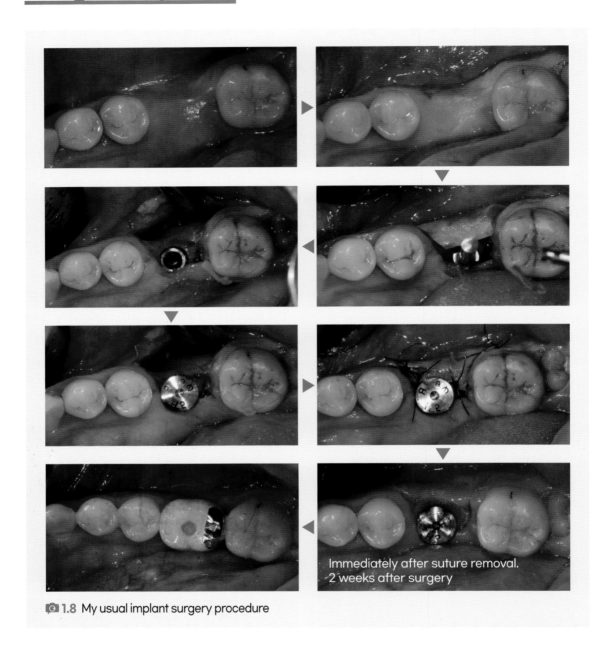

Immediately after suture removal.
2 weeks after surgery

📷 1.8 My usual implant surgery procedure

After the surgery, the vestibule has been more apically positioned, and the keratinized gingiva has been increased (📷 1.8). Actually, the band of keratinized gingiva was not too narrow, and the vestibule was not too coronally positioned in this case. But I think it's still better to do it like this because you can improve prognosis without putting much effort into it. In the long run, there's no harm in having more keratinized gingiva and deeper vestibul. I don't think this kind of surgery will cause more swelling or make the postoperative pain worse. For postoperative pain and swelling, I think whether papilla is incised or not is a determining factor. By the way, even though there was a second molar, metal occlusion on the distal aspect of the implant crown was done. I really don't know why since this is a very old case. I probably made a mistake.

Youngsam Flap case 2

Let's take a look at another mandibular first molar case (📷 1.9). Actually, there are many good cases, but unfortunately I don't have complete sets of intraoral pictures for many of them. So, I feel bad that I cannot show you all the good cases in this book.

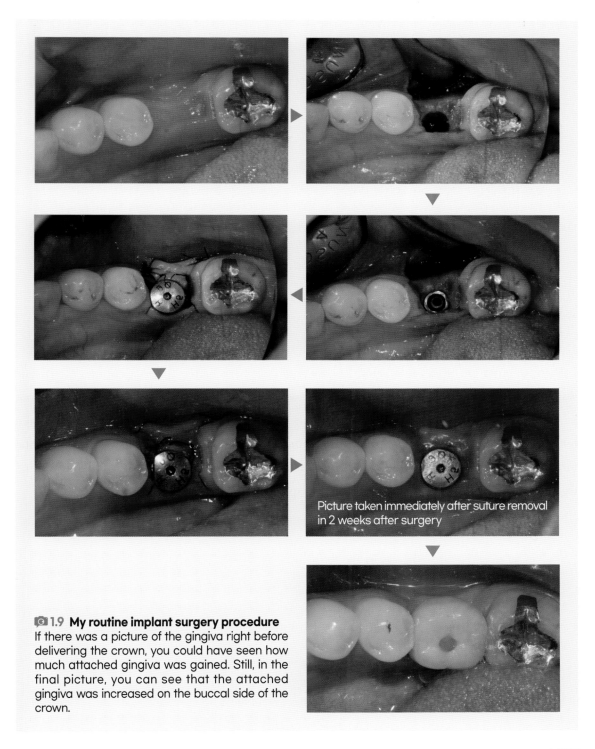

📷 1.9 **My routine implant surgery procedure**
If there was a picture of the gingiva right before delivering the crown, you could have seen how much attached gingiva was gained. Still, in the final picture, you can see that the attached gingiva was increased on the buccal side of the crown.

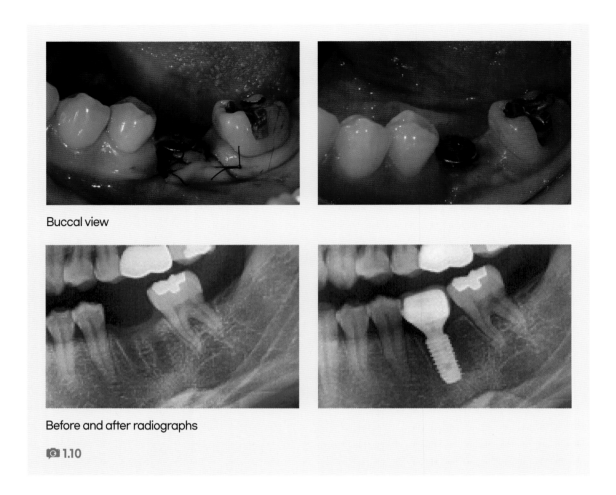

Buccal view

Before and after radiographs

📷 1.10

The case in 📷 1.10 makes me regret that it would have been better if the flap on the mesial side was larger and more apically positioned. Usually, when this happens, you may have done it without paying attention, thinking that this is enough, or you may have not made the mesial vertical incision long enough due to the mental foramen. Sometimes, I make shorter incisions if I think the mental foramen is too close . Also, in the case of a recent tooth extraction, the crestal side of gingiva is too thin to push and hold the attached gingiva in the apical position like COE-PAK

Youngsam Flap case 3

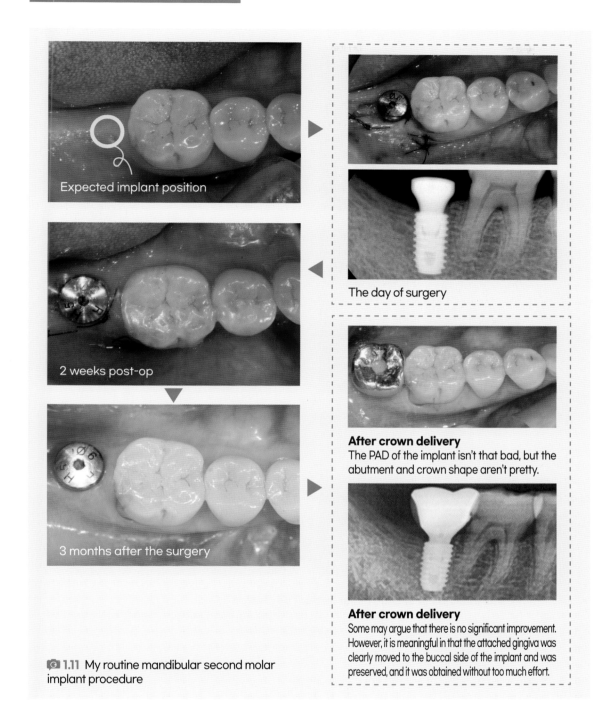

Expected implant position

The day of surgery

2 weeks post-op

3 months after the surgery

After crown delivery
The PAD of the implant isn't that bad, but the abutment and crown shape aren't pretty.

After crown delivery
Some may argue that there is no significant improvement. However, it is meaningful in that the attached gingiva was clearly moved to the buccal side of the implant and was preserved, and it was obtained without too much effort.

📷 **1.11** My routine mandibular second molar implant procedure

For the distal side of mandibular second molar cases, rather than making a distal vertical incision, a slightly curved incision towards the ramus from the distal aspect of horizontal incision is usually made. And this distal portion of the flap is loosely sutured or even left as it is without any sutures (📷 **1.11**). When the keratinized gingiva is really narrow, or when the apically repositioned flap keeps moving coronally, I usually try to hold down the flap as far apart as possible, sometimes even using the Louis button.

Youngsam Flap case 4

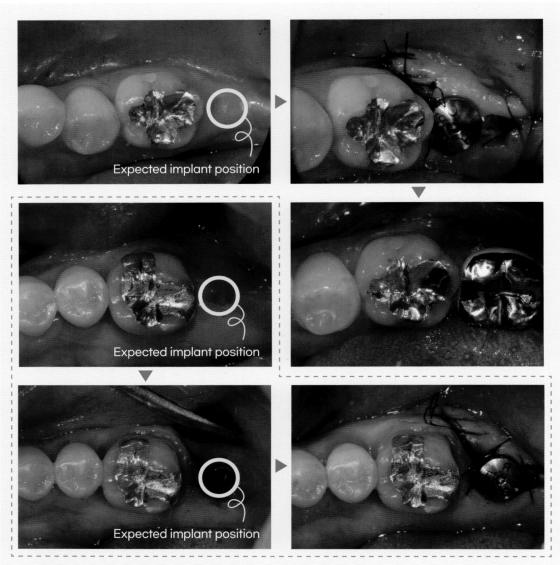

Expected implant position

Expected implant position

Expected implant position

📷 1.12 My usual mandibular second molar implant procedure
It's just a record of my daily surgeries. In both cases, the photos were not completed. The important point is that the sutures are similar as if they were the same case.

Since most of my implant cases have been done the same way, there were not that many pictures taken (📷 1.12). In order to record a complete set of pictures of one case, I need a good patient who agrees to take pictures and a restorative dentist who is willing to take pictures at every step. Anyway, the key is to use the keratinized gingiva like COE-PAK that pushes the buccal gingiva towards the vestibule.

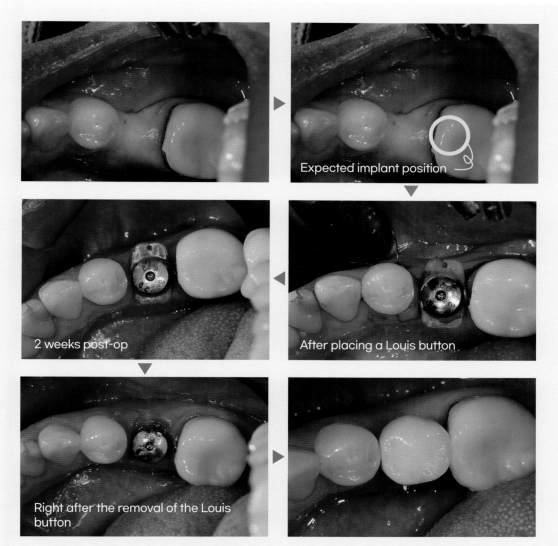

📷 1.13 A case in which a Louis button was used on mandibular first molar site
This is a case that has been around for over 10 years, and whenever I see it in a lecture, I am impressed.

There is a product called Louis button from Dentis (📷 1.13). It is difficult for beginners to make this type of incision, but it is even more difficult to suture. Especially when gingiva has thin phenotype, it often gets torn when suturing. In this case, with or without sutures, a Louis button can be used to press and hold the gingiva apically. The price is about $10 each, and there are several sizes to be compatible with most implant systems. Although it is a premolar case, you can see that the vestibule has become deeper after the surgery.

It can definitely be used in actual clinical practice, and if you are a beginner, it is very useful for mandibular second molar cases. Beginners are not good at suturing the Young Sam Flap in the mandibular second molar region, and they are usually not able to secure and stabilize apically repositioned flap well.

Youngsam Flap case 5

📷 **1.14** is a mandibular first and second molar case. When both first and second molars are extracted together, the keratinized gingiva is absorbed very quickly towards the extraction sockets and the vestibule follows probably because the surrounding tissue that holds the vestibule is also lost. As shown in 📷 **1.14B**, when you imagine the ideal position of the implant on the gingiva before surgery, you can tell that almost no keratinized gingiva will be present on the buccal if flapless surgery is done. If you look at the post-op pictures, you can see that the keratinized gingiva and vestibule were recovered at least to the pre-extraction level.

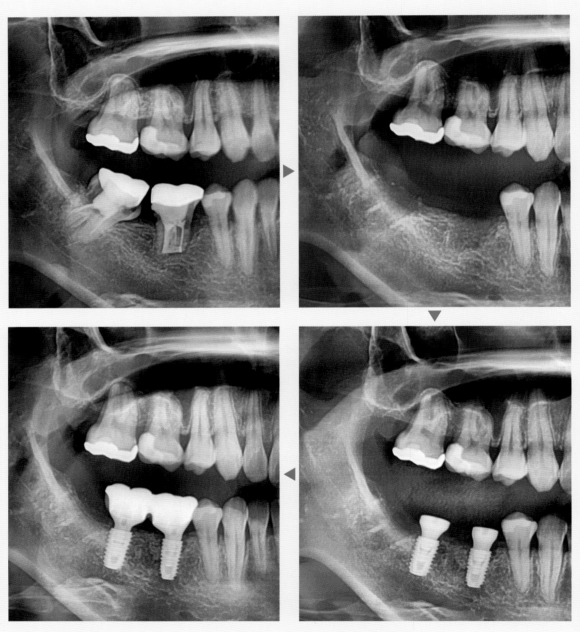

📷 **1.14A** Mandibular first and second molar implant surgery using a Louis Button

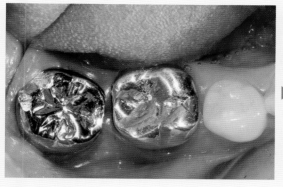

Pre-extraction

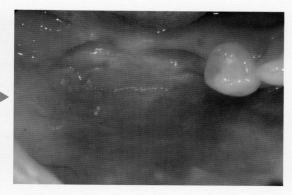

Post-extraction

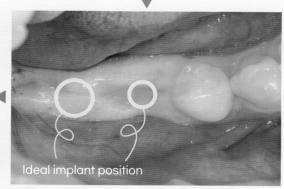

After anesthesia

Ideal implant position

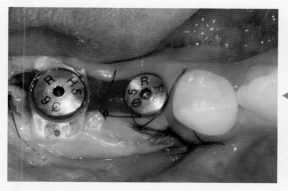

Right after surgery

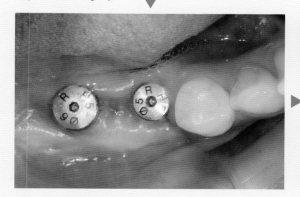

Buccal view after crown delivery

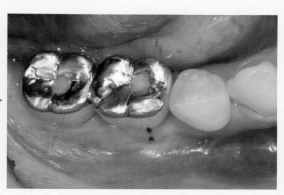

📷 **1.14B A case in which a Louis button was used for mandibular first and second molar implants**

Youngsam Flap case 6

I use the same technique for maxillary first molars as well (📷 1.15). You can see that the vestibule has already been coronally positioned not too long after extraction. By the way, I almost always use Young Sam flap for both maxillary and mandibular molars. But as you go toward anterior from the maxillary molar region, there are many variables to consider such as high smile line and cosmetics even for maxillary premolars. So, different flap designs can be used for these areas.

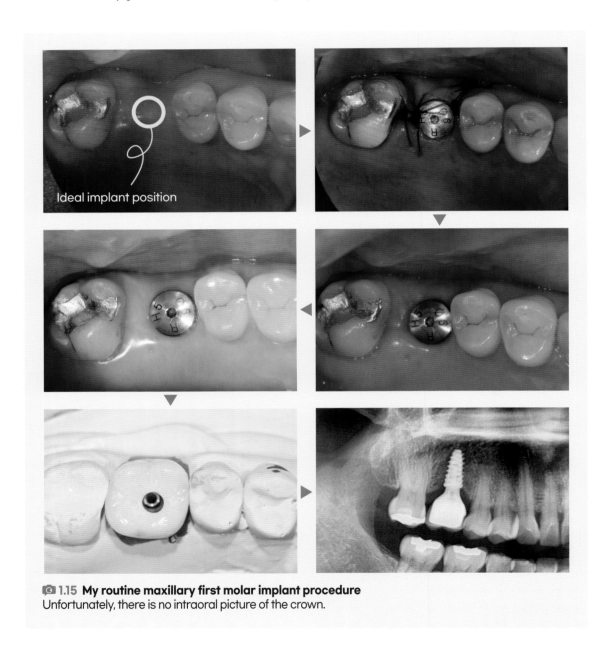

📷 1.15 **My routine maxillary first molar implant procedure**
Unfortunately, there is no intraoral picture of the crown.

Youngsam Flap case 7

If you look at 📷 1.16, you can see that the vestibule has become deeper. As usual, implants were placed after the Young Sam flap. It can be seen that the vestibule has deepened on the buccal and the keratinized gingiva has also been improved. Of course, there are opinions that this is not necessary, but **this can be done at no cost and is not too difficult**, so there is no reason not to do this.

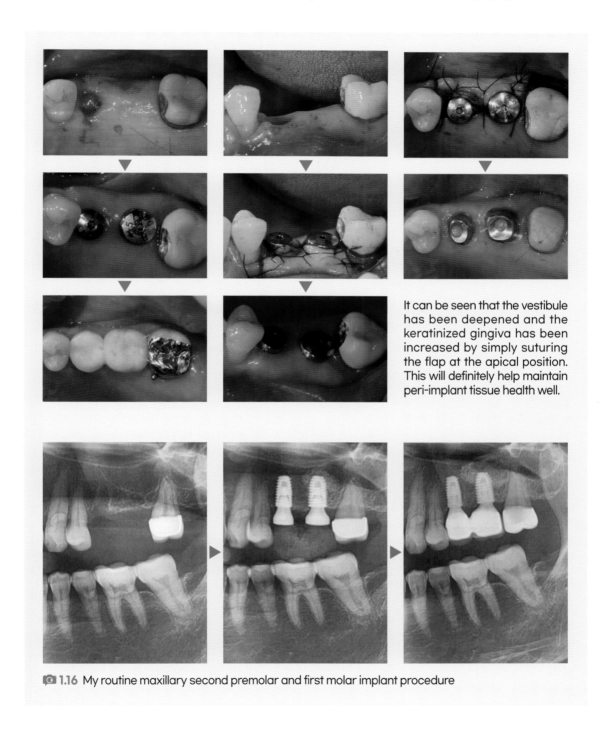

It can be seen that the vestibule has been deepened and the keratinized gingiva has been increased by simply suturing the flap at the apical position. This will definitely help maintain peri-implant tissue health well.

📷 1.16 My routine maxillary second premolar and first molar implant procedure

Youngsam Flap case 8

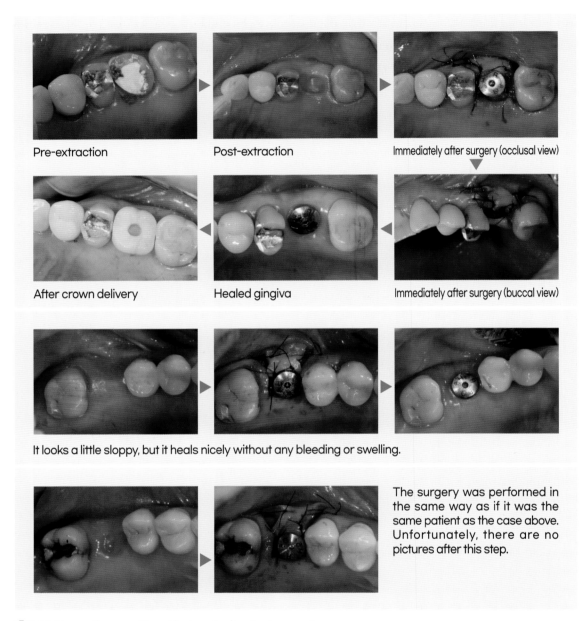

Pre-extraction

Post-extraction

Immediately after surgery (occlusal view)

After crown delivery

Healed gingiva

Immediately after surgery (buccal view)

It looks a little sloppy, but it heals nicely without any bleeding or swelling.

The surgery was performed in the same way as if it was the same patient as the case above. Unfortunately, there are no pictures after this step.

📷 **1.17 My routine maxillary first molar implant procedure**
In fact, it would have been much nicer if 2-3 mm of the coronal portion of the flap had been cut out in a half moon shape. I'm thinking of changing my habits a bit in the future: preserving the vestibule and keratinized gingiva, but cutting off unnecessary portions. But sometimes, when you try to cut a little bit, it gets cut too much. So, I just go back to my old habit and repeat the cycle endlessly.

In 📷 **1.17** cases, the vestibules were not coronally positioned much, so it would have been nicer if the flaps were cut a little and sutured. But because of my darn habit, I always do it the same way.

There is "the principle of suturing" that I always emphasize during live surgery. **"Suturing is not attaching the buccal flap to the lingual gingiva, but attaching it to the buccal bone."** However, no matter how much I explain it, beginners try to do the former even by pulling the buccal flap over the healing abutment. You should always keep this principle in mind. Again, the principle of suturing is to attach the flap to the buccal bone. So, there is no need to worry about the tissue being not closed tightly or anything like that. It's all filled up by secondary intention.

Usually, during live surgery, if there are no special requirements, almost all the posterior cases are done using the flap design shown above which my faculty members started to call it "Young Sam flap". Because of them, my students started to call the flap design "Young Sam flap" as well. So, we just decided to call it "Young Sam flap".

As in the case shown previously, the gingiva becomes thicker toward the maxillary posterior region, and the distal of maxillary second molars is not easy to manage for beginners. In addition, because of the thicker gingiva, healing by secondary intention happens slower. However, considering that maxillary implant cases usually need one more month of healing period compared to mandibular ones, slower healing does not seem to affect the timing of final impression significantly. If there is enough keratinized gingiva on the buccal, it is easier to suture by cutting a small amount of the gingiva around the healing abutment. Also, in the maxillary second molars, the depth of vestibule is usually good as well.

Anyway, there are so many poorly done flapless guided surgery cases posted on social media. I don't understand why they want to get rid of that precious keratinized gingiva. It hurts my heart as much as if I prep a healthy tooth.

There are many wonderful cases in which the attached gingiva was increased and the vestibule was deepened only with the Young Sam flap, but since I am a busy private practitioner, I feel bad that I cannot take as many clinical pictures as I want.

When multiple implants are placed or when cosmetic outcome is a main concern, as long as the vestibule and keratinized gingiva are maintained well, I also use various types of incision designs and suturing techniques. However, such flap management has already been discussed in many books, so I do not cover it much in my book. We will only briefly describe the Palacci flap, which is often useful when multiple implants are placed.

Palacci Flap

It is called Palacci flap or Palacci technique because it was designed by a French periodontist, Patrick Palacci. Actually, many dentists who have never learned this flap design often do this naturally from their clinical experience. So, even though they use this technique, surprisingly many of them still do not know the name of this flap design. In live surgery, Palacci flap is taught as an example of other flap designs to distinguish the Young Sam flap from them. Of course, it is rarely performed unless the attached gingiva is very abundant or if the surgical site is in the aesthetic zone. Here is an example of the Palacci flap that was done in my live surgery.

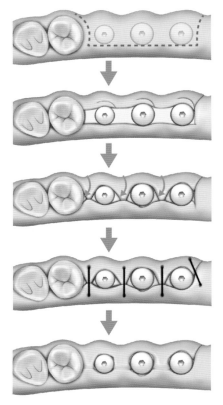

Schematic for Palacci flap

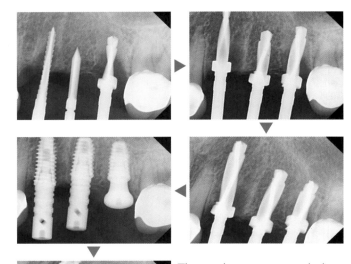

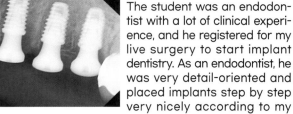

The student was an endodontist with a lot of clinical experience, and he registered for my live surgery to start implant dentistry. As an endodontist, he was very detail-oriented and placed implants step by step very nicely according to my instruction. After the placement, I left the operating room to see other students, and the rest was guided by Dr. Jungpyo Hong, a graduate of Heidelberg dental school in Germany.

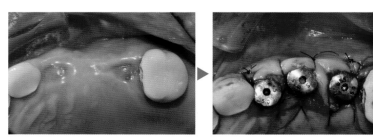

Immediately before surgery (2 months after teeth extraction)

📷 1.18

Clinical picture of Palacci flap
Although it is not shown well in the photo, the palacci flap seems to be more effective here because the mesial flap design was too palatally positioned and there was a large gap between the healing abutment of implant #24 (#12 U.S.) and the palatal gingiva.

It's embarrassing, but let's take a look at some of my mistakes.

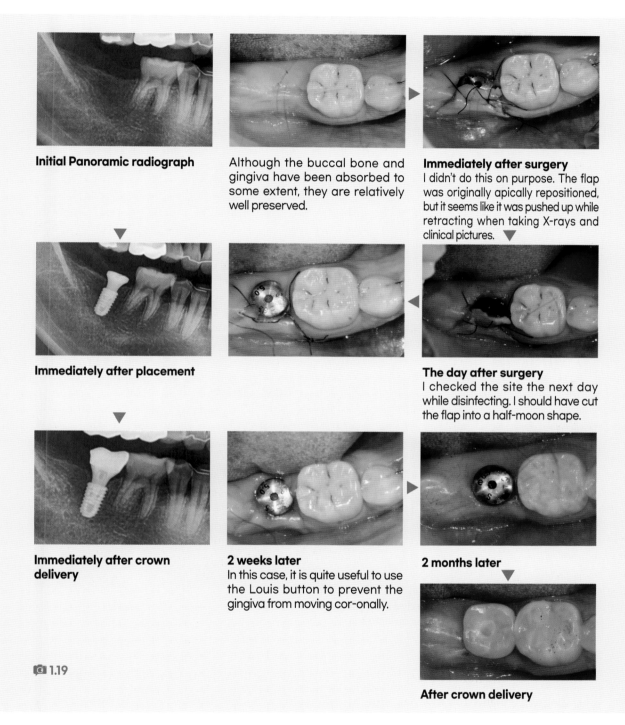

Initial Panoramic radiograph

Although the buccal bone and gingiva have been absorbed to some extent, they are relatively well preserved.

Immediately after surgery
I didn't do this on purpose. The flap was originally apically repositioned, but it seems like it was pushed up while retracting when taking X-rays and clinical pictures.

Immediately after placement

The day after surgery
I checked the site the next day while disinfecting. I should have cut the flap into a half-moon shape.

Immediately after crown delivery

2 weeks later
In this case, it is quite useful to use the Louis button to prevent the gingiva from moving cor-onally.

2 months later

1.19

After crown delivery

Nothing is perfect, but the great thing about this Young Sam flap is that it doesn't cost money or requires any extra effort. If you do not cut the keratinized gingiva but make a habit of doing some sort of vestibuloplasty on the buccal side when placing implants, the prognosis of the gingiva and implants can be very good in the long term, and cases that require FGG due to mucogingival defect can be reduced significantly.

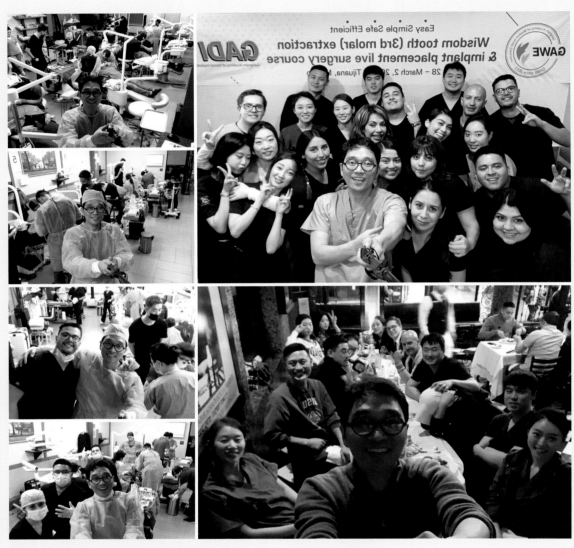

📷 1.20 **Pictures from my first Mexico Live Surgery (February 2019).**
They are the same pictures I posted on Instagram.

These are pictures from February 2019, when I had my first live surgery course in Mexico (📷 1.20). Spending three nights and four days with young dentists was really dynamic and interesting. During the day, we worked hard doing surgeries and in the evening enjoyed delicious Mexican food and tequila at different restaurants every day. The picture at the bottom right is the restaurant at Caesars Hotel, where Caesars salad was first made. Right next to our dining table, the chef made Caesars salad himself, so everyone was busy taking pictures. The people I took pictures with are beloved students who claim to be my sincere followers. Now, most of them are faculty members and have been helping with my course since then.

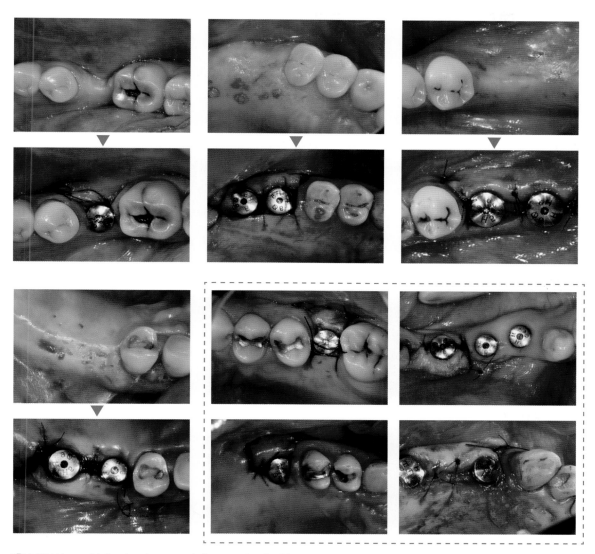

📷 **1.21** We couldn't take pictures of all cases, but looking at the pictures we took, all cases were done by using Youngsam flap. When you go back to your own practice, you can do whatever you want, but my principle is that when you learn from me, you should do everything my way.

Let's take a look at some cases from my first live surgery in Mexico (📷 1.21). I teach that **it is as important to revisit the surgery he or she did as it is to do the actual surgery.** So, I invited staff members from Korea to the course in Mexico to take clinical pictures for all cases. To commemorate the first live surgery in Mexico, I organized the pictures myself. From the second time on, the staff members organize and send emails to our students after the course, so the students can post their cases on a Facebook live surgery group.

If you look at the cases, you can see that most of them were done by incisions and sutures that I teach. For their first incisions, I marked the incision lines by making little dots on the gingiva with a periodontal probe just like the connect the dots. Most of the sutures were done in my way. You can go anywhere else and do whatever you want, but in live surgery I always follow the principle of "Under my roof, my rules."

Let's take a closer look at Dr. Yoon's case. 📷 1.22 and 📷 1.23 are his first and second implant cases. I think they were very well placed for the first implant he did in his life. Let's look at the second case. Wherever I teach, if there are no X-rays of at least four specific steps, I remove implants no matter how well they are placed. It can be seen that this case followed the process well.

In any case, the worst suturing causes the flap to climb up and cover the healing abutment. As mentioned earlier, sutures should attach the flap to the buccal bone, not to or over the healing abutment. When sutured like 📷 1.23 and 📷 1.24, most of the precious keratinized gingiva is absorbed.

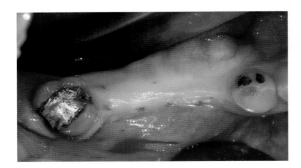

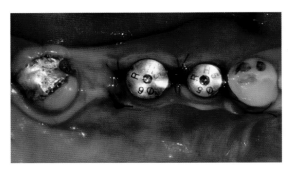

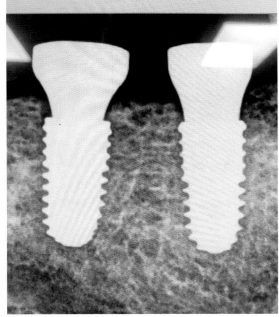

📷 1.22 **Dr. Yoon's first implant case**

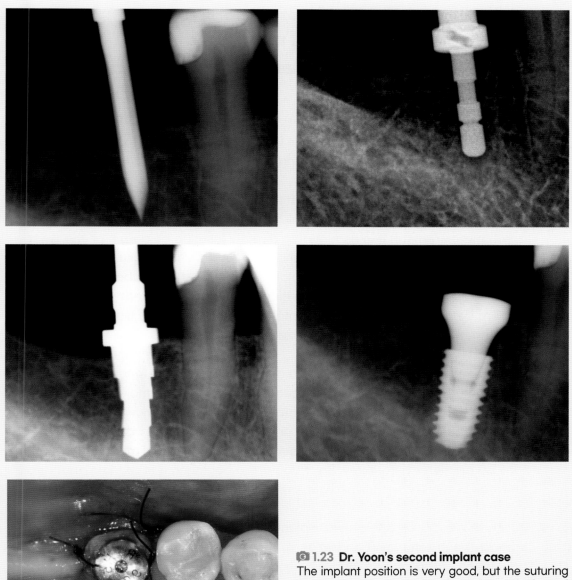

📷 1.23 **Dr. Yoon's second implant case**
The implant position is very good, but the suturing is poor. Sutures should attach the flap to the buccal bone, not to the healing abutment. The purpose of suturing is to gain the attached gingiva by repositioning the vestibule as apical as possible.

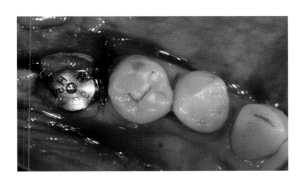

📷 1.24 **Poor suturing seen in another case**

Note : Four radiographs that must be submitted when placing an implant during my live course.

1. First, insert the lance drill about 5 mm and take an X-ray. You don't have to go deeper than this. This is because the lance drill is not about looking at depth, but about looking at "position, spacing, and angulation".

2. The second one is an X-ray taken after the twist drill. Although it varies from company to company, most companies use a 2.0 mm (diameter) drill for initial depth measurement. It is essential to directly insert a guide pin or the twist drill with depth markings into the osteotomy. At this time, it is not necessary to drill as deep as the size of the implant to be placed. That's because we are just trying to get an idea of the position, angulation and depth (PAD). Once you are satisfied with the PAD and make sure that it is safe from anatomical structures, you can start using full-size drills.

3. The third one is an X-ray taken with a drill that has one size smaller (diameter-wise) than the final fixture to be placed. This way you can make any changes or corrections if needed before the final drill. Taking an X-ray with the final drill is meaningless because the position or direction cannot be changed anymore. If you place a 5.0 diameter implant, there are many intermediate drills to reach that 5.0 diameter osteotomy. So, if you are a beginner, it is recommended to take one or two more intermediate X-rays for those wide implants.

4. Last one is an X-ray after implant placement. When placing implants, I usually stop at the crestal level and take an X-ray. This way I can still change the angulation of the implant fixture if needed while placing it more subcrestally. You always want to take an X-ray of the implant fixture before placing it to the full depth. If you place a fixture to the full depth and reserve it to fix the angulation later, you will lose its initial stability for sure. And you can also take one more X-ray once the fixture is completely placed and a healing abutment is on. From this X-ray, you can check and see if the healing abutment is properly inserted with no gaps. I usually don't take this X-ray because I believe that feeling a sudden stop through tactile sensation is more accurate than radiographs to check that. There are many cases that look like healing abutments are all the way in with no gaps radiographically but actually they are not. But still, in the live surgery, the required final X-ray is the one with the healing abutment on. In my practice, I take a panoramic radiograph as the final X-ray to check everything.

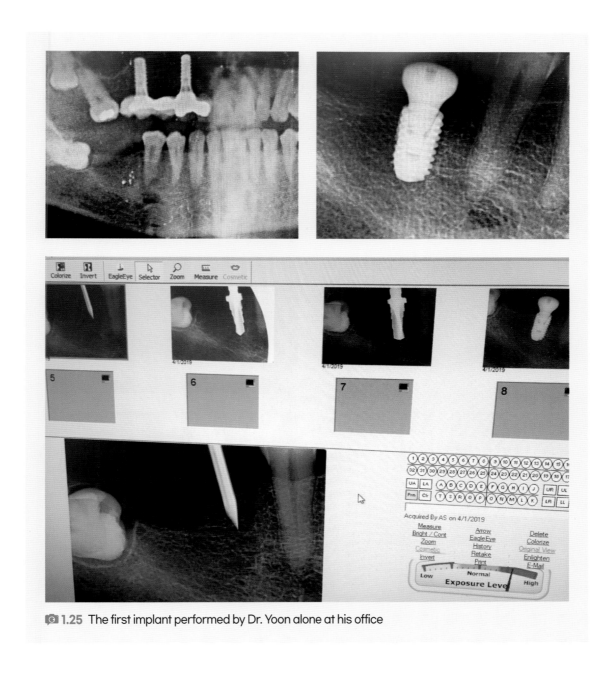

📷 **1.25** The first implant performed by Dr. Yoon alone at his office

This is a picture that Dr. Yoon sent right after returning from the first live surgery course in Mexico (📷 **1.25**). He did it all by himself, and I was so proud of him. I found out that an X-ray for measuring the depth was missing (the second one from the four mandatory radiographs), and he explained that it was taken, but the staff seemed to have deleted it or did not save it. And I also pointed out that the healing abutment was not completely engaged. You must feel a sudden stop when tightening healing abutments. Beginners are not good at making incisions, so there are many cases where healing abutments get caught around the gingiva and do not get engaged well. Anyway, in live surgery, **I think it's more important to teach my students to keep the same protocol for most of the surgical procedures**

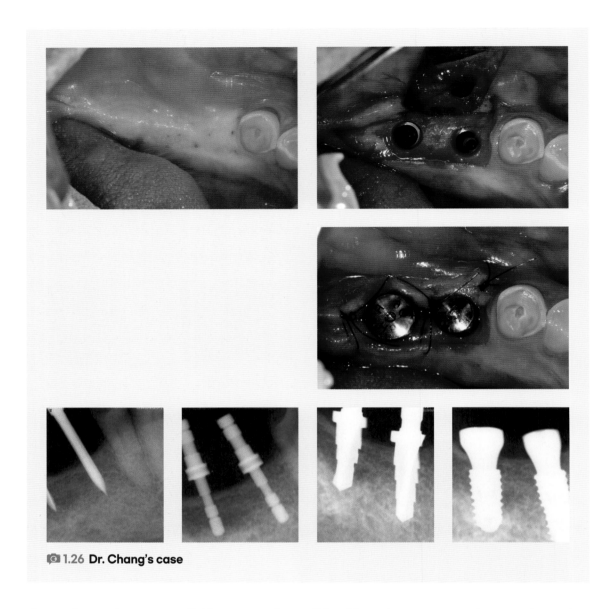

📷 1.26 **Dr. Chang's case**

than to do actual surgeries well. That means they will be able to do surgeries on their own later when they go back to their practices. Dr. Yoon's skill has improved so much since then, and he knows my implant philosophy better than anyone else, so he has been coming to my live surgeries in Mexico as a faculty member.

This is a case of Dr. Chang in Seattle. Since she only did flapless guided surgeries before the course, she was not confident in making incisions. So I marked big incision lines by making dots on the gingiva with a probe (📷 1.26). However, the horizontal incision line that she made was a little too lingual than the line that I marked. If the direction of the blade was perpendicular to the bone rather than just vertical from above, the incision line would move more towards the buccal. Also, if the distal vertical incision line was slightly curved from the distal side to the buccal side and extended to the mucosa, the oral vestibule would have been deepened and the attached gingiva would have been more

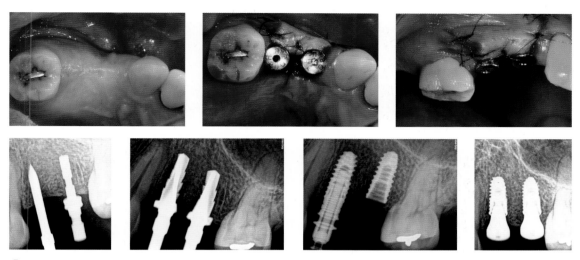

📷 1.27 **Dr. Lee's case**

preserved. Again, sutures should attach the flap to the buccal bone, not to the healing abutment. But in this case, the flap was pulled a little too much to the lingual. However, I still like this case because it follows many of my implant techniques.

This is a case of Dr. Lee in Texas (📷 1.27). He had enough implant experience and was already great even before my course. This is a case that I am very grateful for because he tried to follow my instructions exactly even though he was used to different techniques from his previous courses and experience. As we can see from the picture on the right, the disto-buccal portion of the flap was folded. Since there is enough keratinized gingiva on the buccal, it's not a big problem. But I'd rather cut it out, fill the papilla with the palacci flap, or extend the vertical incision for more apical repositioning. If you look at the first X-ray, you can see that he checked the depth and position together using a lance drill and a guide pin since there was enough bone. And we can also see that the healing abutments were not fully screwed in.

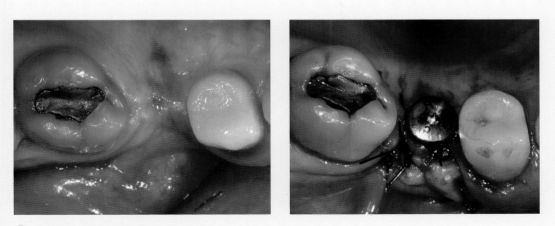

📷 1.28 **Another case from Dr. Lee**
Although it was cut a little bit in the picture on the right, it can be seen that about 4 to 5 mm of keratinized gingiva was formed on the buccal side of the implant.

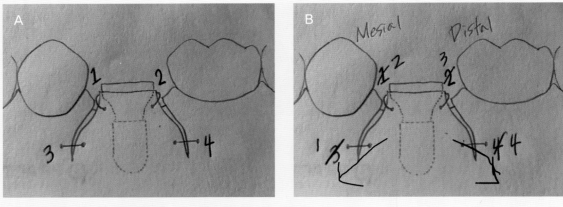

📷 1.29 Youngsam flap suture sequence drawn by Dr. Lee

After the course, he drew a picture himself and asked me about suturing order as in 📷 1.29. I am so envious of dentists with such skillful dexterity. I usually do it like 📷 1.29A. In some cases, no. 4 in the figure is not sutured. In cases where the mesial aspect of the surgical site is aesthetically important or the keratinized gingiva is insufficient, sutures such as 📷 1.29B are used to bring the flap as apically as possible. So, the suturing order varies from case to case.

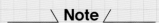
\ Note /

Probably it's because the circumstances of dentistry in Korea and the United States are very different, but I felt that Dr. Chang was much better at general extractions and alveoloplasty than me, except for wisdom teeth and implant surgeries. In Korea, there are very few young edentulous patients because dentists don't just extract teeth due to the patients' financial status and request. However, it is very different in the U.S., and I don't want to make any comments here. Anyway general dentists in the U.S. tend to do a lot of relatively extensive oral surgeries. Looking at Dr. Chang's cases, she seemed to have better skills than mine. She understands my philosophy and style well, so she often comes to my live surgery courses as a faculty member.

With Dr. Lee

Dr. Joung Lee in San Antonio, Texas is currently playing the most important role as a right-hand man in my live surgery course in Mexico. He is very thorough and meticulous, so he lectures on anterior implants and how to make a temporary prosthesis immediately after anterior implant placement. He has been instructing students very well in all cases strictly following my techniques and philosophy. 😍

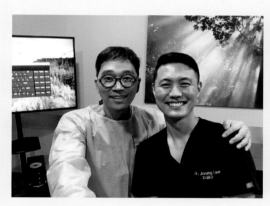

with Dr. Joung Lee

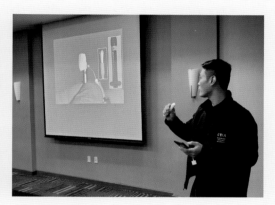

Dr. Lee lecturing

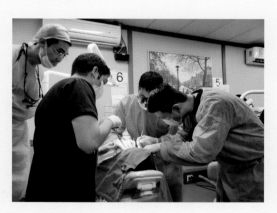

Dr. Lee instructing

With the graduates of my first Live Surgery course in Mexico who believed in and supported me. I miss you all so much! 😭

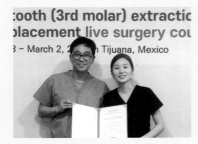

Dr. Addie Chang

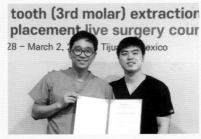

Dr. Jongho Yoon

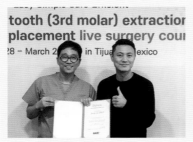

Dr. Joung Lee

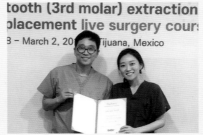

Dr. Juli Kim

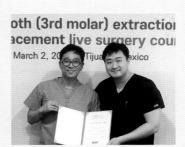

Dr. Leo Choe

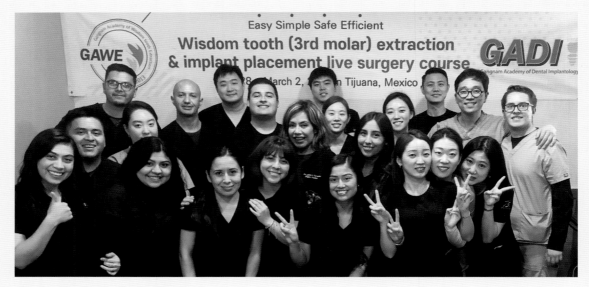

📷 1.30 **1st graduation ceremony**
I would like to express my sincere gratitude to Dr. Adriana Cervantes at Clinica my dentist in Tijuana, Mexico for her support and hospitality for my live surgery courses thus far. I wish you all the best and ask for your continuing support. 😍

Le quiero agradecer a la Dra. Adriana Cervantes de Clínica my dentist en Tijuana, México. Gracias por darnos la permissión a usar la foto, apoyar nuestro curso, proveer la clínica. Espero seguir esta relación amigable. Gracias.

"It's not important that I'm right,
but it's more important that
we are happy together."

● Haemin Sunim ●

Dr. YOUNGSAM KIM'S

CLINICAL NOTES

EASY SIMPLE SAFE EFFICIENT

MASTERING DENTAL IMPLANTS

The Essential Elements for Success in Dental Implants

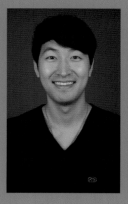

Dr. John Yun

Dr. Youngsam Kim is a good friend and colleague who has always been as approachable as this book is. 'Mastering Dental Implants' is an easy-to-read implant overview that covers most of the fundamentals required to perform implant dentistry comfortably and predictably. He is not shy about sharing his honest opinions and experiences on controversial topics and encourages us to think once again. The environment and circumstances in many countries in which we practice our dentistry may be different, but I appreciate his effort to keep implant dentistry as easy, simple, safe, and efficient as possible.

Dr. John Yun graduated from the University of Toronto's Faculty of Dentistry. Dr. Yun and his team of dentists run multiple offices in Ontario. His primary focus is Implant surgery and Cosmetic restorative dentistry. Dr. Yun is a past and present member of Ontario Dental Association, Academy of General Dentists, International Association of Orthodontics, American Academy of Implant Dentistry, and American Academy of Cosmetic Dentistry.

Bone Grafting in Implant Dentistry
No free lunch

6-1 Membrane

6-2 Bone Graft Material

6-1
Membrane

Mastering dental implants

Membrane

The use of membranes in implant dentistry has always been controversial. First, let's start by answering the question, "Is membrane really necessary in implant surgery?" In early 2000 when I was heavily training in implantology, most membranes were non-resorbable, and many were reinforced with titanium. It must have been due to the fact that long and large diameter implants were preferred at that time. However, as times are changing, trends are also evolving. And as I often say, **"The market always follows the direction the public wants."** Now, let's take a look at the flow together.

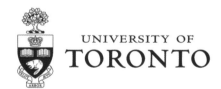

UNIVERSITY OF
TORONTO

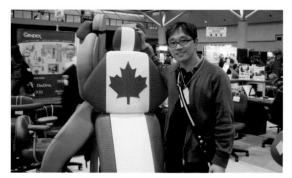

📷 1.1 **At the dental exhibition held in Toronto, Canada, in May 2006**

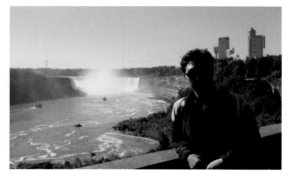

📷 1.2 **At Niagara Falls in Oct 2005**
My life in Canada - studying on weekdays and traveling on weekends.

When I was studying at the Department of Periodontology at the University of Toronto, Canada, in the fall of 2005, one of the professors made a wise statement with a hint of complaint, **"The best membrane is the periosteum."** Since dental research has become commercialized and is funded mainly by large corporations, it has become increasingly difficult to find pure unbiased literature. Because of his unpopular opinion that the periosteum is the best membrane, his research could not get any corporate sponsorship, and he never got invited to give lectures at conferences. On the other hand, commercialized professors got the corporate funding for their research, had their papers published in a prestigious journal with the help of large corporations, and were offered to give lectures in various dental meetings. However, as a scholar, he refused to follow them, and all he could do was make that statement with bitter emotion. I am not certain I fully understood what he said due to my poor English, but I still remember his words. Had I known that I would be giving lectures and writing books like this, I should have taken a picture with the professor at that time.

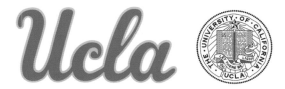

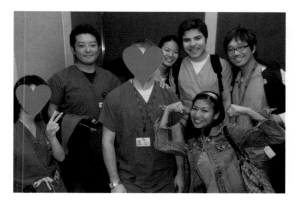

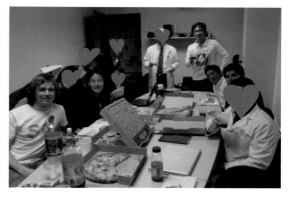

📷 1.3 **With 3rd year Periodontal residents at UCLA in March 2008**

📷 1.4 **After periodontal lecture in March, 2008**
We were treated with pizza by the professor.

On the other hand, when I was at the Department of Periodontology at UCLA from 2007 to 2008, one of the professors emphasized the importance of membrane in bone grafting procedures to prevent the ingrowth of soft tissue into the graft material. As a result, it was a common practice for Periodontal residents to use membranes in their grafting procedures. They were also encouraged to try as many different materials as possible in a generous amount during their training years. It was a refreshing experience for me as I had a habit of using only the necessary amount of materials where I absolutely needed them.

South Korean dentists are not easily impressed when they see international dentists performing surgeries, regardless of how famous they are. This may be because they have already witnessed the professors at the local universities and many other colleagues around them performing surgeries at a very high level. When I was at UCLA, there were two residents per year, a total of 6 residents in the Department of Periodontology, and they were all unique surgeons. Among them, two of the 3rd year residents were exceptionally skilled, probably because they were in their final year in training. Still, they were remarkably better surgeons than other residents, in my opinion.

Once, I observed one of the third-year residents performing a lateral window sinus elevation. Usually, at the UCLA Periodontal department, they would insert a considerable amount of allograft material when performing a sinus graft. In my practice, even back then, I did most of the sinus elevation with crestal approach simultaneously with short implants, so I was not used to this type of practice. Since the resident and I attended the professor's lecture about the importance of barrier membrane, I asked if he would be placing a membrane in the sinus. And his answer was typical, "yes if the sinus membrane tears, no if it doesn't." So I reminded him, "Didn't the professor say you would get soft tissue invagination without a membrane?" My English was not fluent enough to carry a deeper conversation, so we both laughed it off and ended the conversation.

Anyway, I prefer not to use a collagen membrane whenever and wherever I have a clean, intact periosteum. I believe the membrane not only compromises blood supply to the graft and interferes with healing but also increases the cost of the surgery, complication, and failure rate without any particular benefit.

I remember attending a lecture about the importance of the periosteum. It was a lecture about medication-related osteonecrosis of the jaws (MRONJ), and the message of the lecture could be summarized as "You do not need to worry as much as in the past." In the lecture, we were shown the recovery process of the patient whose mandible was resected due to MRONJ, which showed spontaneous new bone formation. This healing process was different from other mandibular resection cases, such as in malignancy, most likely because the MRONJ resection cases left the periosteum intact. Although the periosteum does not make bones by itself, it can be interpreted that it plays a crucial role in bone formation. I believe most of my colleagues would agree.

In fact, there are a lot of new collagen bone materials in the market right now, and if you formally ask the company for the instruction, they will tell you that it can be used without a membrane. Is it simply because it is a lump of bone? Surely the collagen between these bone particles would not prevent the soft tissue ingrowth. And I do not think all those dentists who actively supported the use of the membrane previously used the membrane only to hold the bone particles together. I've seen the developer of OSTEON™ 3 Collagen from Dentium, which I am currently using, use it comfortably without a membrane during live surgery.

Let's look at one of my cases (📷 1.5). My implant surgery protocol is always the same, but this case is particularly well documented. A membrane is unnecessary in cases like this where the periosteum is cleanly peeled off. The patient returned to the hospital two years after surgery, and a CT scan was

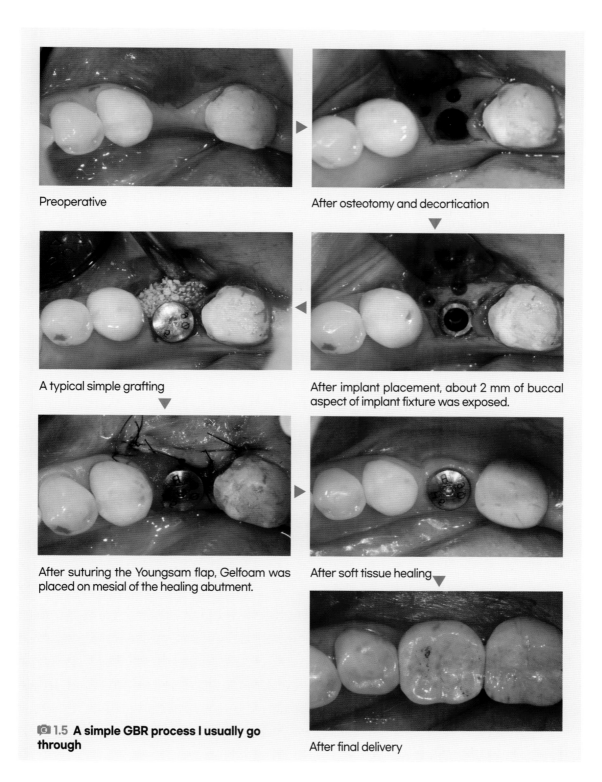

Preoperative

After osteotomy and decortication

A typical simple grafting

After implant placement, about 2 mm of buccal aspect of implant fixture was exposed.

After suturing the Youngsam flap, Gelfoam was placed on mesial of the healing abutment.

After soft tissue healing

📷 1.5 **A simple GBR process I usually go through**

After final delivery

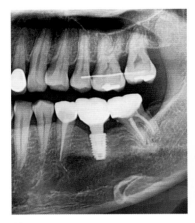 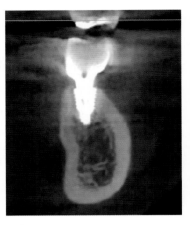 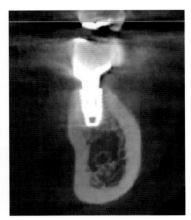

📷 1.6 CT cross-section taken 2 years after treatment

taken to confirm the presence of the buccal bone.

In 📷 1.6, you can see that the graft is well maintained without any unusual findings. My preference is a small amount of Xenograft in this type of case. Since the implant fixture was OneQ from Dentis, I used Obisbone from Dentis (BCP synthetic bone 80% β-TCP + 20% HA) under the principle of using products from the same company.

I often run into cases with a similar type of buccal defect because I place the implant in a prosthetically correct position rather than wherever the bone is. The defect itself is not a big problem, but I like to cover the exposed threads with a graft like this. And I do not feel the need to graft **more than 2 mm from the implant**. Sometimes, I do not even know if this graft is necessary, but it is something that I do to ease my mind. The only purpose of bone grafting is to prevent resorption, maintain shape, and support soft tissue. Graft material selection will be discussed in the next chapter.

This case started with the inadequate amount of attached gingiva, but I overcame it by simply utilizing Youngsam flap. I would not call it a perfect result, but a decent outcome for the effort put in. The screw access hole can be seen slightly distal than my usual cases, but there is an explanation. If we had adjusted the crown of the mesially tilted 2nd molar, I believe the access hole would have ended up more in the center of the crown. When I treat cases where the distal tooth is tipped mesially, I place the implant at mesial to distal ratio of 6 to 4, meaning slightly distal than the center of the ridge. The reason being the prosthetic doctor may decide to adjust the mesial part of the distal tooth. And in the future, if the patient loses the 2nd molar, the implant for the 2nd molar can be placed straight up, not tilted mesially. That is why I do not place the implant for 1st molar just by looking at the remaining space but rather place it as parallel as possible to the 2nd premolar and as if there will be a proper-sized 1st molar. However, in this case, 2nd premolar also has a distal tilting, further making things seem odd. Hopefully, we will have more discussion in the sequel on how to place implants in these various cases.

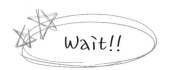

Is decortication necessary for bone grafting?

The debate as to whether decortication of the buccal plate is essential for bone grafting procedures ended a long time ago. Many studies and lectures have said it does not make much of a difference, and I agree. So I do not drill many big holes, but I still prepare two or three habitually. It seems that there is an

Clinical photos from occlusal view

Clinical photos from occlusal view

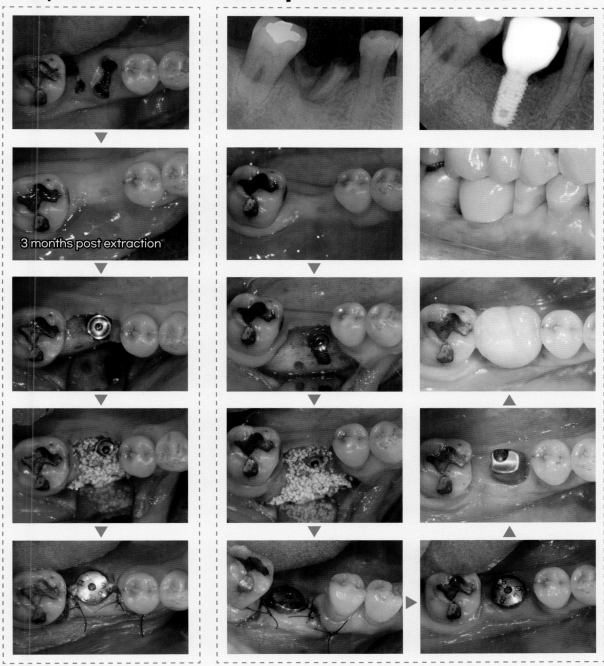

3 months post extraction

anti-slip effect that the bone graft material does not move freely due to the holes and is stably maintained.

The defect is slightly larger in this case, but my protocol is the same as usual (📷 1.7). As you can see from this case, the buccal vestibule has come up to the occlusal surface of the ridge after the tooth was extracted. Usually, I place a healing abutment even with simultaneous grafting, but for this case, I placed a cover screw and buried the implant to prevent the bone particles from escaping with Youngsam flap. It was mainly to take progression photos, actually. On a side note, this patient is an acquaintance of mine who consented to having clinical photos taken, and many photos were taken to document the progression of treatment.

The healing abutment prevents the pressure on the soft tissue and therefore prevents the buccal bone graft from sliding down apically. It also helps to push the vestibule buccally as much as possible. So my preference is to use the healing abutment whenever possible. However, in cases with substantial defect, I will stage my surgeries. I may want to check during the uncovery surgery if there was any movement of the initial graft material and attempt additional grafting at that point. This particular case was the latter. In this case, I achieved excellent results as if I did the minor vestibuloplasty and FGG just by performing Youngsam Flap during the second surgery.

📷 1.8 is panoramic radiographs of the above case, and the last one was taken one year after the final restoration. It can be seen that the opposite side was done in a similar manner.

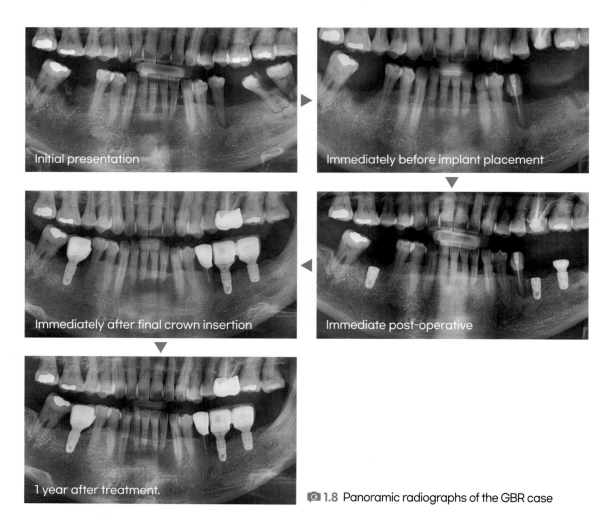

📷 1.8 Panoramic radiographs of the GBR case

Opposite side - 36 37 case

We will also look at implant cases 36 and 37 of the same patient for reference. At the time, I thought the implants were placed deep enough considering the thin biotype, but in hindsight, I feel they could have been placed a little deeper (about 1 mm for 36, 1.5 mm for 37). This case was done 4-5 years ago, but recently I have been placing implants 1 mm deeper than in the past. At 36 site, I was able to gain keratinized gingiva on the buccal side by utilizing the Youngsam flap during the second surgery (📷 1.9), and about 1-1.5 mm of the healing abutment was visible above the gingiva as seen in the buccal view of the second surgery. Nowadays, 5 mm healing abutments are set to be almost flush with the gingiva in the mandible. Again, the flap was cleanly raised with intact periosteum, and therefore no membrane was used in this case.

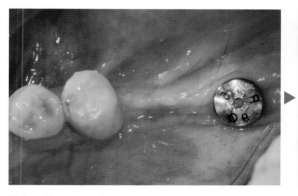

Before the second surgery

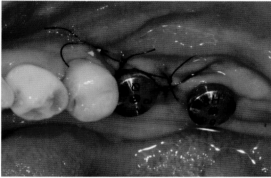

Immediately after the second surgery around 36
I like to perform Youngsam flap during the second surgery to preserve the attached gingiva as much as possible. It is unfortunate to see that some of the previously grafted bone particles escape while raising the flap. Also, in these thin biotype cases, you should always keep in mind that the implant needs to be placed deeper, not just in the proper position and angulation.

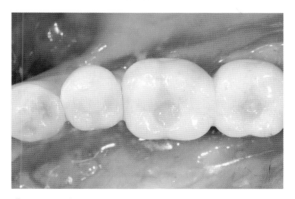

Clinical photo immediately after the final restorations.
It can be seen that 36 implant was placed slightly lingually. I always insist that the implant should be placed in the correct position prosthetically, but it seems that even I tend to lean somewhat towards where the bone is. It is a pity that I forgot to take a clinical photo right before the final restoration to show how well the attached gingiva was maintained with the Youngsam flap.

📷 **1.9 Clinical photos of 36 37 implants**

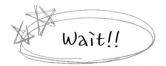

Wait!!

Another thing I would do differently now is the choice of graft material. In the above case, synthetic bone with 80% -TCP was used. However, I recommend using xenograft, which does not resorb and maintains its shape for a long time. And remember to place the implant deep enough.

Case using a membrane 1

This patient is the mother of a close comedian friend of mine. Following photos were taken with her approval and cooperation. I take this opportunity to express my gratitude.

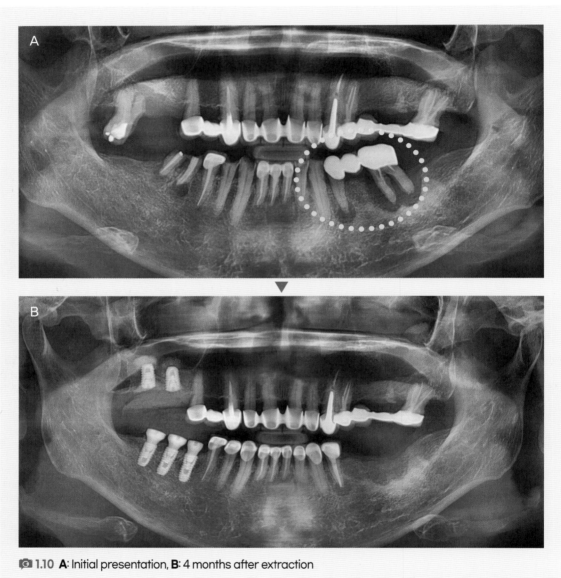

📷 **1.10 A**: Initial presentation, **B**: 4 months after extraction

📷 1.10 shows an initial presentation of a 71-year-old female patient. After extracting 36, we decided to proceed with implants for 35, 36, and 37. And we also decided to remove the over erupted bridge in 2nd quadrant and place implants. The implant surgery was performed four months after extraction, but the socket did not heal very well due to the large size of the initial defect and the patient's age.

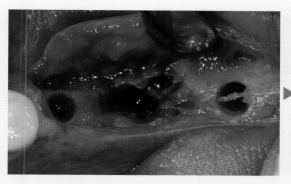

The top of the socket is covered with what appears to be granulation tissue rather than periosteum.

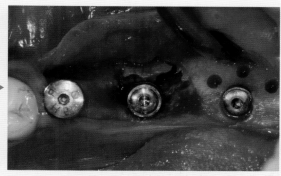

After implant placement, bone grafting was prepared for the 36 defect site and 37 buccal side.

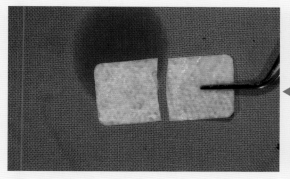

I usually cut a 15 x 20 mm membrane and use it to fit the shape. But my staff took out a longer one and I had to cut it in half.

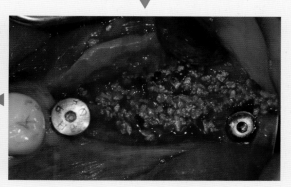

The defect was covered with a bone graft material.

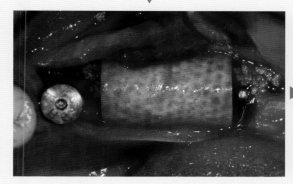

Just covering the area that had compromised periosteum.

🄲 1.11

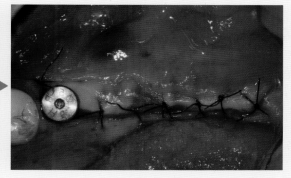

I applied Youngsam flap for 35 and the GBR area was sutured with regular single interrupted sutures.

Therefore, a membrane was used for simultaneous bone grafting with implant placement.

In this case, I used the synthetic bone Ovis from Dentis, the company that sponsors my live surgery courses in Korea, and the resorbable membrane GENOSS from Dentium, one of the most popular membranes in Korea. As you can see from the size of the membrane, it is not covering the entire bone graft material but just covering the top of the socket that was missing the periosteum (🄲 1.11).

The membrane was exposed ten days after surgery (📷 1.12). However, after another week, soft tissue was covering the top of the membrane, and if you look at the photo from the second stage surgery after four months, you can see that soft tissue is firmly formed.

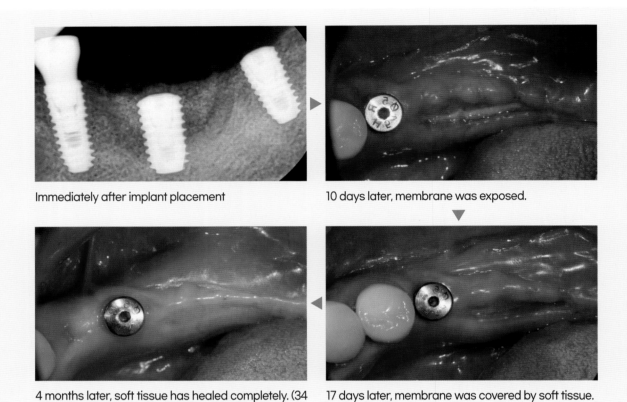

Immediately after implant placement

10 days later, membrane was exposed.

4 months later, soft tissue has healed completely. (34 was extracted due to failed root canal treatment)

17 days later, membrane was covered by soft tissue.

📷 1.12

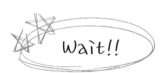

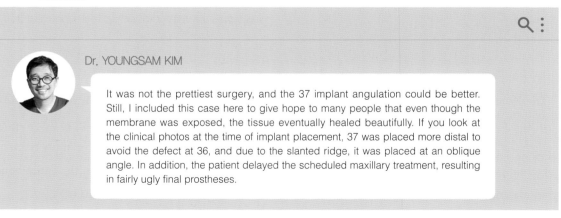

Dr. YOUNGSAM KIM

It was not the prettiest surgery, and the 37 implant angulation could be better. Still, I included this case here to give hope to many people that even though the membrane was exposed, the tissue eventually healed beautifully. If you look at the clinical photos at the time of implant placement, 37 was placed more distal to avoid the defect at 36, and due to the slanted ridge, it was placed at an oblique angle. In addition, the patient delayed the scheduled maxillary treatment, resulting in fairly ugly final prostheses.

However, when I opened the site for the second surgery, the membrane inside remained as clear as it had just been inserted (📷 1.13). However, since it is a resorbable membrane, I assumed it would resorb on its own and only removed the occlusal part of the membrane and completed the uncovery.

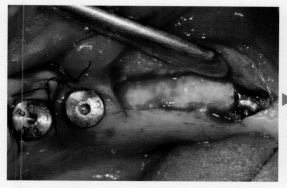

4 months later, 34 implant was placed at the same time as uncovery of 36 37 implants.

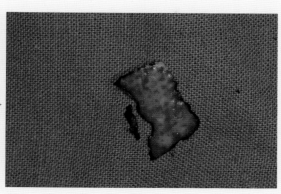

Part of membrane removed ▼

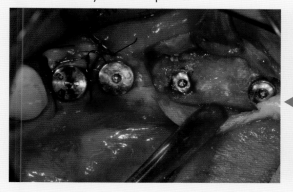

Remove the bone graft material above the fixture to expose the cover screw ▼

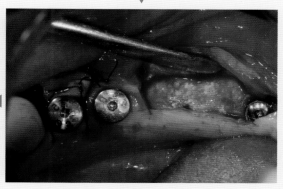

Alveolar bone after membrane removal

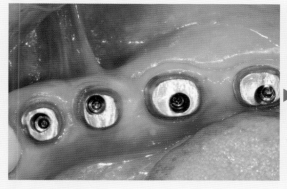

After final delivery
The position of the 37 implant is still disappointing. It should have been placed slightly more mesially, ignoring the 36 bone defect.

📷 1.13

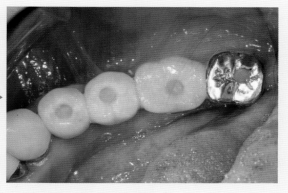

After the abutment insertion
There is no immediate post-operative clinical photo following the second stage surgery, but looking at this photo after the abutment is inserted, you can see nicely formed attached gingiva around the implant using Youngsam flap.

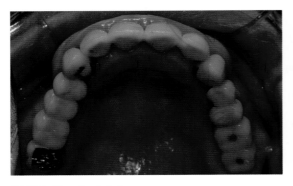
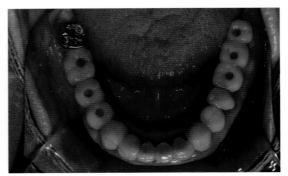

📷 **1.14** After final delivery

📷 **1.14** is the final delivery photo. As the patient refused the treatment of the second quadrant, the occlusal surface was lowered too much, and the occlusal plane on the right side was also slightly lowered as a result. In the case of the right side, since the top and bottom implants were done together, I was not too concerned about the height adjustment. I do not think I placed the implants too shallow, but the final crowns are disappointing. Maybe it was to match the height of the left side. This is an old case, so these are relatively long implants.

Perhaps, if the second quadrant had been treated together, the occlusal plane of the posterior mandible could have been raised, and the crowns could have looked better. Looking at the final height, it is disappointing in many ways. This is why I find prosthetics challenging, and I do not enjoy it.

If you look at the one-year follow-up panoramic radiograph, you can see that the crestal bone is stably maintained (📷 **1.15**). Even after five years, there is almost no change (📷 **1.16**), including the bridge in the second quadrant. I was a little embarrassed to see that the bridge in the second quadrant held up so well because I initially recommended replacing it, thinking it would not last this long. I once again realized that it is always better to observe and treat more conservatively.

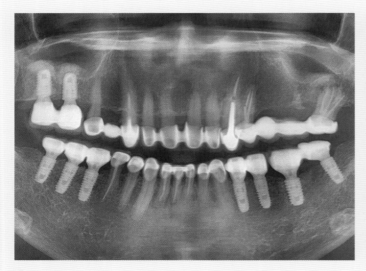
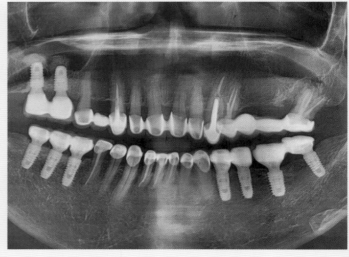

📷 **1.15** 1 year follow up panoramic radiograph after final delivery

📷 **1.16** 5 year follow up panoramic radiograph after final delivery

Wait!!

Which membrane to use?

When I started my implant training in the early 2000s, non-resorbable membranes were popular. Then, around 2005, when implant dentistry was in full swing and block bone grafts and ridge splinting became popular, resorbable membranes seemed to gain popularity. Because the bone itself acts as a tent, there was no need to use a membrane to maintain its shape. As the use of non-resorbable membranes decreased in Korea, imports of these materials were also temporarily suspended. Since I was doing a lot of dental insurance lectures, I was able to find out about the import and registration of these products. Then as we passed 2010, more emphasis was put on placing a shorter implant in the correct position rather than a large diameter and long implant, and the membranes that hold their shapes, such as titanium mesh or non-resorbable membranes, regained their popularity. Nowadays, it is becoming a trend to simplify and minimize the surgery itself, so a standard resorbable collagen membrane seems to be favored unless the tenting effect is required. Even the use of regular titanium mesh has decreased, and in cases with implant placement and simultaneous vertical or buccal grafting, the use of titanium mesh that inserts onto the implant fixture (SmartBuilder from Osstem) is increasing. The goal is to reduce trauma and the number of surgeries as much as possible. There is a lot of debate on whether to use a collagen membrane over the titanium mesh, but my decision always depends on the condition of the periosteum.

What to do if the membrane is exposed?

Depending on the membrane type, some may be fine getting exposed and some are intended to be exposed from the beginning. There is no need for me to know about the things that I do not use, so I will talk mainly about my experiences with the general collagen membranes that I use. When I was studying implant dentistry, I was taught that the collagen membrane should never be exposed. However, whether you are a lecturer or student, you may have been dismayed by the membrane exposure in cases where you thought the surgery went well. I have been there myself. Sometimes, it is fine until the next day, but when the patient comes back in 2 weeks to get the sutures removed, the membrane is exposed. The most crucial thing in grafting, in my opinion, is the blood supply. Many people say that flap tension is the worst, but I believe tension compromises the blood supply and causes tissue necrosis. Even when I thought my periosteal releasing incision was enough to relieve tension, there were times when things didn't go as expected (whether it is better to do the releasing incision before grafting or just before suturing is another topic to contemplate on). Anyway, when I noticed the membrane exposure on the day of the suture removal, I was too busy to redo the grafting, so I asked the patient to come back a few days later. However, when the patient returned, I witnessed the gum completely covering the membrane on several occasions. It is upsetting for anybody to see the exposed membrane after you have worked so hard to cover it. Some may boldly open it up again, remove everything, and re-graft. Or some may not know what to do, so they consult with other colleagues, study and research, just to find out that everything is okay at the next post-op appointment. Through this experience, some would learn that even if the membrane is exposed but without infection, observing without further intervention can often bring out decent results. And eventually, some would attempt to leave the membrane exposed on purpose, as in the open membrane technique. Therefore, I tell my students that it is best to close the flap without tension in the graft, but if the membrane is exposed soon after, think of it as an open membrane technique. And check it frequently but observe and wait.

Case using a membrane 2

When I posted this case of sinus elevation on social media, a colleague asked me if the lower implant case involved GBR (📷 1.17). So, I asked my staff to find the lower GBR case photos, and I uploaded them. It's just a pity that the rest of the photos are sparse.

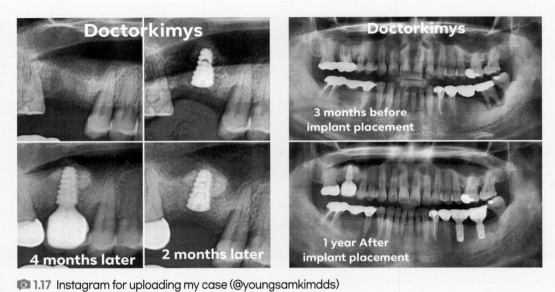

📷 1.17 Instagram for uploading my case (@youngsamkimdds)

The implant surgery was done three months after extraction, but the socket was not filled in sufficiently, as shown in the photo. So xenograft (Cerabone from Straumann) was used to graft the defect, a resorbable collagen membrane (OssGuide from Osstem) was used to cover the graft, and the flap was sutured. It is disappointing to see that the 37 implant was placed slightly lingually where the most bone was. Since the initial stability was adequate, the uncovery was performed a month and a half later. The impression was taken another month and a half later to deliver the final crown.

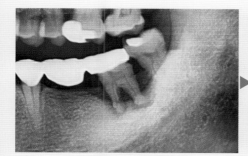

Initial panoramic radiograph before extraction

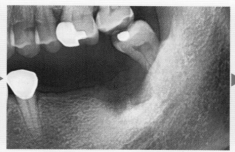

3 months after extraction

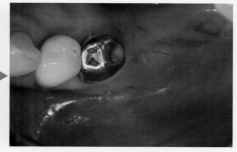

3 months after extraction, immeidately before implant placement

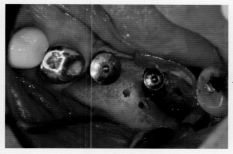

Decortication to prevent bone graft from slipping

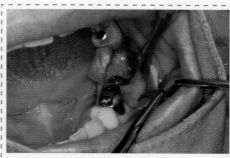

Due to large defect with compromised periosteum, I decided to use a membrane and tucked it on the lingual side.

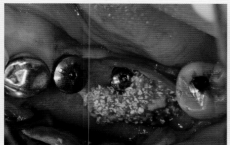

The defect was too large, so an autogenous bone was placed inside and a xenograft bone on top.

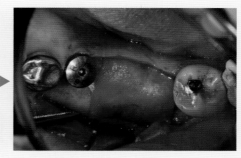

Membrane covering over the graft and immediately before suturing

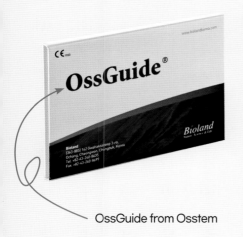

OssGuide from Osstem

📷 1.18

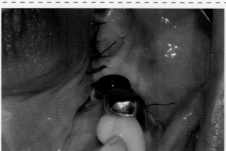

immediately after suturing

As a general rule, I use single interrupted sutures for most cases. I admit my suturing skills are not top-notch. I have a good sense of space, but I do not seem to have much dexterity in this field. So, if I teach the way I do, the students do not have a problem following.

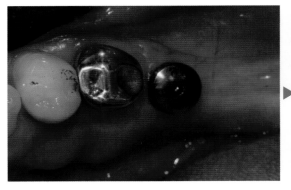

A month and a half after implant placement, just before the second surgery

After final restoration

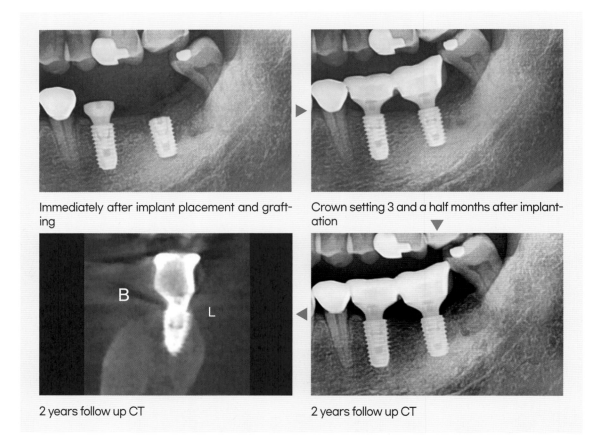

Immediately after implant placement and grafting

Crown setting 3 and a half months after implantation

2 years follow up CT

2 years follow up CT

📷 1.19

I consider complete gingival healing (thickness restored to the same as before surgery) to be crucial, so I tend to do the second stage surgery as soon as possible when staging my surgeries. You can see the beautiful bone formation in a CT scan taken two years after implant placement (📷 1.19). I cannot comment on the bone quality, but it has been maintained well for over four years so far (📷 1.20, 1.21).

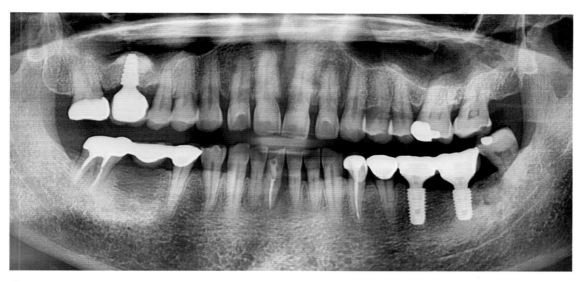

📷 1.20 3 year follow up

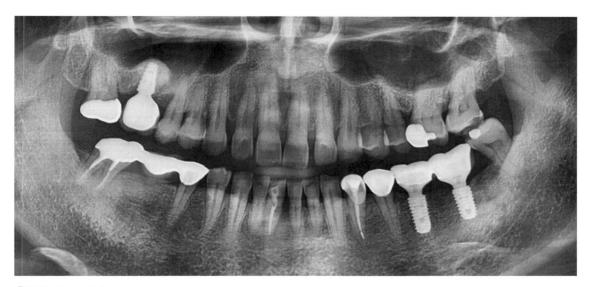

📷 1.21 4 year follow up

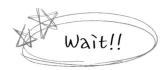
Wait!!

I do not have many clinical photos taken during surgery.

I do not take clinical photos myself diligently, and my staffs take them when they have time. But they are often also swamped. I usually work with three dental hygienists as a team. The last time I checked in April 2021 right before writing this book, I worked 18 days, extracted 463 wisdom teeth, and placed 48 implants in that single month. Considering that I usually do not get to see even half of the patients I used to see because I have to run a live surgery course four days a week, I am simply too busy to take photos. On the other hand, there are many cases where I am too impatient and quick-tempered to take photos in the middle of surgery and want to finish the surgery quickly. So, there are many before and after photos but only few mid-surgery photos. Moreover, Korean patients tend to be very sensitive about taking pictures during surgery. So please forgive the lack of proper procedure photos. Sometimes these surgeries are so common that I feel like photos are unnecessary. That is why most of the well-documented cases are my acquaintances.

When do I place an implant after extraction?

A few years ago, a survey was conducted among Korean dentists about when they prefer to place an implant following a tooth extraction, and most of them answered "about a month and a half" at the time. However, nowadays, I tend to place it immediately as long as I can achieve good primary stability. Placing after a month and a half would basically mean giving enough time for the soft tissue to heal but not the bone. I had done it that way for a while, but not these days. If the bone condition is good and there is no need for a lot of graft during implant placement, the implant can be placed anytime without any problem. However, suppose there was a significant infection with extensive bone loss around the tooth, and it requires a lot of bone grafting at the time of implant placement. In that case, I think it is better to wait up to three months instead, not just for the primary soft tissue healing. The case would most likely be completed in a similar time frame. It is essential to have bone formation to some extent during the healing because this would help achieve primary stability and enable us to place the implant in the correct position. Even so, the most important thing for me is the proper healing of the soft tissue. Especially in the case of the mandibular first molar, the soft tissue at about a month and a half after extraction is still thinner than usual. It is not just a matter of thickness but the blood supply may be limited from the soft tissue and mostly comes from the socket below. Therefore, after cleaning out the socket and placing an implant, there are many cases in which the soft tissue necroses and loses more volume after the surgery. Moreover, if a membrane is used, the blood supply is further compromised, and the soft tissue above the membrane may not survive. This is not something I read somewhere, but strictly from my own experience.

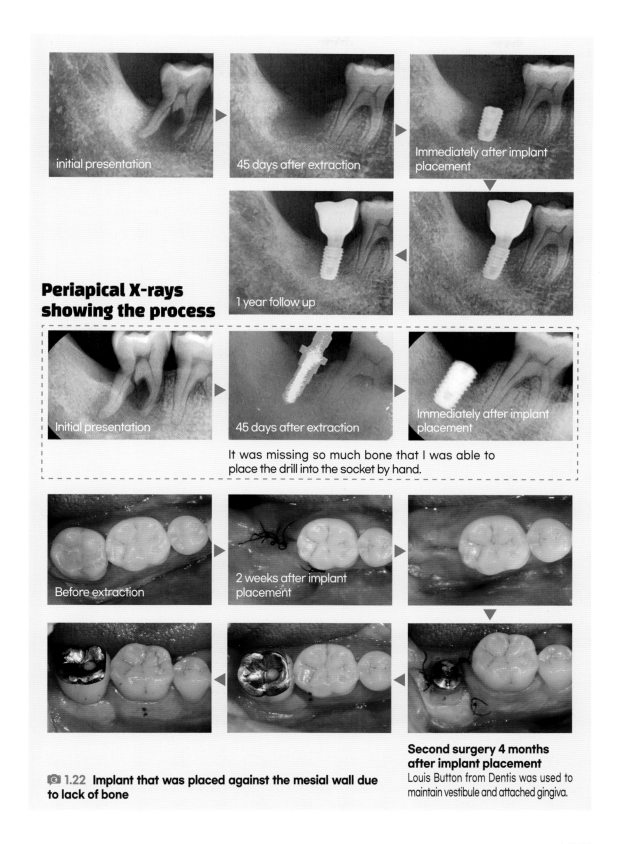

Periapical X-rays showing the process

initial presentation

45 days after extraction

Immediately after implant placement

1 year follow up

Initial presentation

45 days after extraction

Immediately after implant placement

It was missing so much bone that I was able to place the drill into the socket by hand.

Before extraction

2 weeks after implant placement

Second surgery 4 months after implant placement
Louis Button from Dentis was used to maintain vestibule and attached gingiva.

📷 1.22 **Implant that was placed against the mesial wall due to lack of bone**

In 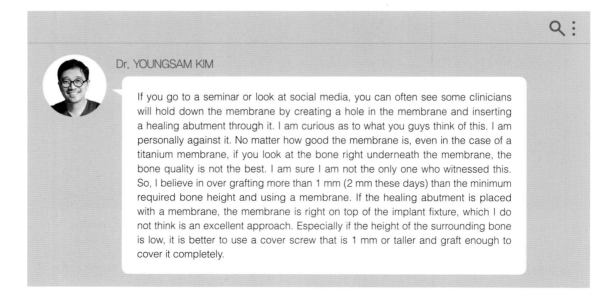 **1.22** case, it was practically impossible to place the implant because our staff booked the surgery appointment too early. We have a lot of patients who would go through extraction and decide whether they want to proceed with implant surgery in the future, and my staff will often automatically set up their appointments in a month and a half. However, there is no way that a case like this would have a socket filled in with bone in a month and a half. The position of the implant is not ideal by my standard. Because it was missing so much bone, the osteotomy sequence involved just one drilling with the final osteotomy drill, and initial stability was extremely poor. I left the fixture against the mesial wall where there was some bone present. Sometimes I prefer a 0.5-1.0 mm high cover screw, but I used a regular cover screw for this case because I was concerned about the stability. After scraping off all the granulation tissue, I just placed the fixture by my hand and screwed the cover screw, then decided to close the flap without bone graft or membrane. The surrounding bone was at a higher level than the top of the implant fixture, so it seemed to be in a good position for spontaneous bone formation. Since the bone quality is always the best with the spontaneously formed autogenous bone compared to grafted bone, I do not graft where the bone is likely to develop anyway. The second stage surgery was performed four months later due to poor initial bone condition. During the second surgery, I used the Youngsam flap with Louis Button from Dentis, and achieved the vestibule deepening and increased attached gingiva. It has been three years since the surgery, and I want to bring the patient back for a follow-up, but the patient refuses to come in because it is inconvenient to travel during the pandemic. However, the patient reports the implant is functioning well without any problems.

Dr. YOUNGSAM KIM

If you go to a seminar or look at social media, you can often see some clinicians will hold down the membrane by creating a hole in the membrane and inserting a healing abutment through it. I am curious as to what you guys think of this. I am personally against it. No matter how good the membrane is, even in the case of a titanium membrane, if you look at the bone right underneath the membrane, the bone quality is not the best. I am sure I am not the only one who witnessed this. So, I believe in over grafting more than 1 mm (2 mm these days) than the minimum required bone height and using a membrane. If the healing abutment is placed with a membrane, the membrane is right on top of the implant fixture, which I do not think is an excellent approach. Especially if the height of the surrounding bone is low, it is better to use a cover screw that is 1 mm or taller and graft enough to cover it completely.

Titanium mesh

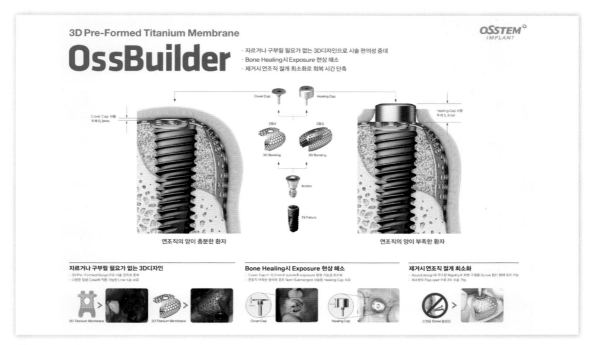

📷 **1.23** Osstem has changed the name of this titanium membrane several times and now calls it OssBuilder. Its name changes so often, so I am not even sure what the current name is. In any case, SmartMembrane, SmartBuilder, and OssBuilder are all the same.

If the ridge is very thin and the narrow span is long, or you need to increase the vertical height, a titanium mesh connected to the implant fixture can be used. Maybe because I am not a meticulous surgeon, using regular titanium mesh in vertical grafting took too long and was difficult, and the results were not good for the amount of effort. Patients also seemed to experience more discomfort. So, I made a tent out of titanium and used it on top of the implant. In 2009, I visited Osstem's headquarters, drew and shared my ideas, and named it "Bone Cover". Later, Osstem made a prototype and gave it to me, and I used it for a while. It is 100% identical to the concept of the Smart Membrane on the market now, and it had the same fixation system using the prosthetic abutment in the early days. These days, they came up with a fixation system designed specifically for Smart Builders, and the usage has improved. Shortly after that, Osstem manufactured and started selling this product. That is why I was not fond of Osstem for a while. Later, I asked them to at least list my name as one of the developers, but the request was ignored. The prototype Osstem made for me at that time was too thick, and you had to bend the curve on the buccal side yourself, so it was challenging to make it smooth and round. And perhaps due to the impurities in the titanium alloys, the bone formation in the mandible was a little slow and had some soft tissue ingrowth. I wish I had been more passionate about communicating with the staff and putting more effort into product development. Later, as I became more recognized as a dentist and I was on good terms with Osstem,

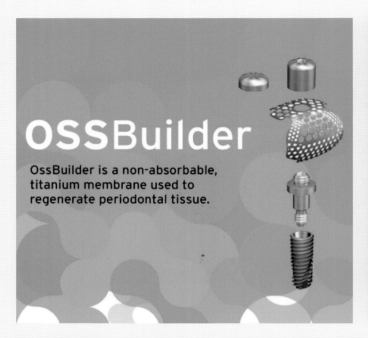

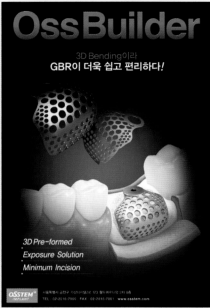

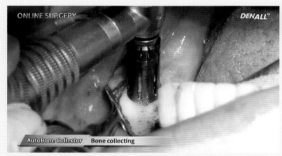

https://youtu.be/ezY8mHIqYSc
The case by the dentist with golden hands, whom I call Yuna Kim of dentistry.

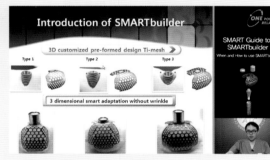

https://youtu.be/kgfTXl3ghBE
Lecture from a rising star dentist who I call a 'trending man'

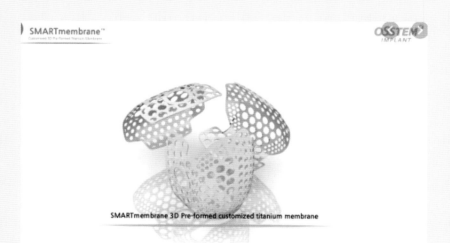

https:// youtu.be/ FnWNmHabKPc
Introductory video on OssBuilder from Osstem.

📷 1.24 **Videos on OssBuilder from Osstem**

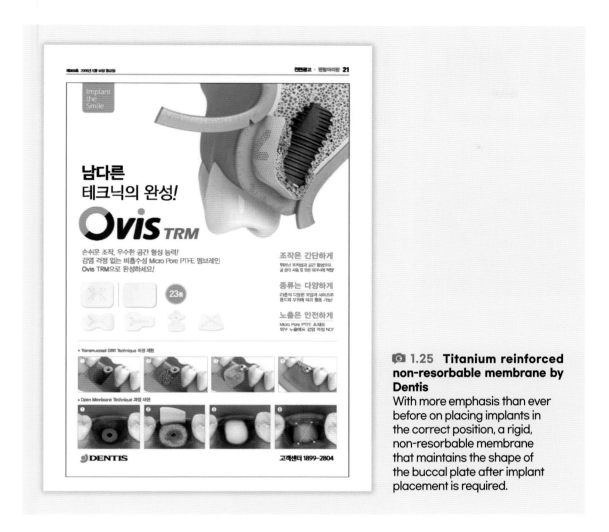

📷 1.25 **Titanium reinforced non-resorbable membrane by Dentis**
With more emphasis than ever before on placing implants in the correct position, a rigid, non-resorbable membrane that maintains the shape of the buccal plate after implant placement is required.

I brought up the story, and they told me that employee had been out of the company for a while and all the records were gone (even though they made the prototype). Anyway, this is the concept I thought of even before these products came out on the market, but now many companies are using titanium mesh this way.

These days, I use only OssBuilder from Osstem sometimes, but the frequency is decreasing with the use of a collagen bone that maintains a proper bone shape relatively well. It can still be useful for vertical augmentation of 2-3 mm. After placing OssBuilder, which is a titanium mesh, there are different opinions among surgeons as to whether or not to use a regular collagen membrane on top of it. But as I mentioned before, I do not use a collagen membrane if the periosteum is cleanly peeled off and only use it if the periosteum is compromised. Instructions are self-explanatory for these titanium mesh type of membrane, so anyone can easily use it just by looking at the product catalog (📷 1.25).

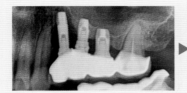

Panoramic radiograph at the time of the first visit

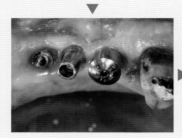

Immediately before implant removal

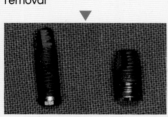

25 implant was left as it was, and only 24 26 implants were removed. Partially, it is because I am very conservative in my treatment planning, and also the patient expressed the psychological burden of having to remove all of them. So I decided not to remove 25 implant, which was in relatively good condition. 25 implant seems to have helped maintain the residual bone as a result.

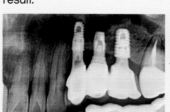

Panoramic radiograph 15 months after the final prostheses.
Vertical augmentation at 24 and also the sinus augmentation at 26 are clearly ossified.

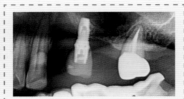

Radiograph 6 months after implant removal

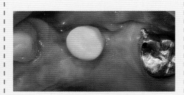

Clinical photo 6 months after implant removal. Severe resorption of buccal bone at 24.

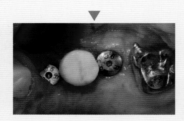

Before the impression

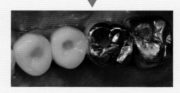

8 months after implant placement and immediately after the final prostheses are inserted.

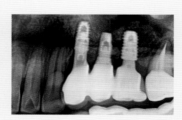

Panoramic radiograph after final prostheses
The prosthetic treatment was completed 8 months after implant placement, not for any specific reason, but because the patient did not visit the clinic on time.

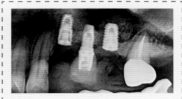

A titanium mesh was used at the same time as implant placement, and the height of the implant was matched to the expected bone height of 25 implant.

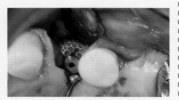

There was no clinical photo at the time of implant placement and grafting, but I found one clinical photo from the day of membrane removal.

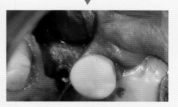

Good bone formation is visible immediately after membrane removal.

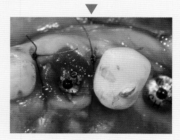

Healing abutment was inserted and sutured.

📷 1.26

Case using titanium mesh 1

Let's look at the case using titanium mesh. I prefer short implants, so I don't get to perform vertical augmentation very often. However, this case had a vertical and severe buccal bone loss, so it was necessary to use the titanium mesh to keep the height of the bone at the same level as the adjacent implant. There was a severe infection around the implants at the initial presentation, but because the patient was busy, we only drained the infection and eventually decided to have them removed. The implant at 25 was not removed and was left in place.

Reason for not removing 25 implant

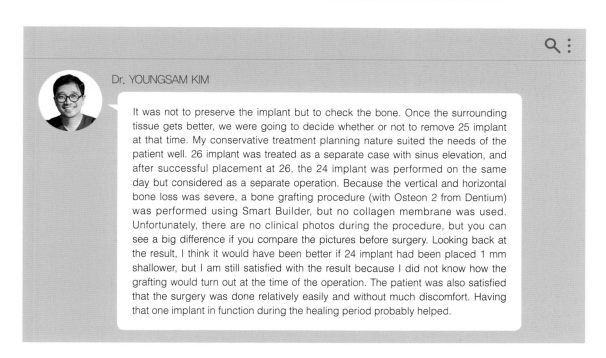

Dr. YOUNGSAM KIM

It was not to preserve the implant but to check the bone. Once the surrounding tissue gets better, we were going to decide whether or not to remove 25 implant at that time. My conservative treatment planning nature suited the needs of the patient well. 26 implant was treated as a separate case with sinus elevation, and after successful placement at 26, the 24 implant was performed on the same day but considered as a separate operation. Because the vertical and horizontal bone loss was severe, a bone grafting procedure (with Osteon 2 from Dentium) was performed using Smart Builder, but no collagen membrane was used. Unfortunately, there are no clinical photos during the procedure, but you can see a big difference if you compare the pictures before surgery. Looking back at the result, I think it would have been better if 24 implant had been placed 1 mm shallower, but I am still satisfied with the result because I did not know how the grafting would turn out at the time of the operation. The patient was also satisfied that the surgery was done relatively easily and without much discomfort. Having that one implant in function during the healing period probably helped.

Case using titanium mesh 2

A 73-year-old male patient came to the clinic complaining of a lot of pain in the lower left jaw. Root canal treatment was attempted at the Endodontic Department, but it was eventually diagnosed as non-restorable, and extraction was performed. It is not visible on the panoramic radiograph, but 36 had severe buccal bone loss. Two months later, implant surgery was performed, but more than half of the implant was exposed on the buccal side. Moreover, the periosteum was compromised, and the area of bone loss was filled with granulation tissue, so a collagen membrane was used. Since the bone loss site was too wide and the bone graft material could not be maintained stably, a titanium mesh

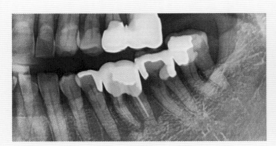

Panoramic radiograph at first visit

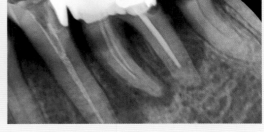

Root canal treatment was performed for 35, but it was eventually determined to be extracted and 4 teeth were extracted from 35 to 38.

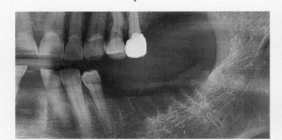

Panoramic radiograph 2 months after extraction

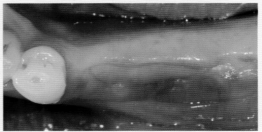

Clinical photo 2 months after extraction.
In the photo, it looks voluminous, but 36 buccal was filled with granulation tissue.

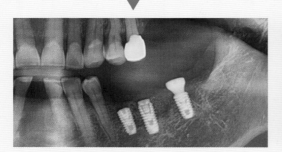

Radiograph immediately after implant placement.
36 Implant is covered with titanium mesh on 1 mm height anchor.

📷 1.27

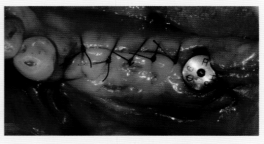

Clinical photo immediately after implant placement.
The thick granulation tissue soft tissue on the buccal side was removed, and the releasing incision was sufficiently performed and sutured.

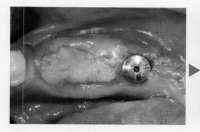

15 days after implant placement and immediately after suture removal.
As expected, the gingiva on the graft material died and the collagen membrane was exposed.

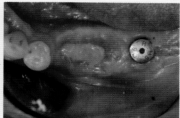

After 11 days, 26 days after implant placement.
Gradual gingival healing over the graft.

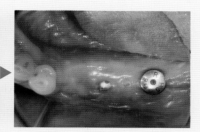

After 30 days, 56 days after implant placement.
The collagen membrane resorbed faster than the speed of gingival healing, so the titanium mesh is visible.

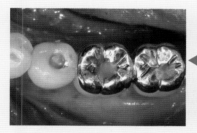

15 months after final prostheses insertion.
It is strange to see that there is still excess resin on the occlusal surface even though it has been in function for 15 months. Did it get replaced recently or did it not function at all? Prosthetics are very difficult!

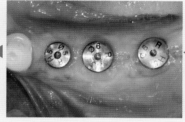

Immediately after impression, 6 and a half months after implant placement.
We could have done it sooner, but we were waiting to do the impression together with the maxillary implants that were placed after the mandibular implants.

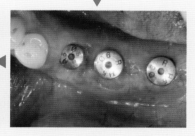

5 months after implant placement.
The sutures were removed after uncovering 35 implant. Unfortunately, there are no photos before or during the uncovery surgery. As I recall, the soft tissue healed over the titanium mesh by itself.

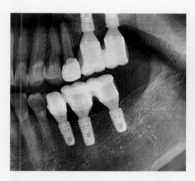

After final prostheses insertion

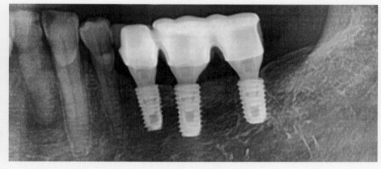

15 months after final prostheses insertion.
The bone height is maintained very well.

📷 1.28

was used, and a collagen membrane was draped over it (titanium mesh - OssBuilder® by Osstem, collagen membrane - Ovis® membrane by Dentis, bone graft material - synthetic bone Q-Oss® by Osstem).

I usually use a 5 mm high healing abutment unless a membrane is used. So, 37 implant received a 5 mm healing abutment on the day of implant placement. However, many people wonder why I did not wait until the uncovery of other implants. It is partially just a force of habit, but the healing abutment can also serve as a reference point later. The new soft tissue at the extraction site is not suitable for GBR. In my experience, this is true, not just in this case, but in most implant surgeries as well. The newly formed gingiva on top of the extraction site receives blood supply mainly from the socket, and this is probably because sufficient blood circulation has not yet been established in the gingiva on the vestibule side. That is why when I place an implant only a month and a half after tooth extraction, I would prefer not to do GBR that relies on the gingival tissue. Instead, I would prefer to place a healing abutment and perform a simple GBR without membrane on the buccal side. In this case, the blood supply must have been interrupted further, especially since all the thick soft tissues on the buccal side were removed using a scalpel. Moreover, since excessive bone grafting was performed with titanium mesh and collagen membrane, no matter how well the releasing incision and passive flap closure were done, there is a very high possibility of necrosis due to lack of blood supply. However, the bone defect was so significant that there was no other option. So, I don't usually use a membrane on a titanium mesh, but I covered the titanium mesh with a collagen membrane with the possibility of exposure in mind.

This patient had severe sinusitis, which negatively impacted the outcome of sinus elevation. The sinus elevation at the extraction sites of 16 26 did not turn out well. It should have been confirmed by CT, but it is probably because the surgery was performed in a state with incomplete healing of the sinus membrane. Synthetic bone Q-oss from Osstem was also used for sinus grafting, but after a long period of time, it does not ossify as pretty as a xenograft but has a partially resorbed candy-like shape. Usually, I use xenograft in Sinus Elevations, so I am not sure why I chose to use synthetic bone in this case... It is a case of many regrets.

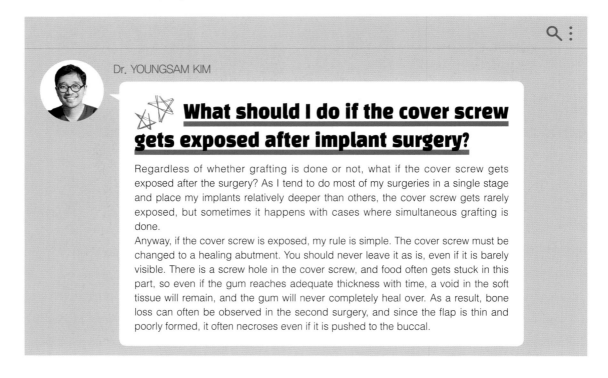

Dr. YOUNGSAM KIM

What should I do if the cover screw gets exposed after implant surgery?

Regardless of whether grafting is done or not, what if the cover screw gets exposed after the surgery? As I tend to do most of my surgeries in a single stage and place my implants relatively deeper than others, the cover screw gets rarely exposed, but sometimes it happens with cases where simultaneous grafting is done.

Anyway, if the cover screw is exposed, my rule is simple. The cover screw must be changed to a healing abutment. You should never leave it as is, even if it is barely visible. There is a screw hole in the cover screw, and food often gets stuck in this part, so even if the gum reaches adequate thickness with time, a void in the soft tissue will remain, and the gum will never completely heal over. As a result, bone loss can often be observed in the second surgery, and since the flap is thin and poorly formed, it often necroses even if it is pushed to the buccal.

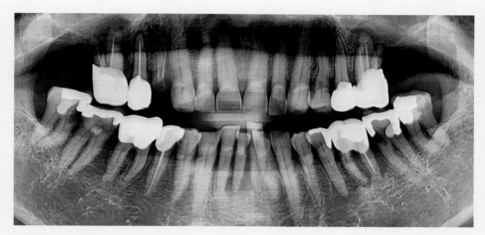

Initial presentation

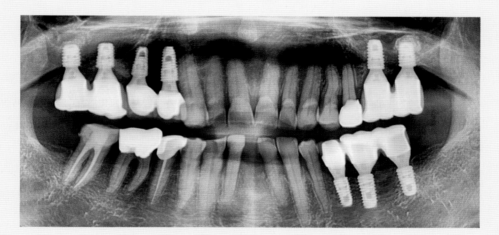

10 months after implant placement, 4 months after final prostheses.

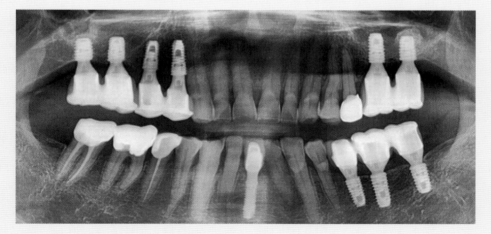

3 year follow up

📷 1.29

6-2

Bone Graft Material

Bone Graft Material

In this chapter, we are going to talk about bone graft materials. I have already talked about it somewhat in the previous chapter, so I will briefly describe it as my grafting style is often simple. Since I like to have my implants short and deep, I tend to worry less about bone grafting than other clinicians. Here is a brief summary of my philosophy on bone grafting:

1. Bone makes bone.
2. Bone graft materials do not turn into bone all at once but slowly change into the bone from the closest part to the native bone (I treat my cases with the assumption that it occurs approximately 1 mm per month). I tell my students to just memorize the following statement. The bone grows at a rate of 1 mm per month, and soft tissue grows at a rate of 1 mm per day. I tell them to memorize it simply, but to be honest, it seems that bone grows slightly more than 1 mm per month, and gum appears to grow slightly less than 1 mm per day.
3. Grafts do not make bone. It only maintains the space.
4. Since bone is formed by 1 mm a month from the native bone, the bone graft material not only maintains the space but also the time for the bone formation.
5. Rather than the bone graft material becoming bone, it is more appropriate to say that the bone permeates through the graft material like water.
6. Bone quality is best when it is made by itself without any grafting
7. Bone created with non-resorbable bone graft material has a weak defense mechanism against infection. However, even if it is vulnerable to infection and bone resorption progresses, the framework remains (based on xenograft).

Therefore, my philosophy for bone grafting is to "use non-resorbable bone graft material but use as little as possible." I try to keep bone grafting as simple as possible. This is because bone grafting should be simple to have fewer complications and a higher probability of success. First of all, it is a waste of time to list and explain the types of bone graft materials. I will write my thoughts assuming the readers know all the different types. The following chart shows the ability of a bone graft material to become bone.

Autograft ❯ Allograft ❯ Xenograft ❯ Synthetic bone

This sequence can be found in any book or lecture. But I don't think I have ever seen clear reasoning anywhere. In my opinion, this order is somewhat abstract. It may be different depending on which material is grafted in which site, and it will even differ depending on the manufacturer. If it is a xenograft, it may be different depending on what kind of animal it is from, and if it is a synthetic bone, it may be different depending on the type and ratio of its components. I'll just share my thoughts on each type of bone graft material here.

Autograft

Harvesting and using the patient's own bone is obviously the most economical. However, instruments used for harvesting and grinding autogenous bone were expensive in the past. These days, technologies for processing and using autogenous bone have developed, but the price is still quite high. For the purposes of our discussion, we will assume we have a small amount of autogenous bone that is ready to use.

I do not intentionally collect autogenous bones. However, suppose I have an autogenous bone that was somehow obtained during surgery. In that case, it is only used to maintain space temporarily, such as the deepest part of the socket or the bottom of the sinus elevation. My philosophy is simple. The body's first signal to the wounded bone is to die immediately. Therefore, even if the wounded bone fragments are collected and grafted, there is nothing to expect other than the ability to maintain a temporary space until it is absorbed. Only autogenous bone can indeed induce bone formation, but time and space must be secured for bone formation. However, autogenous bone is rarely used alone because it is difficult to secure the time. Therefore, it is selectively used only in places that will quickly turn into bone anyway.

I'm not going to discuss ridge splinting or block bone grafting here. I am aware there are situations in which these techniques may be required, but I personally do not use them and think most readers will not need them.

Some say that the bone quality is the best when the autogenous bone is used for grafting, but I believe the bone quality is said to be good because the bone is formed where it was to be formed anyway, and all the autogenous bone is absorbed, and new bone is created. As I write this, I feel a bit sorry for my own bones, as it might sound like I am disparaging autogenous bone. The autogenous bone may, in fact, be the best bone, but it would be more accurate to say that it may not be as important to my style of a surgeon because I only perform necessary bone grafts as minimally as possible.

Allograft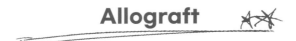

An allograft is bone processed from another human. It mainly refers to demineralized freeze-dried bone allografts (DFDBA). I rarely use allograft these days, so I do not know what is popular. **It is known that allograft has osteoinductive properties and thus helps bone formation, but I have always questioned it.** It is made by processing other person's bones, and the first prerequisite for the processing is that most of the remaining protein needs to be removed to minimize immunological rejection. But how is it supposed to get into another person's body and make bone? Rather than selectively leaving only the BMP in the allograft, I think it might be better to use another type of bone graft material with only osteoconductive property and add the BMP. When I searched the papers on the osteoinductive property of allograft, I could not find anything convincing, and most of them were very old. **Many believe it because it has been said for a long time.** Nowadays, I see many other colleagues who are also skeptical about this.

The biggest problem with the allograft is that most of it gets resorbed after a reasonable amount of time. It may vary from product to product, but you can see it disappearing almost formless after a few weeks. In the case of an immediate implant following a tooth extraction, I have seen many instances in which the graft material was placed in the gap, whether it is in the alveolar bone or soft tissue zone. The belief was that the bone under the crest would become bone, and the bone above the crest would become soft tissue, and so on. If a non-resorbable bone is placed, particles will remain in the soft tissue after the gums are healed, so it seems that allograft is preferred. Allograft can be placed in the gap without great care, but if you are using non-resorbable material, it is necessary to insert the bone right up to the crest and seal it well to prevent it from leaking out. This is probably the most tricky part.

Regardless of whether it becomes bone or not, the biggest advantage and disadvantage of the allograft is that it is resorbed relatively quickly. Therefore, it may be suitable for places where the bone is going to form anyway, but it is not very good for areas such as outside the cortical bone, where it takes longer to become bone, or for areas that need to resist resorption in the future. As a result, I eventually stopped using it because it did not fit well with my philosophy of using the minimal amount of material for absolutely necessary grafts.

In the early days, I used to use allograft materials from various companies until about ten years ago because of their claim to be effective in bone grafting. However, there were many cases where it had already resorbed when I revisited the site for the second surgery. Especially in the buccal region of the maxillary anterior teeth, most of the material appears to resorb before new bone is formed. And

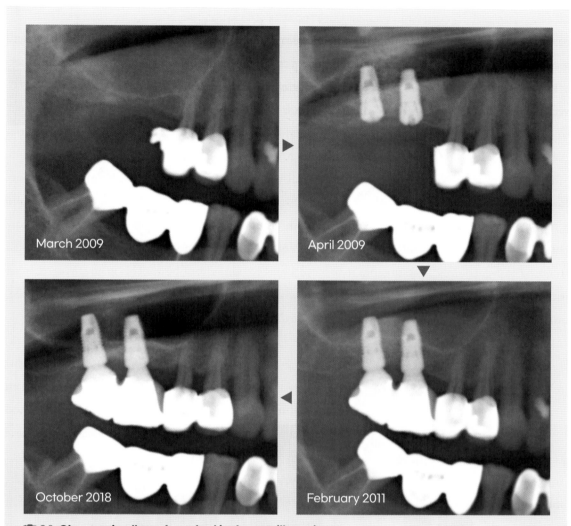

📷 2.1 Changes in allograft grafted in the maxillary sinus.
An allogenic FDBA cortical chip bone material was used in lateral window sinus elevation. You can see it is almost gone in a few years.

March 2009

April 2009

October 2018

February 2011

even in the extraction socket where the jump gap is relatively large between the immediate implant and buccal cortical bone, like in the maxillary canine site, if the jump gap is grafted with allograft, you can see the resorption of buccal cortical bone and grafted bone with time. Allografts may have secured space, but it does not seem to secure time.

There have been some putty-type allograft bones in the market. In the past, OrthoBlast was popular for a while and then disappeared, and in North America, you have AlloOss Allograft Putty and MinerOss Putty, which are bone putty that can be injected into the sinus. I am very much against this. Bone putty material prevents the native bone cells from permeating into the graft, but it also resorbs after a while. In addition, if the sinus membrane is perforated when the putty-type bone is placed into the sinus, the material is not easily removed. If you use particulate bone, most of them will drain through the ostium, but bone putty will not.

Xenograft

Bio-Oss is the most popular example of xenograft. Since it is from a different species or animal, xenografts are processed to remove all the organic components but maintain the mineral component to provide an osteoconductive matrix. It has been observed in many cases where the graft material does not resorb over time and maintains the framework.

That is why I use the xenograft bone material the most. As mentioned earlier about the short implant, there is no need to place very long and large diameter implants, and thus it does not require a lot of bone. I believe that a bone graft of 2 mm around the implant is sufficient. There are many patients who function with implants with threads exposed outside the bone, so I do not see the need to do extensive, complicated surgeries to achieve a massive amount of bone. This is not to say that we should cut corners. I practice implant dentistry with high standards and always strive for excellence, but you can say that where I put emphasis may be different from others.

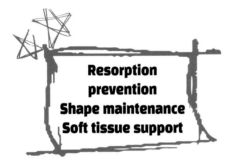

Resorption prevention
Shape maintenance
Soft tissue support

Bone grafting is done not to turn into bone. The role of bone graft material, in my opinion, is to **prevent resorption, maintain shape, and support soft tissue.** Of course, the three may sound like the same thing, but I emphasize this because they have subtle differences.

In a typical scenario, I would place the implant in the correct position and depth, and wherever some threads are exposed vertically and buccally, I would use xenograft to graft around it. **I consider it sufficient to place the xenograft material 1-2 mm higher than the implant platform and about 2 mm thick horizontally.** Since we are assuming that bone forms 1 mm per month, we proceed with prosthetics considering that bones will be adequately formed in two or three months.

So even in the case of vertical dehiscence of the buccal side, the xenograft bone is grafted with a 2-3 mm thickness. I hardly over-graft. The larger your graft is, the longer it takes to become bone, and if the bone graft is too large, there is a possibility that the graft may even give up on becoming bone (I know this is not very scientific, but I could not find a better way to describe it).

As you may have guessed, I only use xenograft for maxillary sinus elevation these days. There is no need to raise the sinus too much because I am not using long implants. So, how about if the implant is placed in the extraction socket? I leave the deepest part of the socket as it is since it will fill in with bone naturally, but if the buccal plate is thin, the plate may resorb much faster than the rate at which the bone is formed, and I may lightly place xenograft between the implant and the buccal plate. If you place too much xenograft inside the socket, the bone quality around the implant may not be ideal, so I tend to put the bare minimum.

Degree of bone resorption

I consider xenograft bone the best option for shape maintenance, so how about looking at the ratio of remaining bone graft material in the bone in general?

Xenograft > Synthetic bone > Allograft > Autograft

In general, most people would agree on the above order. Myself and everyone else say the same thing. Many research data and clinical reviews show that xenograft particles remain almost intact even after some time. That does not mean it has not disappeared at all. Some of it probably has resorbed, but it does not seem so because the scaffold remains.

Autogenous bone resorbs the most. As mentioned earlier, the body needs injured or separated bone to die quickly to make room for new bone. That is why autogenous bone particles will die and resorb. However, depending on the case, if a large piece of bone is stably fixated, it may survive through a simultaneous process of resorption and ossification. Once it heals and hardens, it will be impossible to distinguish whether it is the grafted bone or new bone, so you may say none remains. It may be more appropriate to state that autogenous bone has a faster resorption rate rather than that the remaining ratio is low. However, looking at the block bone grafts I've done in the past, I witness that the shape is well maintained, but I do not know how to interpret it. Maybe I should not make such a statement about autogenous bone.

Allograft has the 2nd fastest resorption rate. There are many types of allografts, but they all resorb whether DFDBA or FDBA. That is also the case in my experience. But the resorption rate is so fast that it is often surprising. Many people use FDBA cortical chip for that reason, but ultimately there is no significant difference, so I rarely use it. Its clinical use is decreasing in Korea, but it is being used a lot in North America. It seems that novice clinicians tend to use it without putting much thought into it. But anyone who has ever used an allograft in a buccal defect and ever opened it again will be terrified to use it again. I did not have to go through many of these horrible experiences myself because once you experience it a couple of times, you do not need to keep trying. Once, I had grafted allograft in the jump gap between a thin cortical bone and an implant following immediate implant placement in the maxillary canine. When I opened the site for the second surgery, I saw that the cortical bone was completely gone along with all the allograft material. Using an allograft may not be the only reason for the results, but I have never used an allograft since. The case was completed after re-grafting xenograft over the implant that was exposed on the buccal side during the second surgery.

Lastly, there is a synthetic bone between xenograft and allograft. In fact, synthetic bone can vary depending on the composition and ratio. There may even be some that are less resorbable than xenograft. Of course, since they are not usually made with such composition and ratio, most of them fall in the same order as above. Now, let's talk about synthetic bone.

The biggest drawback of xenograft such as Bio-Oss is that it is too expensive. There are more economical domestic options out in the market, but if you get burnt in a few cases, you will realize that cheaper does not always mean better. Knowing the method of processing the xenograft is one thing, and **the manufacturers perfecting the processing technology is another thing.** Sometimes, I wonder if that is why I have been burnt in the past.

Synthetic bone

As mentioned earlier, unfortunately, implant-related research has long been commercialized rather than scientific. It is almost impossible to see related cases or read the articles without bias. Looking at the order of ability to form bone mentioned earlier, synthetic bone was said to be the worst. Still, there are many cases in which we see drastic bone formation by the synthetic bone, almost as impressive as the healing of the lame man in a prayer hall. There are also many related papers, but I do not see many people genuinely interested in it. Synthetic bone can really vary depending on its composition and ratio. Here we will talk about two of the most commonly used ones.

Hydroxyapatite (HA)

Because it is the main component of tooth and bone, it is a very familiar name to all dentists. No other explanation is needed but just remember this. HA is classified as a non-resorbable bone graft material because of its prolonged decomposition rate and mainly plays a role in maintaining volume in synthetic bone.

Beta-Tricalcium Phosphate (β-TCP)

Since its main components are calcium and phosphate, this serves as a source of raw materials for bone formation. However, it is quickly resorbed due to its fast decomposition rate.

There are different methods to see the resorption rate by ❶ soaking in a solution, ❷ animal tests, and ❸ clinical trials, but the most important thing is when it is absorbed in clinical practice. In the papers that summarized these, it is reported that "In humans, β-TCP is mostly absorbed after 6-12 months". If β-TCP is indeed absorbed at this rate, it should be able to maintain the graft volume initially and gets absorbed at an ideal rate as the new bone is formed.

β-tricalcium phosphate as bone substitute material: properties and clinical applications

Important Content

Unlike bovine-derived grafts, pure β-tricalcium phosphate is mostly absorbed and replaced with the vital bone after six months in animal studies and has the advantage of not having an immune reaction, so it is considered an ideal material for bone grafts.

Journal of Osseointegration. 2010.

Most synthetic bones are mainly composed of the two components mentioned above and are called BCP (biphasic calcium phosphate). If you look at foreign products, there are various types, such as those with natural ingredients, calcium sulfate, etc., but since the two are the main components, I would like to talk about the ratio of the two components first.

I don't have many memories of foreign synthetic bones. It's probably because I often used the Bio-Oss. However, due to my relationship with many vendors, I have used countless materials here and there.

The material that I have used the most and am still using is Osteon of Dentium. I purchased Dentium implants around 2005 and started using Osteon together. I remember that when the flap was re-opened for the second surgery, it felt very different from other bone graft materials. I could not tell if the bone was formed inside, but most of the particles were still visible on the outside, and some came off during surgery. This was perhaps because the Osteon I used at the time was Osteon 1, which consists of 70% of HA, and therefore was hardly resorbable. After that, Osteon 2 was released in 2011 with different ratio of HA and β-TCP, and HA was reduced to 30%. Since then, I have not used Dentium products much, so I hardly used Osteon 2 myself, but it became one of the biggest hits in the synthetic bone market in South Korea. As a result, many similar products followed, mainly those with a HA ratio of 20-30%. So, when I tried similar products with similar proportions, my experience was not too bad. I particularly liked that β-TCP was radiopaque and came out white and pretty on the X-ray when grafted in the maxillary sinus. However, I still prefer and recommend using xenograft in the sinus.

It would be helpful to understand the context of when Osteon 2 was released. Back then, procedures like ridge splinting and block bone grafts were quite popular. As a result, bone materials to temporarily maintain space between block bone and native bone were needed. Therefore, I believe that β-TCP with a slower resorption rate was preferred over other expensive allografts. Since it was the era of large surgery, a huge amount of bone was being used while the price of implant treatment in South Korea was dropping significantly, so synthetic bone became popular as a cost-effective option (only my opinion).

Nowadays, surgeries have become smaller and less invasive, and there is no need for a lot of grafting. So the trend in bone grafting has also changed to prefer a minimal amount of non-resorbable bone graft material. That is why Dentium, which is leading the synthetic bone market, **made Osteon 3 in 2016, which increased the non-resorbable HA ratio to 60%.** You should always take the information distributed by the company with caution, but when used, it actually seems to ossify well and maintains its shape stably. Of course, it remains to be seen whether a high-quality bone is formed and maintained in the long term and is resistant to external environmental changes such as inflammation. As Dentium is leading the synthetic bone market with Osteon, I predict other companies will produce similar bone graft materials with a higher proportion of HA. I often use synthetic bone because of its cost-effectiveness. In particular, bone with high β-TCP, which has a high resorption rate, can be used for socket grafting. However, **if I want to use the minimal required amount in absolutely necessary sites, I would use xenograft with a proven track record.** Currently, A-Oss, xenograft from Osstem, is used the most. If you want to use xenograft, I would highly recommend ones that are proven and validated. If you simply use it because it is cheap or given to you as a free gift, you may experience terrible results.

However, in my opinion, the difference in technology between the companies is not as significant for synthetic bone compared to xenografts. When it comes to synthetic bone, I think of it as salt from a large corporation or salt from a small business; salt is probably salt. However, since synthetic bone is relatively inexpensive, I wonder whether it is necessary to use a cheap one.

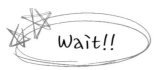

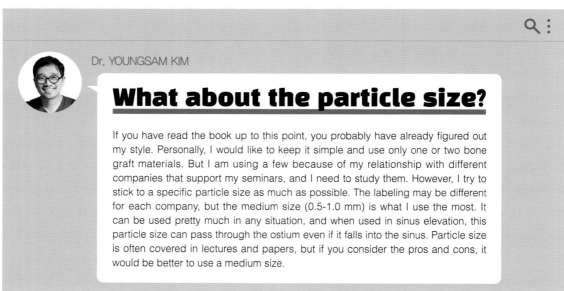

Dr. YOUNGSAM KIM

What about the particle size?

If you have read the book up to this point, you probably have already figured out my style. Personally, I would like to keep it simple and use only one or two bone graft materials. But I am using a few because of my relationship with different companies that support my seminars, and I need to study them. However, I try to stick to a specific particle size as much as possible. The labeling may be different for each company, but the medium size (0.5-1.0 mm) is what I use the most. It can be used pretty much in any situation, and when used in sinus elevation, this particle size can pass through the ostium even if it falls into the sinus. Particle size is often covered in lectures and papers, but if you consider the pros and cons, it would be better to use a medium size.

What about Collagen Bone?

I went to a dental event in 2017 and won a prize for the first time, and it was a Bio-Oss collagen bone. I had only heard of it but never used it. I was comfortable using familiar products, and the desire to try a new product was gradually disappearing. But thanks to the prize, I became curious about collagen bone and wanted to study it further. I bought and tried the Osteon 3 collagen bone, which has 60% non-resorbable HA and maintains its shape like Bio-Oss collagen. Once you use it, you will see that it is easy to manipulate because of its putty nature, but it is not strong enough to prevent deformation by external pressure, so it is not enough to replace block bone or titanium mesh. However, it is definitely easy to handle, and particles are not scattered, so the doctors in my clinic, including myself, are using it more often. I have not used it for a long time, so the long-term prognosis remains to be seen, but I am very satisfied for now.

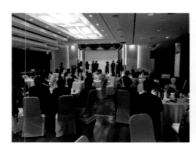 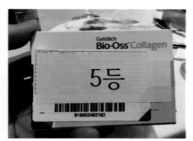 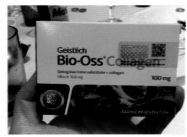

📷 2.2

There is a memorable patient I want to talk about (📷 2.3). When I returned from the United States and went back to work at my clinic, I saw a Caucasian female patient from Australia that I had never seen before. Implant treatment was not routinely done and was still expensive in Australia at that time, so one of the dentists who came to my lecture in Australia told the patient that implants are done well at a relatively lower price in South Korea and suggested she should visit my clinic. I had received a panoramic X-ray from the referring dentist in advance, but the ridge was very thin clinically. The patient said that she would go back to Australia once the treatment was completed and that her tour in South Korea was entertaining and impressive. The cost of three implants in Australia was more than enough to cover her trip and the treatment in South Korea. Although I have to admit my ego took a hit, I gladly proceeded with her treatment.

As expected, the ridge was so thin that all the buccal part of the implants was exposed. Typically, I would have used a titanium mesh (OssBuilder) for this wide and shallowly resorbed bone. However, the biggest drawback of the titanium mesh, in my opinion, is that close monitoring by the operator is necessary. The patient could not decide whether to do the second surgery in Australia or whether to come back to Korea to have the crown inserted, so the Australian doctor only asked for the implant for now. As a result, it was not recommended to use the titanium mesh for a patient who would return to Australia right away. Then, instead of aiming for a risky 100 point score, we placed an implant and grafted the buccal with only the collagen bone to settle for a safe 80-point score. The patient got her second surgery done in Australia and returned to South Korea for impression and crowns. When I contacted the referring dentist in Australia, the dentist said that the threads were slightly exposed at the crest. If there is one thing I regret now, I should have used the healing abutment instead of the cover screw. If so, the bone at the crest would have been better maintained.

However, at that time, I was so focused on making the surgery as simple as possible and trying to minimize any potential problems. If I had done the second surgery, I would have put more effort into securing additional bone grafts and keratinized gingiva. However, the patient was satisfied with the result at the end. For a surgery that was performed without much preparation while also seeing other patients in my busy clinic, I give 80 points for the surgery, but it leaves a lot of regrets. In any case, collagen bone is often useful when it is necessary to maintain the shape of the grafted bone. Sometimes, it is added in the middle of the particles during sinus elevation to maintain the shape. The degree of viscosity that keeps the particles together during manipulation gives great convenience.

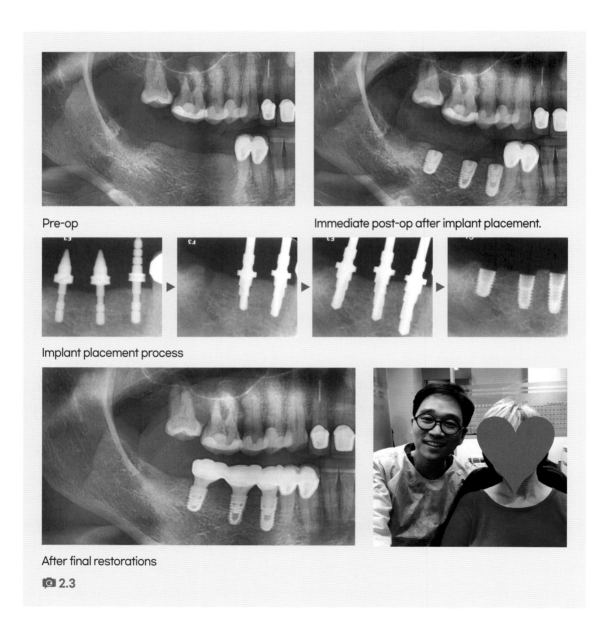

Pre-op

Immediate post-op after implant placement.

Implant placement process

After final restorations

📷 2.3

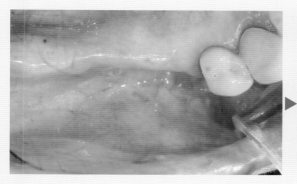

Pre-op

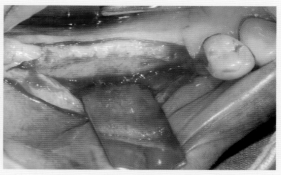

Not only is the ridge thin, but the soft tissue is also very thin. In my experience, Korean patients have thicker gums than others. Not generalizing, but I have seen many Caucasian patients with thin biotype as in the photo. In particular, the thickness of the gums in most patients in Mexico seems to be less than half of the Korean patients. If there are good research papers on gum thickness by ethnicity, please provide recommendations.

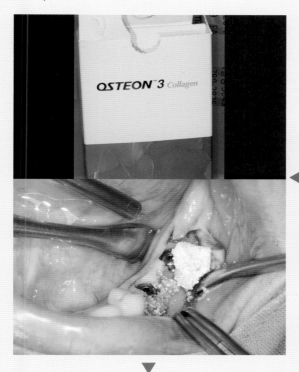

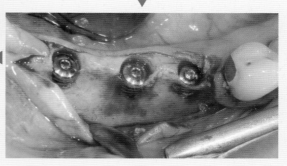

The implant threads are exposed on the buccal side.

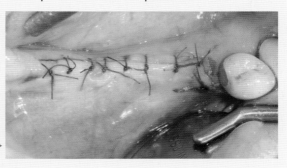

The flap was closed with single interrupted sutures.

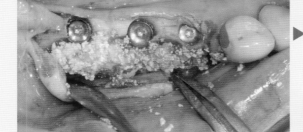

The buccal sides of the implants are covered with collagen bone to a sufficient thickness.

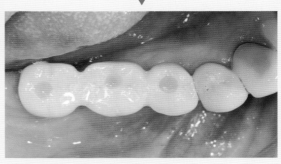

Immediately after final prostheses.

📷 2.4

What about PRF?

If you have read this book up to this point, you would already have noticed. I never use PRF, nor do I recommend it. Since there are many different opinions, I will not discuss it further in this book. Sticky bone is also mentioned often when talking about PRF, but I wonder if it is necessary when collagen bone materials are readily available in the market. Moreover, although sticky bone seems to be stronger than collagen, it is not as viscous, so it tends to fall off like a grain of sand once it is deformed. It seems to me that there is no point in discussing further here, so I will just tell you about a recent case that was ruled as false advertising. 📷 2.5 is page 32 of the illegal medical advertisement casebook. The article in the casebook, "promoting bone growth with autogenous blood for a speedy recovery," was judged as an exaggerated advertisement. The official position of the relevant society referenced in this judgment is attached.

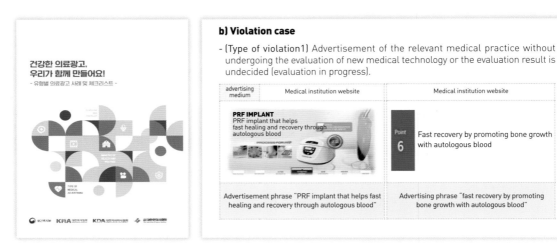

📷 2.5 Source: Ministry of Health and Welfare, and Medical Advertising Review Committee

---

[Korean Academy of Periodontology] 2018

Background

- Platelet rich fibrin (PRF) has growth factors in the granules present in platelets (Weibrich et al., 2002), and many scholars have conducted various experiments under the hypothesis that it will promote soft and hard tissue healing.
- There is a result of promoting the healing of soft tissues (Marenzi et al., 2015), and there is also a report that it helps the treatment of periodontal bone defects (Pradeep et al., 2017).
- There is also a report that the healing time can be reduced when DFDBA and PRF are used together in maxillary sinus bone graft (Choukroun et al., 2006).
- However, it is still the research result of some scholars, and there is no consensus among most scholars that PRF promotes the rate of bone formation and regeneration.
- More studies showing the positive effects of PRF will be required to reach a consensus.

Source: Korean Academy of Periodontology (2018)

⟨The Korean Academy of Implant Dentistry⟩

Before commenting, if you review the literature on PRF, there are still many areas of contention. In summary:

1) Research related to the promotion of bone formation by PRF is basically the literature on whether it is effective when mixed with bone graft material. It is mainly used with xenograft or synthetic bone, and its effect is judged based on the observation results of histological findings. And the results varied with little or no significant difference. Even when it was said to be effective, it was mentioned that PRF 'might have positive potential' in the case of maxillary sinus bone graft. Last year, a paper also mentioned that there was 'no beneficial effect' of PRF when mixed with synthetic bone b-TCP and used for maxillary sinus grafting, where good results are expected regardless of which graft material is used. Therefore, it is difficult to see whether the facilitation effect has been verified when PRF is used with the bone graft material.

2) In addition, there are studies on whether PRF has a facilitating effect on osseointegration as advertised. Most of these studies apply PRF to the jump gap immediately after implant placement following tooth extraction and evaluate initial stability from the viewpoint of increasing ISQ. It has been determined to have the advantage of shortening the loading time in the short term, but the long-term effect has not been proven. In addition, it was reported that the interpretation of the results of the early studies showed effectiveness in increasing ISQ, but in relatively recent studies (RCT) that were designed to be distinguished in more detail, it was reported that there was no additional effect in promoting osseointegration. When performing immediate implants after extraction and evaluating the effect of PRF in promoting osseointegration, it was determined that the use of PRF was irrelevant to the rate of osseointegration.

3) In addition, it seems a bit exaggerated to say that the effect of PRF is due to stem cells. There are still differing opinions on the mechanism by which PRF is effective, but it is determined that PRF helps in stabilization and that the stem cell content is insufficient in terms of the number of cells to have an effect.

4) In conclusion, it can be determined that the current advertisements seem to be misleading as to increase the rate of osseointegration of the implant, but it has not been proven. In addition, cases reported to be effective when used together with bone graft materials are determined to be limited to specific areas such as maxillary sinus grafting. Therefore, some wording corrections are necessary. For example, a phrase about PRF that promotes the healing of bone graft materials is acceptable, but the current phrase is misleading and needs to be corrected.

Source: The Korean Academy of Implant Dentistry

What about Extraction and Socket Preservation?

We can talk about tooth extraction and socket preservation all day, and it will still not be enough. As you have expected, I do not feel the need to preserve the socket. When the implant is placed after socket preservation, you will inevitably have poor bone quality around the implant. Even if the buccal plate is blown away if the graft is performed simultaneously as the implant placement, there will be poor quality bone only on the buccal side, and the rest would be better. It is also clearly more economical (from the patient's perspective) and reduces treatment time. Allografts are often used for socket preservation, but I have seen many cases where they fail to prevent resorption of the buccal plate and disappear altogether. On the other hand, if you use a xenograft bone, the bone quality in the socket will suffer, which is also not desirable. Even after tooth extraction and socket preservation, additional grafting is often required during implant placement surgery. So personally, I am not a big fan of socket preservation.

Of course, I think the best way would be to place the implant immediately after extraction or before the buccal bone disappears. And only use minimal xenograft to graft in the jump gap between the implant and the buccal plate, which is highly likely to resorb. We shall discuss more clinical cases in the sequel.

Jumping distance in implants

If the distance between the implant and the bone is less than 2 mm, you probably have heard that ossification occurs naturally. I do not think it is necessary to look for papers to study this topic. When I searched, most of the papers I found were old, and I could not find any significant results in recent papers. Just to summarize, based on my experience:

- Even if the distance between the implant and the bone is more than 2 mm, bone will fill in if it is going to fill in.
- Even if the distance between the implant and the bone is less than 2 mm, bone will not fill in if it will not fill in.
- The thickness of the buccal plate and the biotype of the surrounding soft tissue seem to be more important factors than the distance between the implant and the bone.
- The buccal plate in maxillary anterior and premolar is hardly bone but just the lamina dura with a thickness of about 1 mm. Since lamina dura receives its blood supply from the periodontal ligament, it is quickly resorbed after tooth extraction.
- When implants are immediately placed following extraction of the maxillary anterior teeth or premolars, it is recommended to graft regardless of the buccal jumping distance.
- I recommend non-resorbable xenograft bone.

I could go on and on about this topic if I wanted to, but I think it may be a little too advanced for the concept of "Easy Simple Safe Efficient" and the purpose of my lecture and this book. In summary, it may come in handy once you have improved your surgical skills and if you need an extensive onlay or vertical grafting. Other than those special cases, I think the current protocol is enough without the need for BMP.

I do not think periodontists are very fond of BMP. Recently, even in the field of basic science, there have been claims that BMP can cause cancer, but there seem to be more research results showing no significant effect at all. Of course, as I have said, the research isn't always pure.

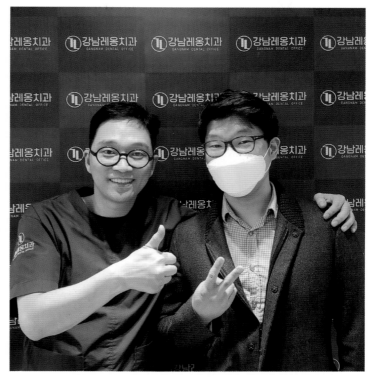

📷 **2.6 With Dr. Young-wook Kim from Wonju Dental Clinic**
A dental colleague's father came to my office to receive implant treatment, but it seemed difficult to place implants for full mouth rehabilitation due to his severe periodontal disease. After discussing with the colleague, we decided to invite Dr. Young-wook Kim to place implants for the full maxillary arch using BMP. I am watching the progress now. It was a commemorative photo taken on the day of the surgery.

I have not used BMP yet because it is costly, and I have not had many issues with my surgery without it. However, I see a huge potential in the future and plan to start using it eventually.

There is one person who helped me open my eyes to BMP, and I will introduce his case here. Dr. Young-wook Kim is the director of Wonju Dental Clinic, and he lectures and stays active in various fields of implant dentistry. After listening to Dr. Young-wook Kim's lecture, I asked for his permission to publish his case in my book.

BMP case by Dr. Young-wook Kim

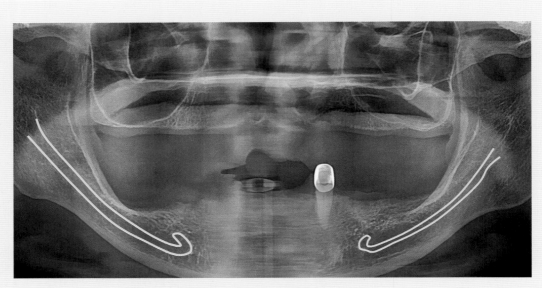

📷 2.7 70 year old female patient. Initial panoramic X-ray

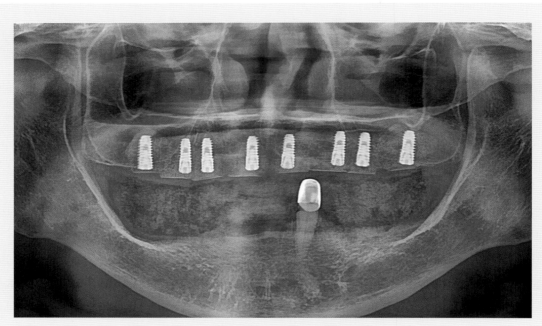

📷 2.8 Immediate post-op after full upper arch implant placement

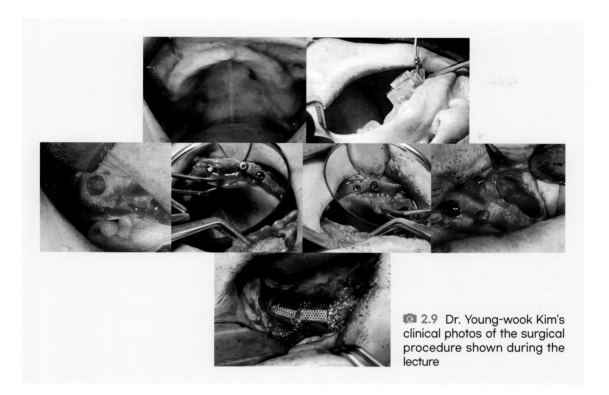

2.9 Dr. Young-wook Kim's clinical photos of the surgical procedure shown during the lecture

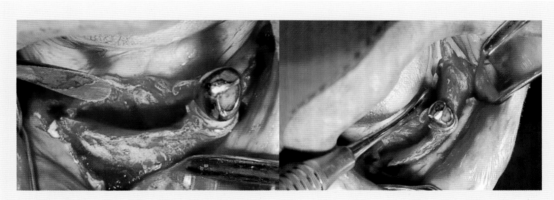

2.10 The mandibular ridge is also very thin.

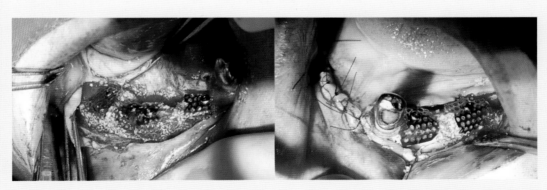

2.11 Vertical and horizontal bone augmentation was performed using the OssBuilder from Osstem described previously.

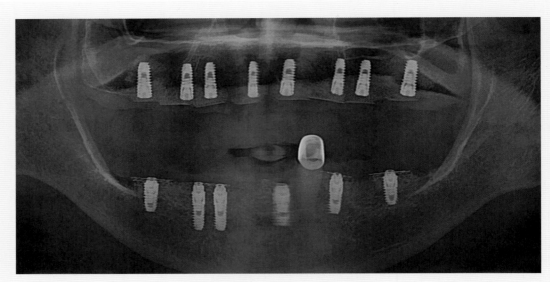

📷 2.12 Immediate post-op panorama

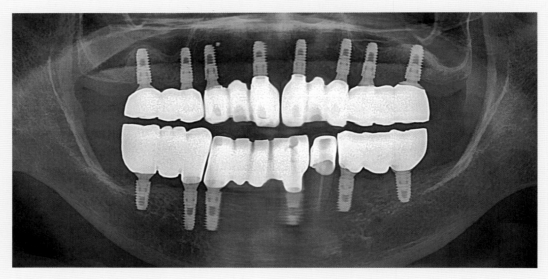

📷 2.13 After final prostheses

Source: Dr. Young-wook Kim of Wonju Dental Clinic

I knew that he was a good surgeon, but he exceeded my expectation. His surgical skill was excellent with or without BMP, but he said frankly that he would not have attempted this surgery without BMP. If I get a chance in the near future, I also plan to use the BMP.

I will close this chapter with a case that demonstrates my typical bone grafting style. The case is my colleague's mother, which was previously discussed in **Chapter 4-2**. Various types of GBR have been implemented for this patient, so this is a good opportunity for me to organize them and post them here.

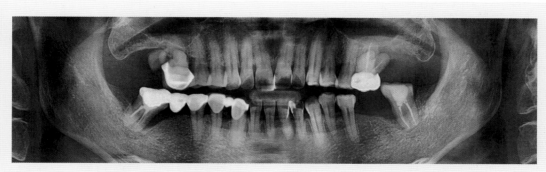

📷 2.14 Panoramic radiograph at initial visit

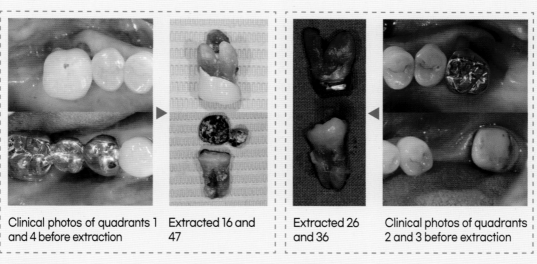

Clinical photos of quadrants 1 and 4 before extraction | Extracted 16 and 47

Extracted 26 and 36 | Clinical photos of quadrants 2 and 3 before extraction

📷 2.15   📷 2.16

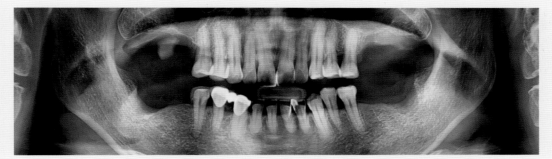

📷 2.17 Panoramic radiograph taken one and a half months after extraction, before we start serious treatment

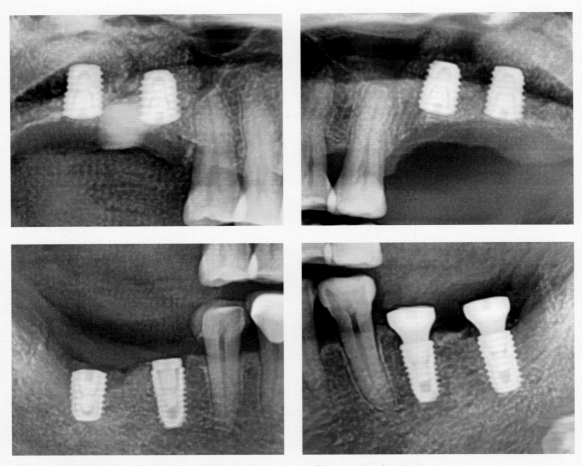

📷 **2.18 Panoramic radiograph of each quadrant immediately after implant surgery**
Single stage surgery for the 3rd quadrant. I would only stage my surgeries when the initial stability is poor, or a membrane is used. 2-stage cases account for less than 5% of my surgeries, so most of the surgeries are performed in a single stage.

Now, let's look at how bone grafting was done in each quadrant. The patient's teeth were in very poor condition at the initial visit to the clinic. Because there were also systemic diseases, her treatment was expected to be complicated. This is a case where the actual implant treatment started after about

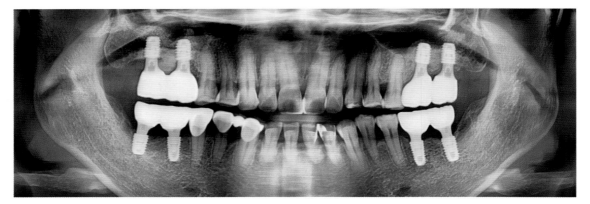

📷 **2.19** Panoramic radiograph taken one and a half months after extraction, before we start implant treatment

four months due to the patient's personal circumstances, and the entire treatment was completed in almost ten months.

▶ **In the 4th quadrant, a titanium mesh and collagen membrane were used with cover screw, then proceeded to 2 stages.**
46 - Titanium mesh (OssBuilder from Osstem)
47 - Collagen membrane (Genos from Dentium) + Xenograft (0.25g of A-Oss from Osstem)

▶ In the 3rd quadrant, implants had good initial stability and were not exposed. Since the bone grafting was only done inside the socket or in the areas with intact periosteum, the membrane was unnecessary, and surgery was done in a single stage with healing abutments.
47 - Synthetic bone around the socket without a membrane (0.1g of Ovis BONE from Dentis, β-TCP 80% + HA 20%)

▶ In the 1st quadrant, implants had poor initial stability. A collagen membrane was used with cover screws, then proceeded to 2 stages.
The upper region of the maxillary sinus grafted with xenograft (0.3-0.4g of A-Oss 0.5g from Osstem) + the lower part of the sinus grafted with synthetic bone (0.5g of A-Oss) + crestal area grafted with xenograft (0.1-0.2 g of A-Oss 0.5 g) + collagen Membrane (Ovis 15 x 20 mm from Dentis)

▶ In the 2nd quadrant, a collagen membrane was not necessary since the periosteum was intact. However, due to poor initial stability, cover screws were used, then proceeded to 2 stages.
The upper region of the maxillary sinus grafted with xenograft (some of A-Oss 0.5g from Osstem) + the lower region of the sinus grafted with synthetic bone (Q-Oss 0.5g from Osstem) + crestal area grafted with xenograft without a membrane

Implants were placed for both sides of the maxilla first because a long healing period was expected after implant placement. Then I placed implants in the relatively easy 3rd quadrant and lastly in the 4th quadrant, which had minimal bone six months after extraction. The 4th quadrant had a long standing bone defect at the mesial of 47, which did not fill in after extraction. Although there were no opposing teeth to use as a guideline and the shape of the bone was irregular, implants were placed by estimating the correct prosthetic position as best as possible. **Chapter 4-2** describes this case, so let's look at the implants in the 4th quadrant that were placed last.

After the implants were placed, the top 4-5 threads of 46 implant, which was about half of the

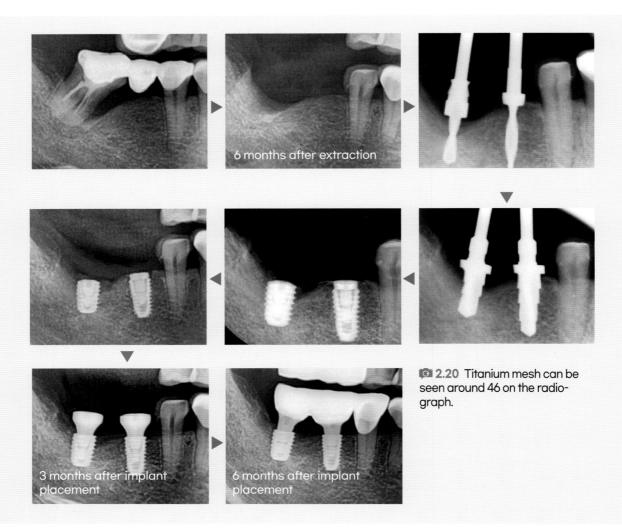

6 months after extraction

3 months after implant placement

6 months after implant placement

📷 **2.20** Titanium mesh can be seen around 46 on the radiograph.

fixture, were exposed on the buccal side, and 2 threads of 47 implant were exposed on mesial and buccal sides. Since the bone loss was severe both horizontally and vertically, it was decided to use titanium mesh. 46 was grafted on the buccal side with a titanium mesh. Since 47 had a sufficient distal bone height and the mesial and buccal sides were tented by the mesh from 46, it was grafted (with 0.25g of A-Oss from Osstem + GENOSS membrane from Dentium) without a mesh and sutured. In retrospect, I think it would have been better if it was placed with a 1 mm height healing abutment or placed the fixture 0.5 mm deeper. However, I thought it went relatively well for a short time spent on the surgery. It is a pity that I could not take a photo after using the titanium mesh.

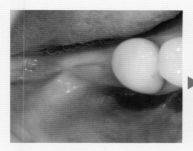

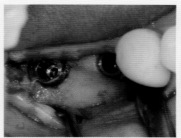

At the 46 side where the bridge pontic was, you can see that a lot of the buccal bone was lost.

47 implant was exposed vertically and horizontally, and 46 implant was exposed horizontally on buccal side. After bone grafting, a titanium mesh was placed on 46 and collagen membrane around 47 before closing the flap. I regret not taking pictures of the process.

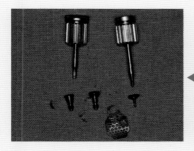

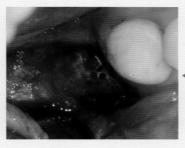

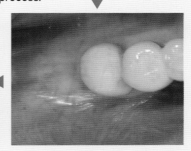

Removed screws and titanium mesh

The flap was raised to check the titanium mesh.

Three months after implant placement, the patient came to the clinic to have the titanium mesh removed.

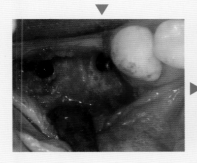

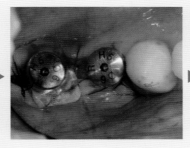

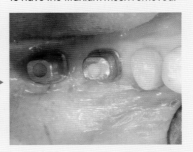

Alveolar bone with titanium mesh removed.
Good ossification is evident.

Louis Button from Dentis was used to help form the vestibule and preserve the attached gingiva on the buccal side of the 47 implant.

Unfortunately, the buccal gingiva is not well visible in this photo right before the final restoration.

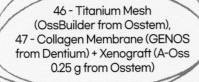

46 - Titanium Mesh (OssBuilder from Osstem),
47 - Collagen Membrane (GENOS from Dentium) + Xenograft (A-Oss 0.25 g from Osstem)

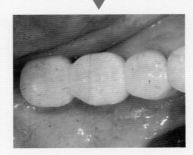

Clinical photo immediately after final restoration

📷 2.21 **4th quadrant surgery**

I have a lot of patients who are dentists or family members of dentists. It is nice to be recognized for my skills by fellow colleagues, but I often run into a dilemma when I want to take clinical photos. When I removed the mesh after three months during the second surgery, I could not take proper photos using an occlusal mirror but managed to take at least a few shots from my eye level. Abundant bone formation was visible. Then the case was completed following the routine protocol. As mentioned earlier, the gingiva at 47 kept coming up towards the occlusal and was pressed with Louis Button. You can see half of it remaining later, but the distobuccal gingiva does not look great. It would be nice to have a mechanism that continues to push the tissue buccally until the crown is inserted.

On the other hand, if you look at the 3rd quadrant, the case was done in a usual manner.

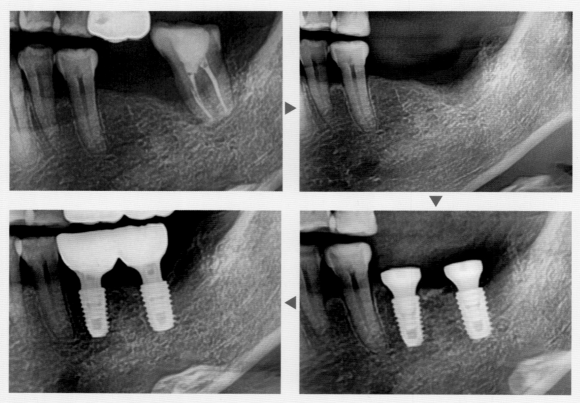

📷 2.22 Panoramic radiograph of the progress in 3rd quadrant

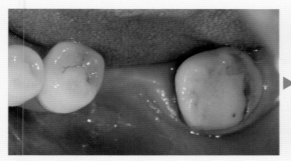

Pre-treatment clinical photo

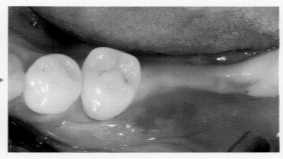

4 months after extraction

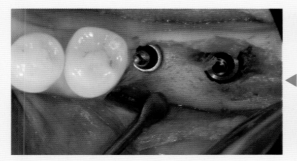

Immediately after implant placement

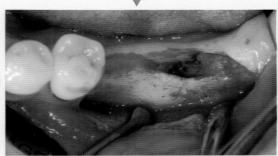

Immediately after incision

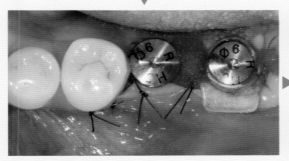

Immediately after suturing

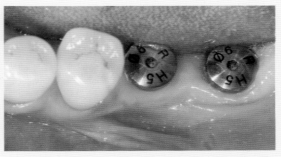

After 5 months of implant placement, a beautifully formed attached gingiva can be seen with a simple Youngsam flap.

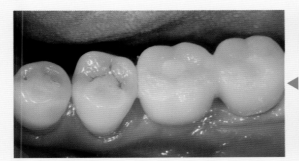

After final insertion

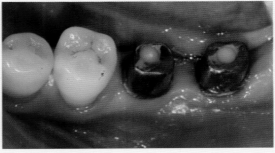

Before final insertion

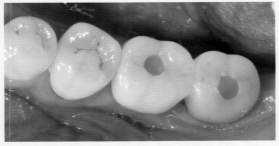

2.23

9 months after insertion

After implant placement, 36 implant threads were not exposed on the buccal side, but some cortical bone fractures can be observed. At 37 site, the implant was pushed slightly towards the buccal and twisted in the final placement due to the extraction socket. When placing the implant in such an underfilled socket, the bone density of the socket area and the rest of the cortical bone is so different that it is not easy to align the implant placement direction. Thinking about it now, if the coronal part had been removed slightly more (Ankylos method), it would have been possible to prevent the fixture from getting pushed towards the buccal direction.

In this case, after the bone graft (Ovis Synthetic bone from Dentis), it was sutured without a membrane. I cannot remember why I used synthetic bone that resorbs. It was probably because I primarily used it to fill the 37 socket. I regret and wonder how it would have been if xenograft was used for the 36 buccal side. Although it was grafted in a minimal amount, it felt like the graft had slipped a little because I did not drill decorticating holes. You may see some dentists doing very extensive grafts even for this kind of case. They say it is to aim for perfection, but surgery becomes more difficult for both provider and patient, and it is questionable if the bone grafted in that way has a better long-term prognosis or is more resistant to peri-implantitis. So, I will continue to pursue the goal of keeping grafts to a minimum. Looking at the clinical photo four months after tooth extraction, you can see how quickly the vestibule comes up to the occlusal surface.

Looking at the CBCT...

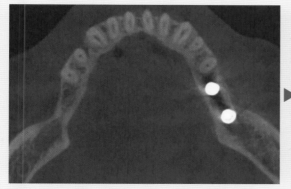

Image of the mandible prior to 4th quadrant surgery (1 month after the 3rd quadrant implant surgery)

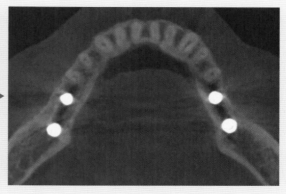

6 months after implant placement, immediately after final crowns

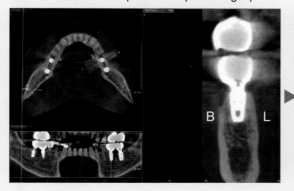

CT image 7 months after implant placement where 36 buccal bone was very thin and slightly fractured

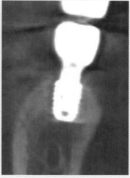

6 months after implant placement, cross section images of 46 and 47 implants, respectively. On CT scan, you can see nicely formed bone around the implant.

A radiopaque object is observed in the cheek of 1st quadrant.

📷 2.24

If you look at the before and after CT scans, bone formation can be seen on the buccal side of the implant. The radiopaque object between the 1st quadrant implants seen in the panoramic radiograph is presumed to be some kind of material in the cheek (I am not sure what it is, but it is thought to be some kind of cosmetic implant).

The maxilla was all treated with sinus elevation via crestal approach. Here is a look at the overall tissue management process for your reference. I perform the surgery in a simple manner that even a novice clinician can do, so anyone can follow it and maintain the quality of implant surgery with ease. The simpler the operation, the less likely it is to fail.

Clinical photos of the progress in 1st quadrant

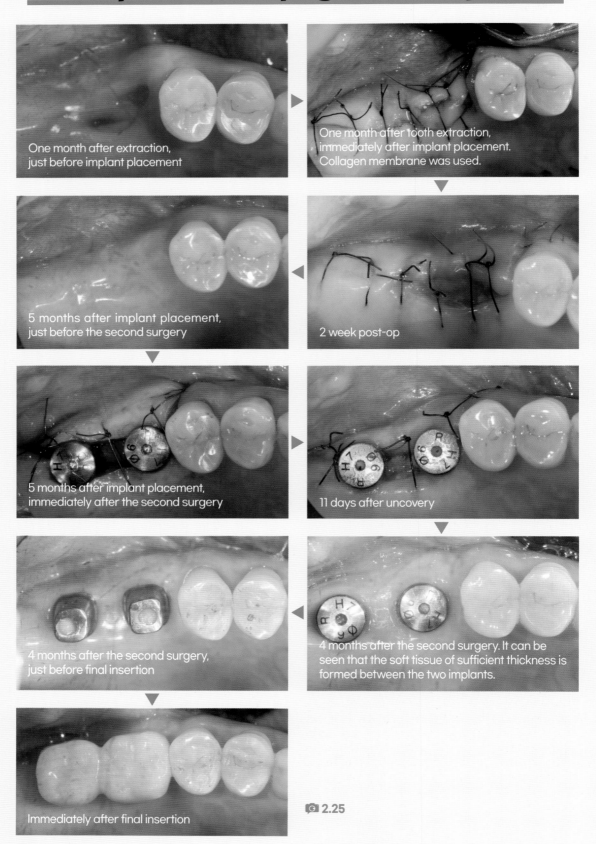

One month after extraction, just before implant placement

One month after tooth extraction, immediately after implant placement. Collagen membrane was used.

5 months after implant placement, just before the second surgery

2 week post-op

5 months after implant placement, immediately after the second surgery

11 days after uncovery

4 months after the second surgery, just before final insertion

4 months after the second surgery. It can be seen that the soft tissue of sufficient thickness is formed between the two implants.

Immediately after final insertion

2.25

Clinical photos of the progress in 2nd quadrant

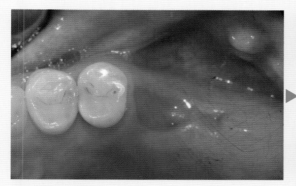

1 month after extraction

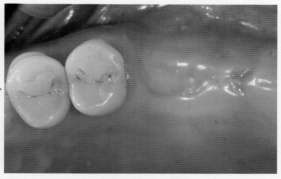

2 and a half months after extraction

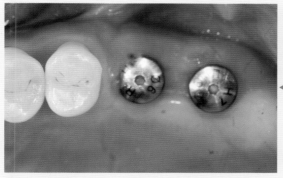

1 month and 2 weeks after the second surgery
The soft tissue was not sufficiently formed between the two implants. The abutment and crown should be designed with proper soft tissue healing in mind.

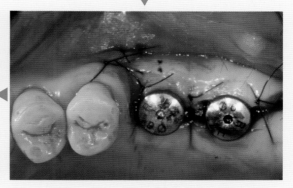

3 and a half months after implant placement
immediately after the second surgery. No photos immediately after implant placement.

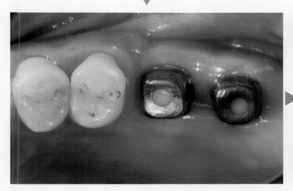

1 month and 3 weeks after the second surgery, just before final insertion. If the impression is taken shortly after the second surgery, it should be clearly communicated to the technicians that the thickness or shape of the soft tissue has not been restored to normal. Otherwise, they will only take the soft tissue at the time into consideration and compromise the crown shape.

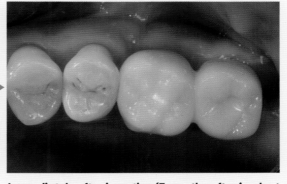

Immediately after insertion (5 months after implant placement)

2.26

9 months after treatment completed in 1st and 4th quadrants (11 months after final insertion in 2nd and 3rd quadrants)

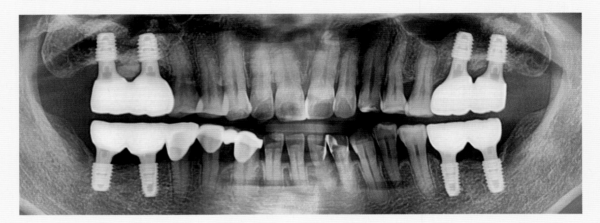

📷 **2.27 Panoramic radiograph 9 months after final insertion on the right side**
The object between the right maxillary implants is some kind of cosmetic implant in the patient's cheek. In the case of the left maxillary implant at 26, the amount of remaining bone after extraction was minimal, and vertical bone loss was severe, so the implant was placed a little deeper on purpose after sinus elevation. However, the second surgery became challenging due to surprisingly good bone formation. After the final insertion, I am not satisfied with the position or shape of the implant. Had I known that the bone would form this nicely, it would have been better if I placed it slightly shallower or attempted to place it in a better position. I was overly focused on achieving initial stability, which was a challenge itself.

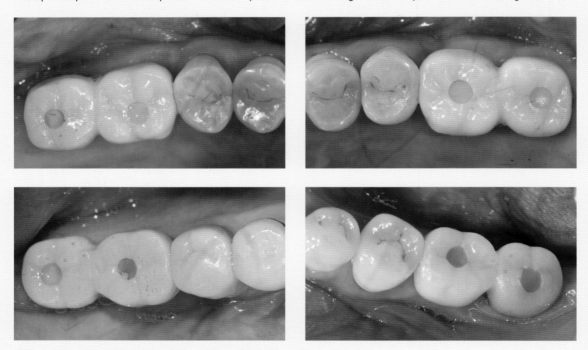

📷 **2.28 Clinical photos 9 months after final insertion**
They are in a relatively good position considering there were no opposing teeth, and the implants were placed with existing premolars as the only reference. Although my surgery may not be flashy or fancy, I can assure you that it is simple and has a good prognosis. I believe that anyone can achieve similar results if they focus on placing the implants where they should be prosthetically instead of making the surgery big and beautiful. Moreover, although guided surgery is becoming more common these days, do not think of guided implants as flapless surgeries, but more as well-made surgical stents. You need to raise the flap and try to preserve the keratinized gingiva and vestibule.

30 month follow up

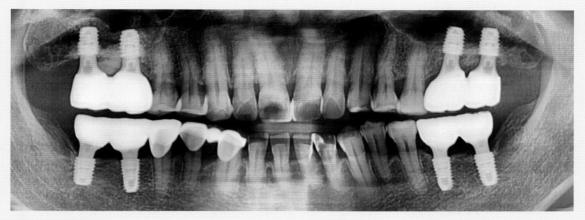

📷 **2.29** **30 month follow up panoramic radiograph.** The bone level is constantly and stably maintained.

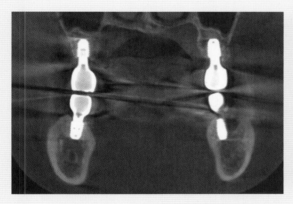

📷 **2.30** **Coronal section of most distal implants at 2nd molar sites**

It can be seen that the bone is still well maintained. Especially in the upper jaw, it seems to be maintained overly well. My goal is 2 mm around the implant fixture.

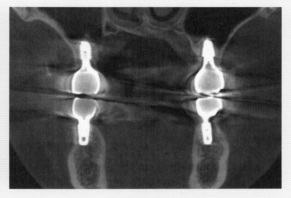

📷 **2.31** **Coronal section of implants at 1st molar sites**

The bone is still well maintained but it is disappointing to see less than the 2nd molar sites. I wonder if the non-resorbable xenografts placed in the maxilla initially was pushed toward the 2nd molar sites and the synthetic bone that was placed next accumulated in the 1st molar sites. I also wish I could have grafted more bone around 46 implant by spreading the titanium mesh buccally.

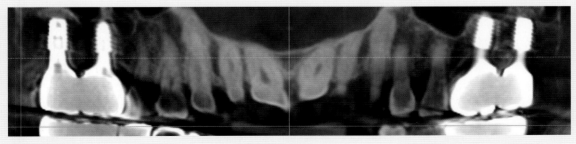

📷 **2.32** In the panoramic radiograph, the space between the implants looked a little empty, so I found a sectional image from the CT showing between the implants. The bone is adequately formed, however my guess is that it look radiopaque due to the contrast with the remaining xenograft material now that the synthetic bone with high resorbable β-TCP component is resorbed. If autogenous bone or highly resorbable synthetic bone is mixed with xenograft bone, the sinus bone graft site has appearance that is lumpy as you see here. If I had to do it again, I would have used a slightly smaller amount of only the xenograft bone.

Dr. YOUNGSAM KIM'S

CLINICAL NOTES

EASY SIMPLE SAFE EFFICIENT

MASTERING DENTAL IMPLANTS

The Essential Elements for Success in Dental Implants

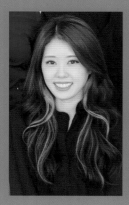

Dr. Chungmi Kim

I was very fortunate to meet Dr. Youngsam Kim early in my dental career. Following his protocols built from his experience, my skills as a clinician improved significantly. I graduated from University of Texas Health Science Center at San Antonio dental school in 2014. Practiced as an associate for 3 years and decided to open up my own practice near our start-up church our family decided to attend. I got married in 2017 and I opened a start-up practice in July 2018 in McKinney, TX and had my first child in August 2018. During this time, I felt like I was falling behind. Of course I still have a lot to learn, but through Dr. Youngsam Kim's wisdom teeth removal and implant lectures, I regained my confidence as a clinician. It's a blessing to have a good mentor to share your passion.

Abutment Selection and Crown
You are stuck with me!

7-1 Abutment and Crown Shape

7-2 Why Screwmentable?

7-1 Abutment and Crown Shape

M a s t e r i n g   d e n t a l   i m p l a n t s

Ideal Shape and Contour of the Abutment

So far, we have looked at very important factors that influence implant success. Proper position, angulation, and depth of implant placement, grafting bone material and soft tissue... Yes. So far these are the surgical aspects of the implant. But over the years, as I placed implants, the most disappointing factor for me has been the selection of wrong prosthesis rather than the wrong surgical procedure. Incorrect abutment selection and prosthetic technique seems to have a greater effect on implant failure. I don't restore implants, but once I saw how the abutment-crown was delivered I nagged about replacing it. If surgery goes well, you must place well fabricated prosthesis.

These are my old implant cases I recently ran across and noticed how I had selected wrong abutments (📷 1.1). These three cases are more than 10 years old and I had to re-implant two of them and replace the entire abutment-crown on the third one because the crown had fractured.

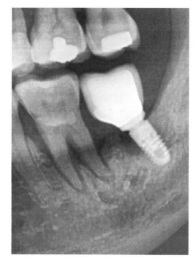 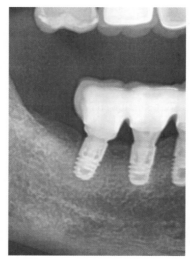 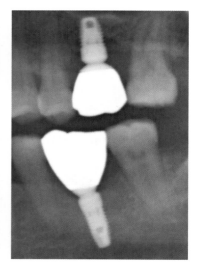

📷 1.1 Cases of poorly selected abutments

One day, I was listening to a lecture by an orthodontic professor, and the professor introduced me to a thesis that he stumbled upon by chance in the library. It was a Quintessence magazine entitled "peri-implantitis: the disease of the future". This paper concluded that an effective treatment for peri-implantitis has not yet been devised and concluded that prevention is the only solution.

As I mentioned earlier, there is one thing worth noting about the Ankylos implants. That is,

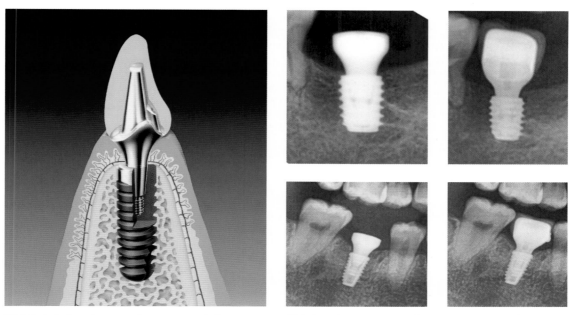

📷 1.2 Ankylos abutment known to optimize gingival health

📷 1.3 When concave and long shaped abutment is selected

periodontally, it is very stable. Why? First of all, because the internal friction angle is so small that it almost becomes cold welded resulting in no marginal gap or movement. However, I also mentioned that there may be some problems if the angle is too small, so if you do not remember, please revisit **Chapter 2-3 Classification and Understanding of Abutments**.

And the key is the elongated C-shaped concave abutment. The concave abutment means that it can hold more gingival tissue. In most cases, implants are smaller than teeth. Therefore, the crown part should be widened, and the question of in what shape does it have to be widened should be considered. This is how I'll describe after thoughtful consideration. **"You have to fill it with as much gingiva as possible."** So, the implant restoration should extend straight out of the implant platform with a smooth surface and widens as it protrudes out of the gingival tissue to create an S-line restoration. Not only people like the S-line, but the abutment looks most beautiful with the S-line. Osstem and Dentis recently released an abutments with C-shaped concavity like the healing abutments that transition into S-shape to the correct cervical tooth anatomy. Of course, these cases are custom abutments, but eventually, technicians will have to get used to these designs. As I said before, in order to achieve S-line,

📷 **1.4** Daily Dental article (March 5, 2020)

the abutment must have sufficient running room.

Let's take a look at the research paper published by prominent professors in South Korea.

This paper summarizes that there was an increased incidence of peri-implantitis if emergenc angle was greater than 30° with convex emergence profile compared to emergence angle of less than 30° with concave emergence profile.

In summary, the incidence of peri-implantitis was the highest (46.6%) in implants with a convex emergence profile and an emergence angle of more than 30°, whereas only 2.4% incident rate was noted when the emergence profile was concave and an emergence angle was less than 30°.

In addition, as a result of comparing the risk factors of peri-implantitis, risk of peri-implantitis

occurrence was 7.04 times higher when the contour of the implant restoration is convex compare to concave restorations. The risk of occurrence was 3.8 times higher when the angle of emergence profile of the implant restoration was greater than 30° compared to the ones with less than 30°. In particular, it was reported that the risk of peri-implantitis was 35.74 times higher when the implant restoration was convex with an emergence angle of 30° or higher compared to the ones with concave contour with an emergence angle less than 30°.

In conclusion, convex implant restoration and implant restoration with an emergence angle greater than 30° are not good for gingival health because they are impinging on living space of the gingival tissue and complicates hygiene and causes peri-implantitis.

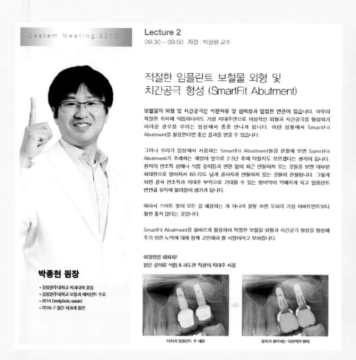
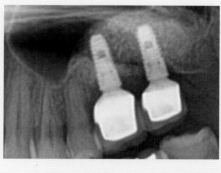
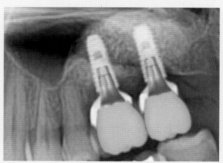

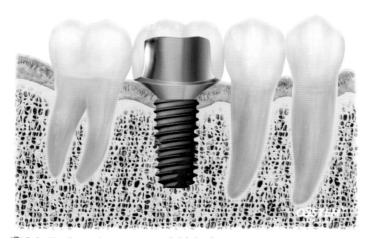

1.5 Dr. Jonghyun Park's abstract (Osstem Symposium 2017 Abstract)

When I was giving a lecture at the 2017 Osstem Symposium, another lecture was being held by Dr. Jonghyun Park in the next room (**1.6**). He is my favorite, both personally and academically. He also places and restores implants and he typically uses Osstem Tissue Level (SS2) implants for molars. The point of Park's lecture was that "shallow placement of implant and the use of large diameter abutments should be avoided".

1.6-1.8 are images created by Dr. Jonghyun Park in collaboration with Osstem. I'm using this image with Osstem's approval on this book. They are very well explained images. **1.6** is the worst example of implant abutment-crown.

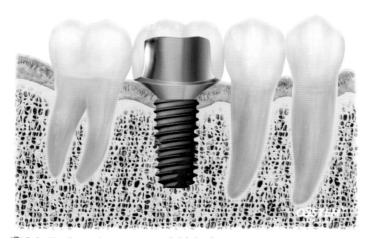
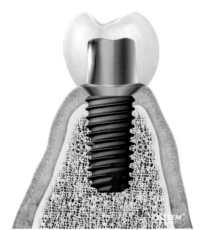

1.6 Shallow placement and thick abutment

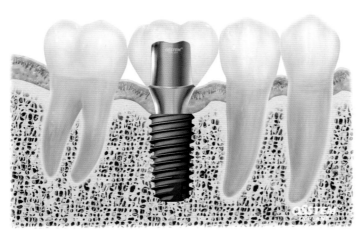
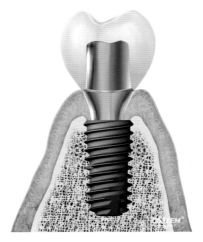

📷 **1.7** Relatively well controlled implant depth and abutment selection

📷 **1.7** is a good case for a fairly well selected abutment.

📷 **1.8** depicts how it is better to make an S shaped abutment-crown by deeply placing the implant to allow ideal soft tissue remodeling. If somebody tells me to redraw this picture, I would make it closer to the natural tooth by increasing the height discrepancy between mesiodistal and buccal and make peri-implant soft tissue thicker.

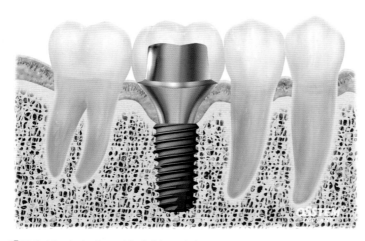
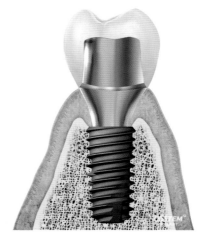

📷 **1.8** Ideal abutment height and shape

Stock abutment selection

Not only the dentist, but the lab technician must understand the ideal abutment-crown shape and contour for healthy implant and peri-implant soft tissue. Usually, it is not so easy to send a patient back home just because I'm not happy with the way abutment-crown is are made, especially those patients who expect to walk out with a tooth. I explain it like this: **"Don't thicken the abutment, thicken the gingiva"**.

I do not restore my implants, they are restored by a prosthodontist. I know that most dentists in South Korea place the abutment into the fixture and make an impression at the abutment level. However, I do impressions at the fixture level and send them to the laboratory for production, but since there are so many of them, I do not select custom abutments each time, but send a lot of stock abutments and the technicians select the ones that fit the model and make them. Most dental offices will run like these except for those with less volume of implant cases.

Here are my poorly executed implant cases (📷 1.9). All of these cases are more than 10 years old, so it seems that I, too, lacked this concept at that time. Even if the prosthodontist had made it that way, it should not have been delivered. I started placing the internal friction type around 2005-2006

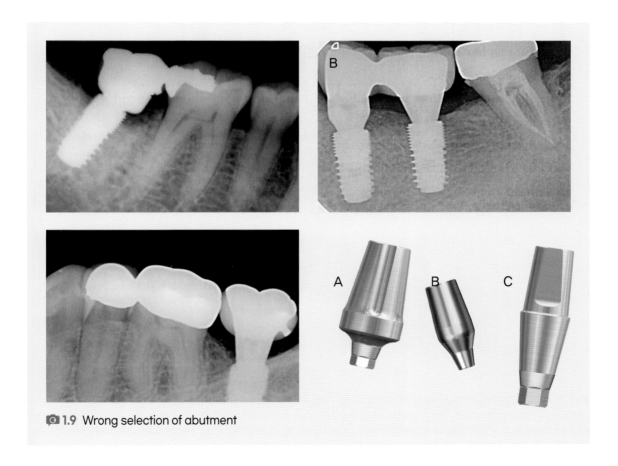

📷 1.9 Wrong selection of abutment

and I started placing a lot of them at the end of 2008 and so that was the period where both the prosthodontist and I had limited understanding of restorative concept. How could I have delivered this type of implant restorations?

Most of my implants showing wrong implant restorative concepts are Osstem's GS3 implants because it was the first bone level internal friction type implant I placed the most in the beginning. It has been almost 10 years since it was discontinued, so you can tell by looking at the photos that it was placed before then.

There are so many different types of abutments (📷 1.10). The left is a stock abutment manufactured by Osstem and has concave C shape similar to a healing abutment. If you have to use a stock abutment, why not use something like this? My younger brother is my lab technician and despite how much we discuss and argue, you have no idea how often I'm not pleased with his choice of abutment.

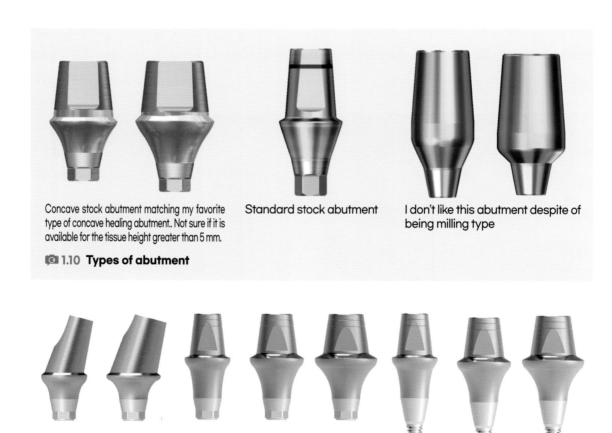

Concave stock abutment matching my favorite type of concave healing abutment.. Not sure if it is available for the tissue height greater than 5 mm.

Standard stock abutment

I don't like this abutment despite of being milling type

📷 1.10 **Types of abutment**

📷 1.11 **An abutment from Dentis that matches the new C-shaped healing abutment**
Starting next month, as a trial, I decided to try them on several cases. Director of Seoul Sunshine Dental and co-author of this book, Dr. Jisun Kim is currently using Dentis SQ implants and newly designed healing abutments and implant abutments (shown above), and he is very satisfied with them. Now is the time to follow the flow of time and use the thin and straight S-shaped abutment.

Cases of incorrect abutment use

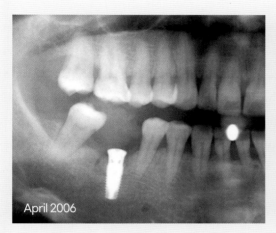
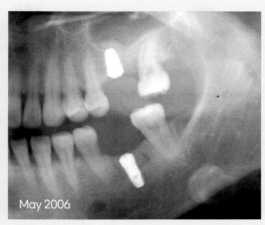

April 2006   May 2006

📷 1.12 My aunt's case (immediately after placement)

This case was done in 2006 when I was in the midst of performing aggressive surgeries (📷 1.12). At that time, I was getting comfortable using the internal friction type as I use Implantium implants from Dentium. You can see that the maxillary sinus was elevated beautifully because I already got accustomed to performing vertical sinus lift by previously using Endopore implants. If you look closely at the panoramic X-ray of the mandible, you can see the traces of ridge splitting on both sides. At that time, I loved to use piezo, so all of the thin ridges either had block bone grafts or ridge splitting procedure was performed.

#46 is a tissue-level implant from DIO Implant. This was my first DIO implant case. This is a poorly placed implant case that I show to explain "why we must use a familiar system". As I got comfortable placing implants, I became bold and didn't find the need to prepare for surgery anymore despite using this system for the first time, and of course I was so perplexed during the procedure. This is my "pickaxe" case ("Pickaxe" implant - unintentionally placing distally angulated implants).

This patient is my aunt, and the surgery was quite successful and she didn't have major problems.

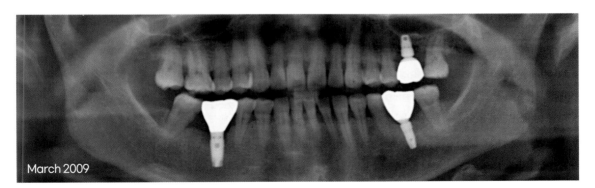

March 2009

📷 1.13

However, since she lived in a rural area, she hardly came to Seoul after abutment and crown delivery, and three years later, I referred her to my colleague in Jeonju.

There is no panorama immediately after seating the abutment-crown but there is a panoramic X-ray that was taken 3 years after seating (📷 1.13). Image quality is different compared to the previous one (Pointnix) since its Sirona line Been using Vatech for the last 7 years. Despite the amount of bone loss noted around the 46 and 26 implants, the patient did not complain of any discomfort. Since the patient is my aunt, I decided to replace them one by one at free of charge. In 2009, the price of gold had already skyrocketed, so it was not a loss for me either, as the previous implant restoration was removed and the gold sold was more than enough to pay the lab fee.

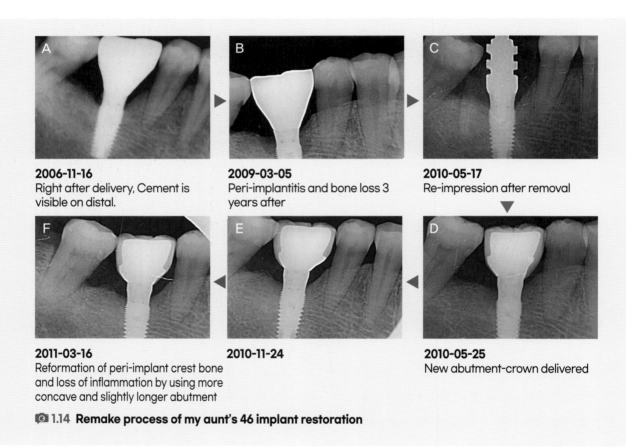

2006-11-16
Right after delivery, Cement is visible on distal.

2009-03-05
Peri-implantitis and bone loss 3 years after

2010-05-17
Re-impression after removal

2011-03-16
Reformation of peri-implant crest bone and loss of inflammation by using more concave and slightly longer abutment

2010-11-24

2010-05-25
New abutment-crown delivered

📷 1.14 **Remake process of my aunt's 46 implant restoration**

Even in 2006, implant restorations were fabricated by the prosthetic department (📷 1.14). He is a talented dentist, but he is not spendthrift like me and due to his frugal nature, he tries to save if possible by using a stock abutment. So, in 2006, a large crown was placed over the solid abutment. Since it was a tissue-level implant, the shape of the abutment or the crown didn't look too bad, but you can see that cement is left behind on the x-ray (📷 1.14A). Peri-implant soft tissue was often inflamed due to deep crown margin (📷 1.14B). In 2010, it was removed and the stock abutment with higher margin was used, and by doing so inflammation disappeared and crestal bone was completely regenerated as shown (📷 1.14C, D). Other than routine non-surgical scaling and prophylaxis, no surgical bone grafting or periodontal surgery was performed (📷 1.14E, F).

After seeing improvement in gingival health just by replacing abutment-crown of the lower implant, I decided to replace 26 abutment-crown as well.

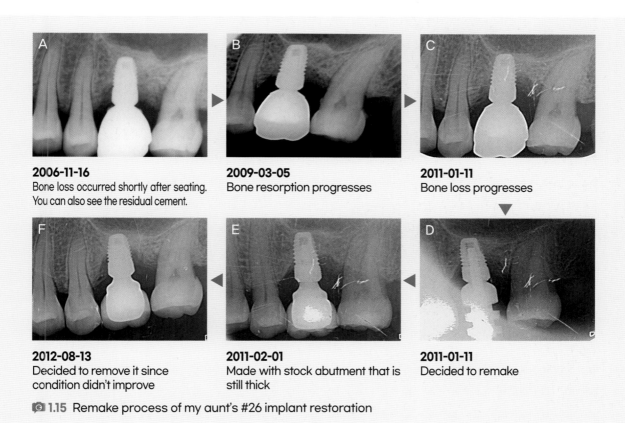

2006-11-16
Bone loss occurred shortly after seating. You can also see the residual cement.

2009-03-05
Bone resorption progresses

2011-01-11
Bone loss progresses

2012-08-13
Decided to remove it since condition didn't improve

2011-02-01
Made with stock abutment that is still thick

2011-01-11
Decided to remake

📷 **1.15** Remake process of my aunt's #26 implant restoration

It was only then that I began to realize the importance of the abutment and crown shapes (📷 1.15A, B). In 2011, new crown was fabricated by re-impressing despite of poor implant condition (📷 1.15C, D). Since the patient was my aunt, I decided to just deliver and monitor the prognosis and remove the implant if needed.

36 showed no bone resorption, but the lower implant also frequently swelled and caused discomfort (📷 1.16). Because the patient was in her 60s, she said that she felt uncomfortable around the implant if she was tired or if her immune system weakened. Once the abutment was removed, I noticed that the abutment was very short, and who knows how long those food debris has been in there and I even noticed possible cement. So, I came to the conclusion that the implant crown margin should not be placed too subgingivally. Be sure to use screwmentable abutment and crown with shallow margin, and if cement cannot be removed, you must unscrew the abutment-crown to completely remove cement prior

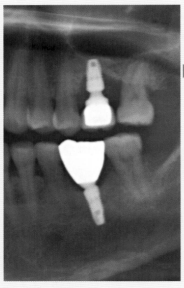

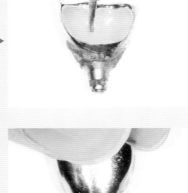

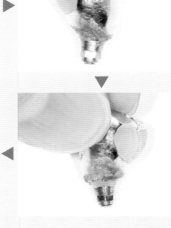

Soft tissue inflammation around 36

Residual cement and plaque

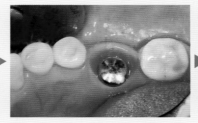

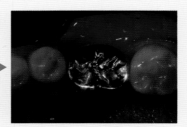

After abutment-crown removal

After removal, impression was taken and healing abutment was placed

New implant restoration

📷 1.16 **Remake process of my aunt's 36 implant crown**

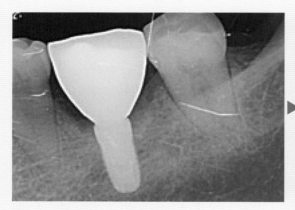

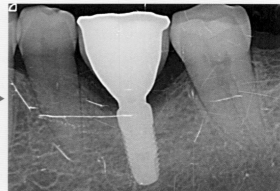

PA prior to removal (2011)

PA with new restoration (2011)

📷 1.17

to applying final torque.

Just by removing the abutment-crown and inserting healing abutment, you can see the extra space where it was previously occupied by the implant restoration. What a shame that I could have saved some money by using less gold back then.

I never thought I would ever write a book about implants, so it never occurred to me to take many clinical photos. Although the angulation of PA is not good, a rough comparison is possible, so let's compare standard PAs taken (📷 1.17). You can clearly see that a thick gingiva is formed around the implant with a new abutment and crown.

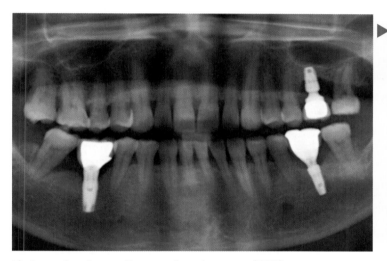 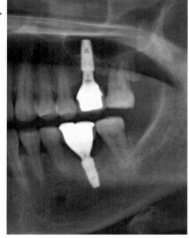

First remake of crown 5 years after placement (2021)

Re-implantation after #26 removal (2013)

📷 1.18

So basically implants placed in 2006 were replaced one by one annually 4 years after placement; it shows the importance of the restoration as much as the placement (📷 1.18). We can suspect failure of implant 26 due to a manufacturing defect of implant despite poorly designed abutment-crown with residual cement since Dentium implant products were being recalled for a while at the time and also because subtle crestal bone loss was noted prior to abutment-crown delivery.

I ended up asking my colleague in Jeonju to remove implant 26 since my aunt was getting old to travel and I was getting old too. I'm not a big fan of the implant he placed since implant size is too long and placed too deep, but you can see that the abutment-crown was beautifully done. He is famous for seeing family, friends and acquaintances of a dentist who left Jeonju due to his well respected treatment planning skills and tooth preparation skills.

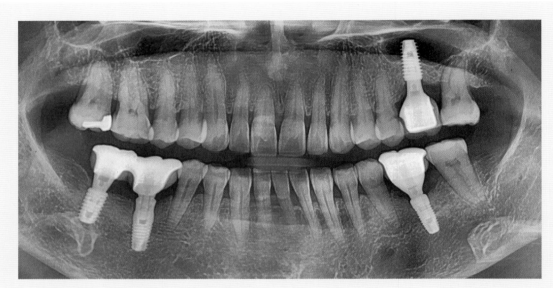

1.19 Panoramic X-ray taken on May 22, 2021

In the process of finishing this book, I begged my aunt in the countryside to come to Seoul once more (1.19). She continues to use the implants well even after 15 years of placement. Recently, I was told that in the process of placing #47 implant, implant crown of #46 was removed and new splinted crowns were fabricated. However, the choice of the abutment for the 46 tissue level implant is disappointing. Since I placed DIO tissue-level implant 15 years ago, either he did not understand the concept of restoring tissue level implant or he did not have the right product to restore.

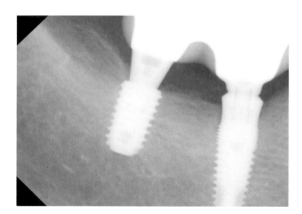 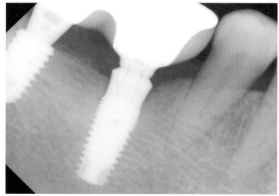

1.20 If you look at this standard X-ray, the abutment chosen does not cover the upper beveled portion of the tissue level implant. If this type of abutment was used, the crown should extend to cover the upper beveled portion. Of course it would have been more ideal if an abutment that covered the upper beveled portion was used and placed supragingival crown margin.

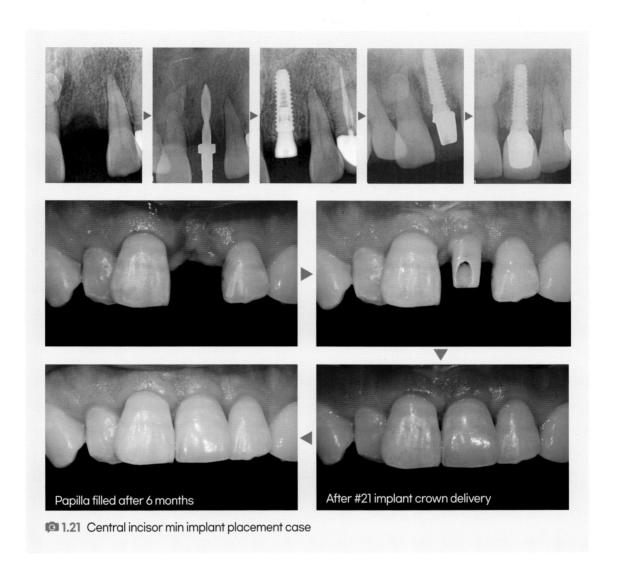

Papilla filled after 6 months

After #21 implant crown delivery

📷 1.21 Central incisor min implant placement case

This is a case seen in **Chapter 3-2**, in which 3.5 mm platform implant was placed at the maxillary central incisor site (📷 **1.21**). It appears to be placed slightly buccal, but you can see that peri-implant soft tissue was remodeled beautifully without black triangle. However, in fact, soft tissue was not initially formed like this nor was not remodeled with a temporary crown. Permanent abutment and crown was delivered and black triangle was naturally filled in. Of course, prosthodontists can perform procedures to preserve papilla and do gingival remodeling procedures, but they are not routinely performed in South Korea due to low cost of implants in the country.

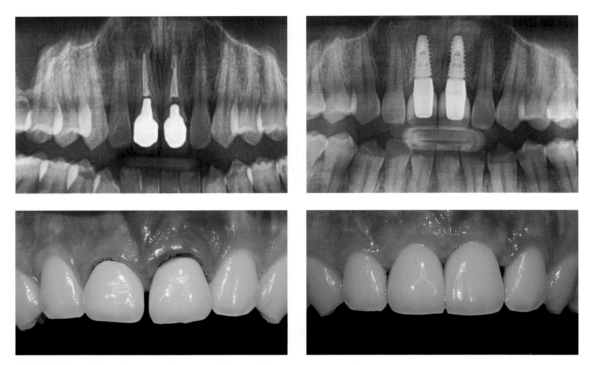

📷 **1.22** Black triangle formed between 21 and 22

Here is another case (📷 **1.22**). It is unlikely that soft tissue will fill in the embrasure space in the future. I don't understand why the prosthodontic department made it this way and the patient immigrated after restoration so I was never able to find out what happened to his black triangle. However, I think that the black triangle probably did not and will not disappear. So, now we will have to consider how to fill the papilla around the implant.

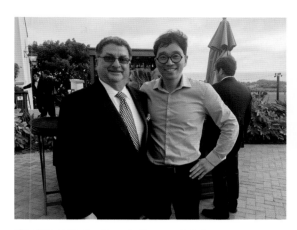

📷 **1.23** With Dr. Dennis Tarnow in LA

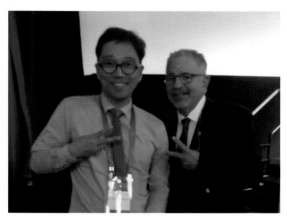

📷 **1.24** With Dr. John Kois in Las Vegas

Two masters appear here (📷 **1.23, 1.24**). There have been many additional studies that came out recently, but in the end, they do not deviate much from the framework established by these two dentists. Let's take a look at their views. Let's look at the famous paper 《The effect of distance from the contact point to the crest of bone on the presence or absence of the interproximal dental papilla》 that put Dennis Tanau to stardom (J periodontol. 1992).

This paper investigates the presence or absence of papilla according to the distance between the crestal bone and the interproximal contact of natural teeth. In almost all cases where the distance between crestal bone and contact point are less than 5 mm, it was reported that the papilla fills the embrasure space. I've heard of "Tanau's 5 mm rule" for a very long time. However, although it is a famous paper but this research was conducted on natural dentition, and the paper only talked about the distance between the crestal bone and the contact point. Therefore, it seems insufficient to use the results of this paper as a sole criterion for the formation of interdental papilla in implants. This person has been to South Korea several times as an overseas guest speaker, and I remember seeing a seminar promoted in the form of 'Dennis Tanau Denies Himself' on a promotional poster. Perhaps I'm assuming that these concepts are changing to a modern concept.

Let's look into John Kois's lectures and papers in order to consider interdental papilla formation in implants and to resolve black triangle issues since his paper considers various factors. It is a famous paper entitled 《Predictable single tooth peri-implant esthetics: five diagnostic keys》 (Compend Contin Educ Dent. 2001). Although this paper discusses about the anterior region where aesthetic factors are important, I think that these considerations presented can be applied to posterior implants as well.

In this paper, the five most important key factors for performing esthetic anterior implants are described as follows.

1. **Relative tooth position**
2. **Form of the periodontium**
3. **Phenotype of the periodontium**
4. **Tooth shape**
5. **Position of the osseous crest**

📁 1.1 Peri-Implant Esthetics

LOW RISK		FIVE DIAGNOSTIC KEYS	HIGH RISK
More Coronal or Lingual	1	Tooth Position/FGM	More Apical or Facial
Flat Scallop	2	Gingival Form	High Scallop
Thick	3	Phenotype	Thin
Square	4	Tooth Shape	Triangular
High Crest	5	Osseous Crest Position	Low Crest
More Likely to be Favorable		OUTCOME	More Likely to be Unfavorable

Source: Kois JC. Predictable single tooth peri-implant esthetics: five diagnostic keys. Compend Contin Educ Dent. 2001 Mar;22(3):199-206.

Looking at 📁 1.1, it has been showen that esthetics for anterior implants are more predicable when the tooth is positioned more coronally or lingually, when the gingiva is less curved and flatter, when the gingival biotype is thick, when the tooth is more square in shape, and when the alveolar crest level is higher. Additionally, this paper also **considers the type of implant, the design, whether or not alveolar preservation surgery was performed, and whether or not the provisional crown was manufactured as the important factors,** but they are not classified as the main factors that can predict the results of anterior esthetic treatment.

In the case of John Kois' thesis, various factors are discussed, but the most important factor in dentistry so far has been the distance from the level of alveolar crest to interproximal contact point of the tooth. In addition, I think the thickness of the gingival tissue and the shape of the teeth are the factors that should be considered additionally.

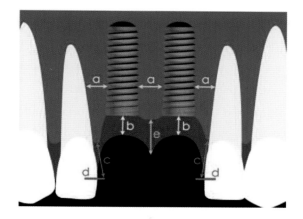

📷 **1.25** Interdental Papilla related diagram from ITI treatment Guide

📁 **1.2 Esthetic Risk Analysis**

Esthetic Risk Factors	Level of Risk		
	Low	Moderate	High
Medical status	Healthy, co–operative patient with an intact immune system		Reduced immune system
Smoking habit	Non–smoker	Light smoker (<10 cigs/day)	Heavy smoker (>10 cigs/day)
Patient's esthetic expectations	Low	Medium	High
Lip line	Low	Medium	High
Gingival biotype	Low scalloped, thick	Medium scalloped, medium thick	High scalloped, thin
Shape of tooth crowns	Rectangular		Triangular
Infection at implant site	None	Chronic	Acute
Bone level at adjacent teeth	≤5 mm to contact point	5,5 to 6,5 mm to contact point	≥7 mm to contatct point
Restorative status of neighboring teeth	Virgin		Restored
Width of eden	1 tooth (≥7 mm)	1 tooth (≥7 mm)	2 teeth or more
Soft tissue anatomy	Intact soft tissue		Soft tissue defects
Bone anatomy of alveolar crest	Alveolar crest without bone deficiency	Horizontal bone deficiency	Vertical bone deficiency

Source: ITI Treatment Guide (2009)

Earlier, we talked about Straumann implants, which can be said to be the best implants in the world. It is a fact that everyone knows that ITI (International Team for Implantology) is the basis for the theoretical background of this Straumann implant. Let's take a look at the 2009 ITI Treatment Guide from him. There are quite a bit of related researches to these, but most of them are based on external hexa type implants that are not used as much anymore nowadays. The research paper published in 2009 must be quite meaningful with relevant data since Straumann started producing bone level internal friction type implants in 2007. Since everyone is smarter than me, if you skim through the table, you will understand it fairly well. This paper does not conclude with a specific millimeter, but only considers the problem as a high or low probability.

According to the various papers and my experience, I concluded that the distance between implants should be 4 mm, not 5 mm, in order for the interimplant space to be completely filled with the gingival tissue. However, one cannot and should not make all cases as 4 mm. There are incidents where gingival tissue fully fills between implants even when they are more than 7 mm aparts.

Personally, **I think the phenotype of the periodontium and the tooth shape are important patient factors.** Of course, thick gingival phenotype will fill in better than gingival phenotype, and square shaped teeth will fill in more than triangular shaped ones. By performing enameloplasty for the triangular shaped teeth or by making a new restoration, one must change the tooth to a square shape since it is impossible to change the patient's gingival phenotype. Of course, the overall cost must also be considered as well.

I performed a lot of anterior esthetic cases until 5 years ago and I found myself applying the same concepts of preventing a black triangle to implant cases. If the distal tooth is tilted mesially in the posterior region, it is not a bad idea to perform enameloplasty on the mesial surface. If it has severe mesial inclination or has carious lesion, MO inlay or crown is fabricated at the time of implant impression. However, implant manufacturers, implant design, immediate placement, use of temporary teeth, and socket preservation do not have any effect on black triangles according to the aforementioned John Kois' paper.

Although it was not included in John Kois' five diagnostic keys for predictable single tooth peri-implant esthetics, I believe that the abutment-crown design is also a very important factor for the long-term health of the peri-implant gingiva, and that long-term health is directly related to esthetic success. The abutment must extend straight out of the implant platform but widens as it protrudes out of the gingival tissue for gingival health.

So the verdict is that a implant restoration must be S-shaped.

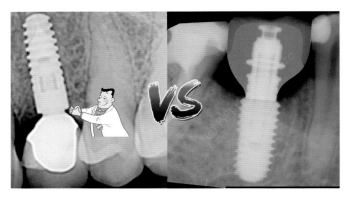

📷 **1.26 From the Facebook page of Dr. Steve Chang in Canada** It is emphasizing that the abutment must be thin.

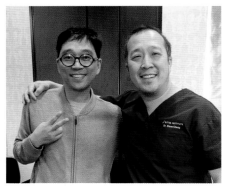

📷 **1.27** With Dr. Steve Chang in Toronto, Canada

I was impressed by a Facebook post by Dr. Steve Chang, and I ran into him when I went to

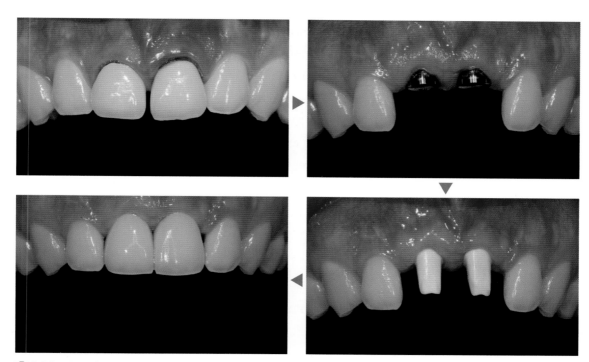

📷 **1.28** The abutment-crown fabrication process for black triangle case mentioned in the text

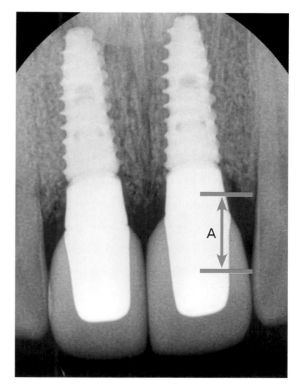

Toronto, Canada to lecture. Wherever I go, most of the knowledgeable dentists with skilled hands are more often than not, Korean dentists. Anyways, the key is that the abutment should be thin.

Let's look again at the case I mentioned earlier (📷 **1.28**). If I had to restore implants even though I do not, I would have shifted midline towards the left by making 11 larger, and also make 21 little bit larger and trim 22 mesial to lower he contact point gingivally.

Papilla would have filled in if the distance of 'A' was 4-5 mm. Or could have shaped the papilla by making a temporary crown with 6-7 mm of the 'A' distance and lowering it until the papilla is formed. Naturally re-shaping gingival tissue like this is called "gingival remodeling" and it's lacking in my cases the most since I do not restore implants.

Abutment diameter selection according to tooth position, assuming the abutment is 3 mm tall

Changes in emergence profile of the implant restoration based on diameter selected

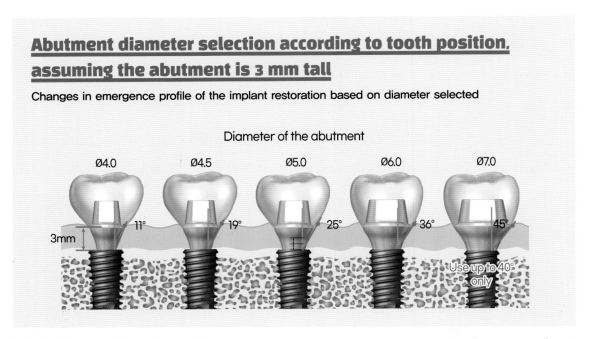

1.29 Based on the contents of Osstem's reference book, emergence profile was drawn according to different abutment diameters.

This is an excerpt from the Osstem lecture material (1.29). In general, it is stating that the emergence angle of the abutment-crown should not exceed 40°, which has become a common concept in general practitioners today. The average recommended thickness of the gingiva is 3 mm and when the 7 mm diameter healing abutment is used in that situation, the emergence angle becomes 45° and so abutment with diameter of 6 mm is recommended. In order to use an abutment with a diameter of 7 mm or more, it seems that the abutment height below the free gingival margin should not be 3 mm but should be more than 4 mm. I know this concept was created by Dr. Ki-Sung Kim, a dentist who is well recognized as a genius lecturer, and it can be said that this content clears up the curiosity of general practitioners. However, since my standard is to use a 5 mm height healing abutment from interproximal gingival level, there will be no issue using a 7 mm diameter abutment for the restoration.

In general, for the gingival health, it is stated that 30° is the most recommended emergence angle as it widens towards the crown. Then, how about the wide mandibular first molar? Let us assume that the mesiodistal width is 11 mm. Assuming it is placed right in the center with the same format as 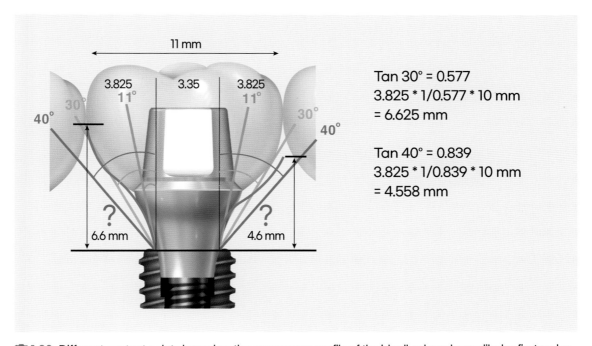 **1.30**, gingival height of abutment becomes 6.6 mm. Assuming 40° of emergence angle, it becomes 4.6 mm. In order to put these concepts into our head, I drew this to be used as rough reference. I have no aesthetic sense at all, so I have to keep looking at this diagram over and over again to get them into my head. What is more important than this is that the emergence profile does not just widens out in a straight line, but it should stretch out thinly toward the top and then widen to the side resulting in S-shape. Roughly think of this picture as a reference guide for us to be able to imagine a crown shape based on implant and different angles.

📷 **1.30** Different contact points based on the emergence profile of the ideally placed mandibular first molar

In fact, I can understand why Osstem is giving this kind of education, but I think it comes from the intention of trying to fix poorly placed implants with rectifiable crowns. As long as the implant is placed in the proper position and depth, there is no need to consider this aspect. So, I overlaid the image of Osstem's Healing Abutment, which I use for the mandibular first molars. It seems a little short, but intraorally inside gingiva, this is enough. The newly relased abutment by Dentist has more ideal height (6.0 mm) with diameter (6.8 mm) and seems to be a better fit when it was overlaid on the image. It appears to be a better match to the crown shape. So, I bought some to use occasionally. As a rule of thumb, I make simple use of instruments and tend to use a 5 mm height healing abutment. Sometimes there is a bridge or a lack of interocclusal space so when 6 mm height healing abutment is used most often than not, it may interfere with opposing dentition. You may think that there is no big difference between the 5 mm height vs 6 mm, but considering the opposing teeth and the available space, 1 mm can make a significant difference. In conclusion, if the distance from the opposing tooth is at least 10 mm, and minimum 5 mm from the interproximal gingival level (minimum of 3.5 mm from buccal), there is no need to worry about all of this.

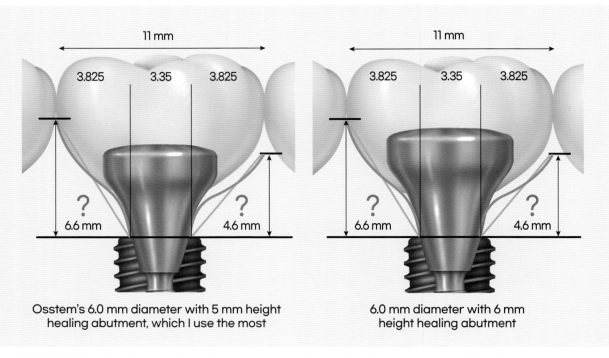

Osstem's 6.0 mm diameter with 5 mm height healing abutment, which I use the most

6.0 mm diameter with 6 mm height healing abutment

📷 **1.31** The healing abutment I use the most was superimposed on the emergence profile of the crown.

That's why I say this every time during my implant lecture. "**In implant, placing is easiest.** So, don't just place it and try to fix it later, **do the easy part twice.**" In other words, if you don't like it, remove it and place it again. As always, even if you dont have more than 10 mm, **keep the length and shape of the abutment consistent, rather reduce the length of the coronal portion of the abutment where the crown seats.**

But what if you weren't able to place the implant at the right position and depth? I set clear principles to the lab technician even though I don't restore implants because I have multiple prosthodontics who restore my implants and at times, prosthodontist changes. Regardless of how the implant is placed, the abutment must extend straight out of the implant plateform and advanced more than 3 mm first and then naturally widen or something. Even if the implant is incorrectly placed, all abutment-crown not designed as described should be returned. The expression 'widen' refers to the angle at which the abutment exits the fixture at 11° or less, and even though it widens outwards at 3 mm point up to 5-6 mm while drawing an S line, the angle from the starting point of the abutment to the crown margin of abutment should not exceed 30°. Moderately deeply placed implant is needed for that to happen. For gingival health, 30° is ideal. For this reason, it is recommended to extend straight up passing minimum thickness of the gingival tissue needed and then make a pontic.

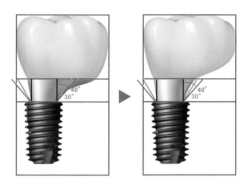

📷 1.32 Emergence angle of abutment must be less than 30° even if implant is not placed ideally. But instead of making it at 30°, I follow the internal angle of the implant, which is 11°, and extend the abutment straight up to 3 mm and then widen to form S-shape. For severely misplaced implants, I request the lab technician to assume that we are making two crowns instead of one as if making a cantilever crown. Of course, there are no cases like this in my practice, but sometimes I have to splint my implant crown with other implants placed elsewhere. So we must fully understand the concept.

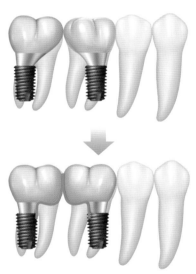

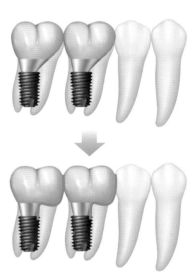

📷 1.33 With the same concept, assume that there are two single crowns in order to have a straight abutment and then splint them. I often request lab technicians to design with the mindset of making a cantilever pontic instead of one crown.

📷 1.34 Similarly, make straight abutments as if they are single crowns and then splint.

Implant prosthesis design of severely misplaced implants were developed by referencing Dental Arirang special lecture column in Feb 2018 by Dr. Kitae Ku, Jungwon Lee, and Dr. Sewook Pyo from Seoul National University Dental Hospital and Facebook cases posted by a doctor who places implants deep.

My abutment replacement case 1

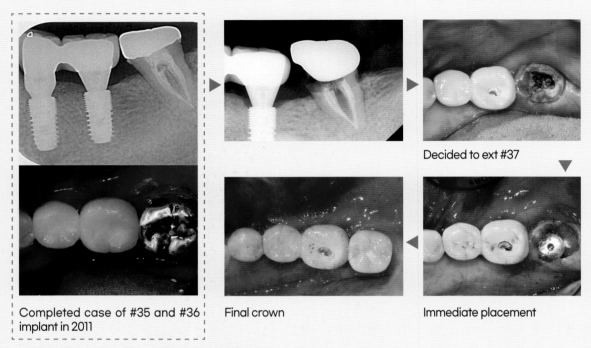

Completed case of #35 and #36 implant in 2011

Final crown

Decided to ext #37

Immediate placement

📷 1.35 Patient with implants placed in 2011 revisited

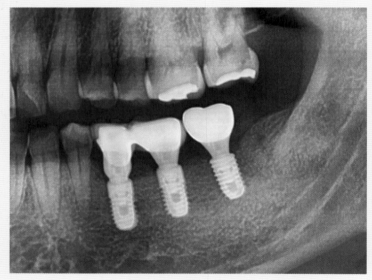

📷 1.36 Immediately after seating 37 abutment-crown in 2020

This is the case of implant 35 we saw earlier where the wrong abutment was selected (📷 1.35, 1.36). After 10 years, 37 was extracted and an immediate implant was placed. You can see the difference between the abutment selected 10 years ago and the abutment used recently.

My abutment replacement case 2

This case was placed in 2009 (📷 **1.37**) by me. I didn't restore the implant, but in 2019, the patient returned to have it recemented because the crown came out. I replaced it at no charge since this patient's entire family has been receiving treatment for a long time since 2002. The old one wasn't screwmentable abutment-crown, so it wasn't easy to remove it, but I am relieved now that I have replaced it. Looking at it now, I wonder what would have happened if the crown had been made a little larger, then the access hole would have been closer to the center. It seems old fashioned to have such a small occlusal table...

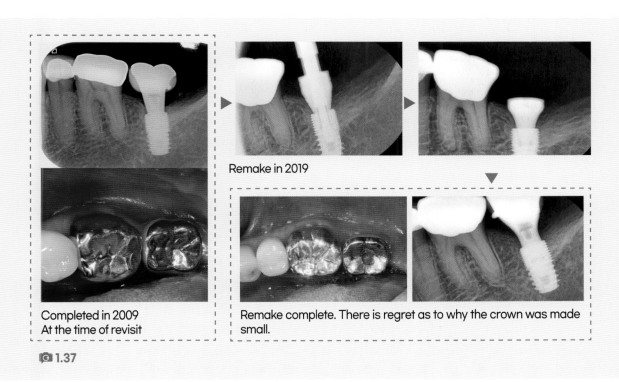

Remake in 2019

Completed in 2009
At the time of revisit

Remake complete. There is regret as to why the crown was made small.

📷 1.37

📷 **1.38** is the patient's current status. The oldest implant is the endopore implant, which was placed in 2005, and it is still in use. Probably because there is no tilting, no micro-gap and no movement since it is splinted. I'm just thinking maybe I'm lucky now.

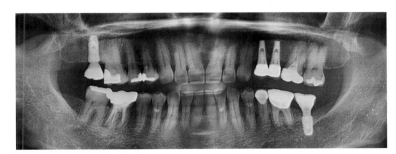

📷 1.38 **Recent panoramic X-ray 15 years after placement**
Placed 17 in 2006, 24 and 25 in 2005, and 37 in 2009

My abutment replacement case 3

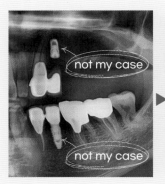 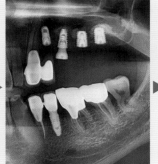 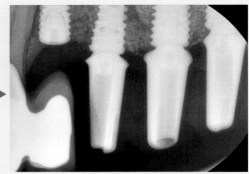

Pre-op   Post-op   First attempt of the abutment delivery

📷 **1.39 Sinus elevation case**

This is the case where I sometimes refer to as the transparent abutment (📷 **1.39**). I just think that 24 implant is amazing. It makes me wonder if the patient paid for the implant or not... After removing posterior teeth on the upper left quadrant, sinus elevation was performed 4 months later and implants were placed. In most cases, I usually place implants as a one-stage surgery with healing abutment. But implant can be pushed into the sinus when healing abutment is used in the area with a minimal crestal height, so the cover screw is used when implant needs to be placed deeper.

I took impression 40 days after the second stage of implant surgery to restore, but the abutment-crown made was so bad that the person from the prosthetic department came to me for a confirmation since they were afraid of being scolded by me. Of course, I told him to remake it. Because the impression was taken shortly after second stage implant surgery was performed, gingival tissue was not fully filled yet, and the technicians contoured the abutment to the height of underfilled interproximal gingiva. Not only for this reason but lab technicians tend to select these types of abutments since it is convenient for them to use deep and wide margin. When the case was sent back for remake, the lab technician asked me how to make it when there was not enough gingival tissue. So I told him to ignore the gingival position and make the abutment so that crown margin is placed at least 4-5 mm away from the fixture platform and the abutment must come straight out 3 mm and then widens 1-2 mm towards the crown margin. Lab technicians are not familiar with the concept of gingival contouring. Especially when the second stage implant surgery is performed the crown shape may not be ideal because the papilla has not been fully filled in yet. The average gingival thickness in maxillary posterior area is 3-4 mm or more and gingival tissue will continue to form and fill in around the abutment design I requested if the implant is placed 1 mm subcrestal at the ideal position.

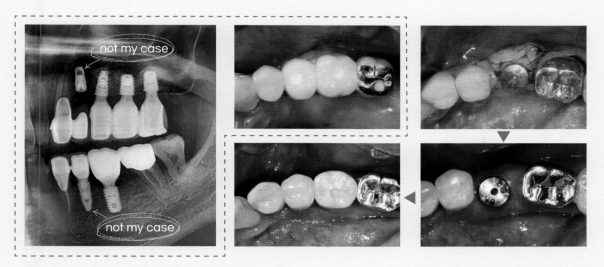

📷 **1.40** Long and thin shape of final abutment   Reference - Clinical photo of #36 implant

📷 **1.40** is a photo taken 18 month after the delivery and the position of 27 access hole is a bit disappointing, but the implant position had to be compromised due to limited buccal bone as shown on the clinical photo. I occasionally had to place an implant like this on upper 2nd molar sites because buccal bone tends to thin out rapidly towards distal, which is not commonly seen on the 1st molar site since 2nd molar is right distal to it. It is also occasionally found in the sinus lift case where the maxillary 2nd molar has been extracted a long time ago. Buccal GBR in this site is not easy either because there is no bone in the maxilla distal to 2nd molar.

Tooth #36 was also non-restorable so it was extracted and an implant was placed. For this lower case, as always, incised keratinized tissue is repositioned and sutured against buccal bone instead of being removed. In my experience, it takes about two and a half months for the mandibular gingival tissue to heal to a normal thickness when the gingiva is separated apart like this, and it seems that it takes about 3 to 4 months for the maxillary posterior gingival tissue to heal fully. As I have already mentioned several times before, most surgeries I do are one stage implant surgeries and one of the reasons is that it takes 2.5-3 months for mandibular gingiva to fully recover to their normal thickness and 3 months for maxillary gingiva. For most part, the healing time of gingiva to their normal thickness is similar to the time it takes for an implant to osseointegrate. This is why I keep emphasizing this concept since most lab technicians overlook the fact that gingival tissue has not recovered to its full thickness and end up selecting a short abutment.

Let's look at the gingival tissue of this maxillary case. Inevitably, due to the elevation of the maxillary sinus through the crestal approach, two stage implant surgery was performed. Usually the final impression is made within a month after 2nd stage surgery. Some dentists impress at 1-2 weeks during the suture removal appointment. It would be hard to find someone who waits several months

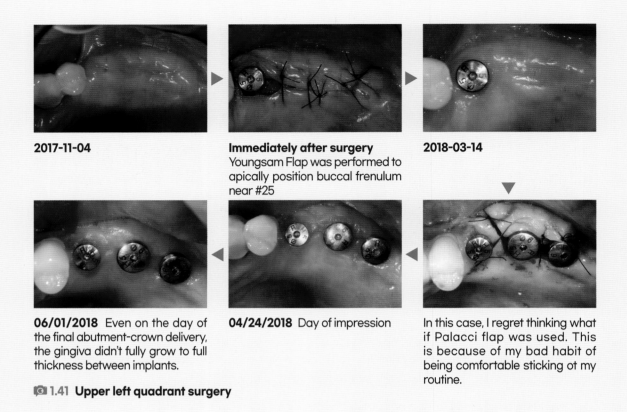

2017-11-04

Immediately after surgery
Youngsam Flap was performed to apically position buccal frenulum near #25

2018-03-14

06/01/2018 Even on the day of the final abutment-crown delivery, the gingiva didn't fully grow to full thickness between implants.

04/24/2018 Day of impression

In this case, I regret thinking what if Palacci flap was used. This is because of my bad habit of being comfortable sticking ot my routine.

📷 **1.41 Upper left quadrant surgery**

for gingiva to fully form after 2nd surgery. So final gingival thickness is predicted and abutment-crown is fabricated just like an anterior case so that papilla can continue to fully form. Second stage surgery was performed 4.5 month afterwards in this case and the flap was left open. Not per se it was left open, the flap was repositioned apically to place keratinized gingiva deep into the vestibule. If the zone of keratinized tissue is wide just like this case, it would have been better to perform a semilunar incision or palacci flap. However since I'm very strict on following the same protocol all the time, I repositioned the flap apically and sutured as I always do. The sutures seem a bit sloppy, but I rarely remove gingival tissue. I have a strange habit of not removing it because it feels like a huge waste. In this case, keratinized gingiva is sufficient and the vestibule is deep, so I think it would have been better if some of the gingival tissue was removed.

I do surgeries because I'm so conservative that I have difficulty prepping the teeth, so of course I would have difficulty removing keratinized tissue since it feels like such a waste. This is my sickness that you will never follow. So, when interdental papilla is not fully matured/filled in to it's normal thickness, instead of using gingival height as reference, instruct lab technicians to have abutment come straight out up to 3 mm and then flares out to crown margin.

Testimonials from doctors who attended implant lecture

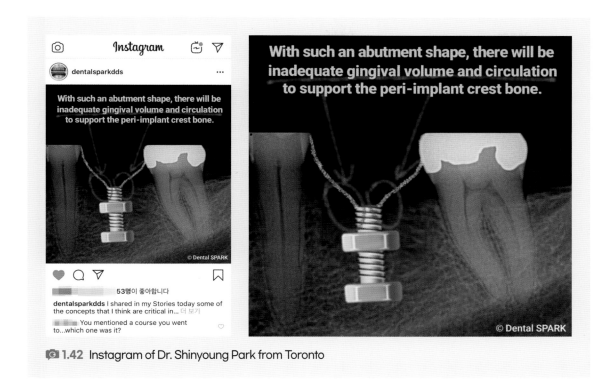

📷 1.42 Instagram of Dr. Shinyoung Park from Toronto

If you are a dentist, I recommend following her (📷 1.42). This doctor attended my wisdom tooth lectures in 2018 and implant lecture in 2019 in Toronto, Canada. After listening to my implant lecture, she liked this portion of my lecture and uploaded it to her Instagram. In fact, I wonder if she learned a lot from my lecture since she already was a very skilled clinician, but she told me that her implants prior to lecture had been pickaxes cases and monkey placing them and it made me feel good. She also participated in my live surgery seminar in Mexico at the end of 2019 with her younger brother.

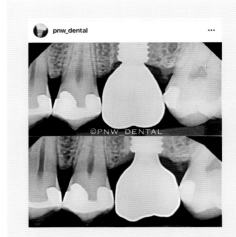
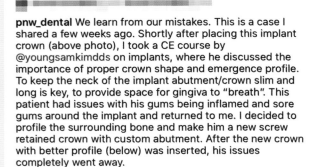

pnw_dental We learn from our mistakes. This is a case I shared a few weeks ago. Shortly after placing this implant crown (above photo), I took a CE course by @youngsamkimdds on implants, where he discussed the importance of proper crown shape and emergence profile. To keep the neck of the implant abutment/crown slim and long is key, to provide space for gingiva to "breath". This patient had issues with his gums being inflamed and sore gums around the implant and returned to me. I decided to profile the surrounding bone and make him a new screw retained crown with custom abutment. After the new crown with better profile (below) was inserted, his issues completely went away.

1.43 Instagram of Dr. Guyan Kim from Seattle

This is a photo posted on the Instagram of Mr. Gyuan Kim from Seattle, USA (1.43). This post is about how he replaced previously restored thick abutment-crown with S shaped abutment-crownafter attending my lecture and it resulted in significant improvement in peri-implantitis. These are the happiest moments from lecturing worldwide.

7-2
Why Screwmentable?

Why screw retained crown cannot be done in internal friction type implant?

In the process of crown fabrication in a dental laboratory, error can be made resulting in a discrepancy when fitted intraorally. We call this laboratory error and it is usually considered to be less than 50 μm, and in most crowns, this error is typically resolved by cement space. Although it may depend on the implant types, I'm thinking that a similar level of laboratory error occurs during the fabrication of implant abutment-crown.

For a reference, according to Karl Mish's book 《Avoiding complications in oral implantology (2017)》, the error is significantly greater in external hexa type implants. According to the contents of this book, implant manufacturers allow a misfit range for abutments or copings, and because of this, misfit rotation of ±10° of abutment or coping can occur inside the implant body itself. Further, if 10° misfit rotation occurs, it results in 99 um of horizontal discrepancies. Also, studies have shown that the plastic castable pattern (used for manufacturing screw type prosthesis) may be inaccurate and may show a vertical error of 66 um.

However, despite the fact that this was published recently, it can be said that they do not match the recent concept since most of the cited papers are from 1996. However It doesn't seem to have a major problem with fabrication of screw type prosthesis on external hexa type implants since misfit error range is considered as normal and accepted when manufacturing external hexa type implants. Also, screw type prosthesis can be used in external hexa type implants because the gap between abutment and implant fixture are recognized as norm from the beginning.

However, since internal friction type prostheses are operated on the premise that there should not be a gap between the abutment and the fixture in principle, it should be approached differently from the external hexa type, which is manufactured under the premise that it does not matter if misfit errors occur. Of course, the master I spoke to recently said that he agrees so he didn't fabricate screw type prosthesis on internal friction type implant, but nowadays it has become so precise that if it is well made, he said it can be delivered without any problem. To summarize my thoughts, it is possible to make a screw-type prosthesis with the internal friction type, but it must be manufactured very precisely, and even a small error may take a long time to adjust and set. In addition, since it remains a permanent error and often appears as a failure of the implant after a certain period of time, I wonder if there is a need to make a screw-type prosthesis. Of course, if you want to make it, you can, but it makes me think 'why do you choose the hard way?' Just make screwmentable crown...

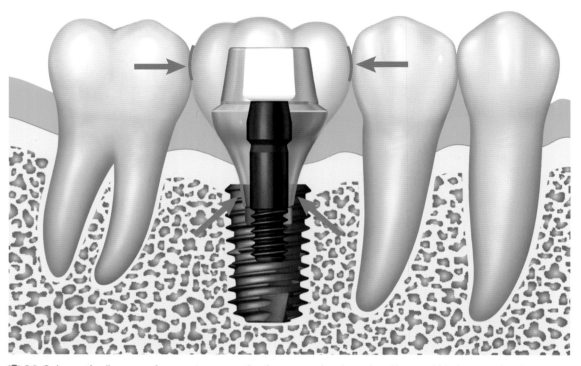

📷 **2.1** Schematic diagram of screw type prosthesis mounted on bone level internal friction type implant

Most of the crowns I use are SCRP (Screw & Cement Retained Prosthesis, Secrewmentale crown), but in the United States, it is common to see internal friction type implants with crowns and abutments attached to them as screw-retained crowns. You can never do this with internal friction type implants.

Let's assume that the laboratory has been making implant restoration where abutment and crown are attached as in 📷 **2.1**. Although not as much as the external hexa type, this is a implant restoration that has no choice but to have errors. First you have to try it on the fixture in your mouth to see if it fits well, then you will have to adjust the interproximal contact marked with the purple arrow to make it fit. Otherwise, the crown will not go in. If so, what would happen to the gap between the abutment and the fixture shown in the blue arrow? If the interproximal contact is adjusted to fit well, all the errors that occurred during the laboratory process and the interproximal contact adjustment will be transferred to create a gap between the fixture and the abutment. Since there is fremitus movements of adjacent teeth, if the laboratory process is relatively precise, you can deliver the prosthesis without problem if you press it to a certain extent and tighten the screw. However, if the laboratory error is large, the blue margin gap indicated by the blue arrow may be significantly large after interproximal contact adjustment. If you tighten the screw right away, it will not have movement initially, but after a short time, micro-movement does occur due to the gap between the fixture and the abutment, which can result in fracture of screw or abutment, crestal bone resorption, tearing of fixture, etc. If such a screw-retained prosthesis is to be used, it should be used only for external hexa type implants that are designed to allow the misfit degree and gap between the abutment and the fixture from the beginning.

I really like Dr. Kiseong Kim's lectures. It feels like he studies and experiences what I'm curious about in advance and lets me know through his lecture. I feel like Dr. Kiseong Kim's lectures are very well organized sparknotes making it easy for students to grasp important concepts summarized based on his experiences. He truly is a "genius instructor". When I listen to his lecture he really scratches the itch in my brain.

Anyways, Dr. Kiseong Kim was mentioning the article 《Comparison of implant component fractures in external and internal type: A12-year retrospective study (J Adv Prosthodont. 2018;10:155-62)》 and that it was drawing the wrong conclusion. In this paper, it is concluded that an external hexa type should be used in the posterior region because the internal friction type (Astra type) abutment fractures easily. All abutment-crown used in this paper were made of gold cast UCLA type. Therefore, I think that either the design method of the thesis is wrong, or it should have been concluded that 'screw-retained crowns should not be manufactured in the posterior region for the internal friction type implants'. Same for the article called 《Cumulative survival rate and complication rates of single-tooth; The same is true for focused on the coronal fracture of fixture in the internal connection implant (Journal of Oral Rehabilitation. 2013 40;595-602)》. Fixture fracture or screw loosening occurred in 41.2% of Astra 4.0 regular size implant placements, but these were all cast-to-abutment types. Therefore, even here, the success rate of implants or the incidence of complications are not important. This article also should have been concluded that screw-retained implant restoration where the abutment and the crown are one piece should never be used.

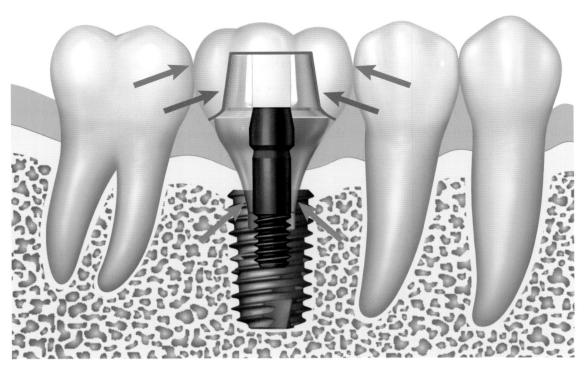

📷 2.2 Schematic diagram of cement retained prosthesis mounted on bone level internal friction type implant

Therefore all of the internal friction type implants I placed are restored with cement retained crown. When I deliver implant restoration, as shown in 📷 2.2, I first mount the abutment well to the implant so that there is no gap in the area indicated by the blue arrow. And then I adjust interproximal contact so that the area pointed by the purple arrow fits passively so that all the errors arising from impression taking and laboratory processes get offset by the cement space indicated by the red arrow.

This is because if the contact point pointed by the purple arros do not fit passively, the patient gets uncomfortable, and if the abutment and the fixture connection point indicated by the blue arrows do not fit passively, everyone gets uncomfortable later. However, in the cement retained crowns, excess cement remains at the crown margin causing peri-implantitis, and when patient returns clinic due to a problem with the abutment-crown or due to any maintenance, it becomes such a hassle to drill a hole into the crown to access screw to remove the abutment. Furthermore, recently I have been more inclined to restore with screwementable type crown where it has an access hole on the occlusal surface for easy access for screw removal since the material of the crown has been changed to zirconia, which is difficult to drill a hole in. In fact, I believe the invention of the screwmentable crown was not just for easy insertion and removal of the abutment and crown later, but more so for extraoral removal of excess cement at the abutment and crown margin after cementation. I also think that this part of the screwmentable crown is one of the biggest advantages, but in everyday dentistry, the process is very cumbersome, so it is not well implemented. I have to ask the prosthetic department to remove excess cement extraorally after cementation since I do not restore the implant, but it doesn't seem to be implemented as I intended. Even if you don't do it that way, you should always keep in mind that there is a high chance of having residual cement remaining at the abutment and crown margin of the implant restoration when the crown is cemented intraorally.

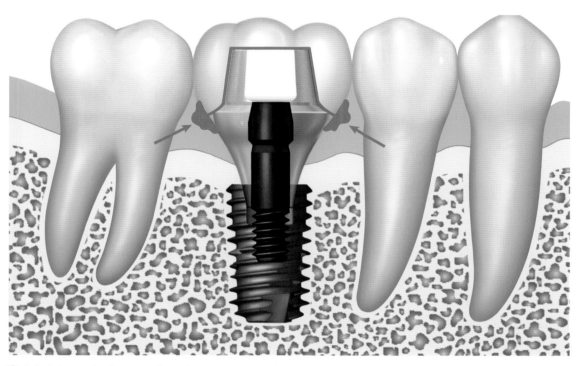

Cement Removal of Screwmentable type Crown

📷 **2.3** Schematic diagram of residual cement remaining when cement retained implant crown is delivered

It is true that dentists in South Korea do not pay much attention to cement removal since in our country the dental hygienists are the ones who remove excess cement. However, as mentioned earlier, the main reason why screwmentable crown is invented is for the complete removal of excess cement.

It is common for a large amount of excess cement to overflow and adhere to the area indicated by the red arrow. After delivering the implant crown in the prosthetic department, I advise them to make a habit of performing standard imaging in lower radiation settings. The same goes for regular check-ups. This is because it's not uncommon to see the remaining cement in some cases at a recall appointment. Nevertheless, keep in mind the excess cement on either buccal and lingual side is not visible on the radiograph.

The radiograph shows excess cement on the mesial. In my experience, most of the excess cement remains on the mesial side. Amount of the residual cement seems quite a bit despite the fact that I

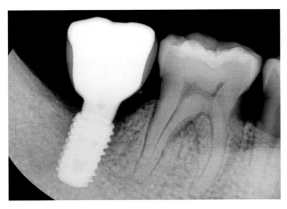
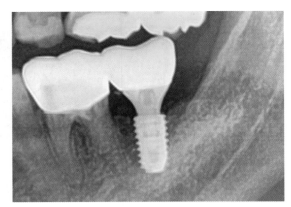

📷 2.4 Residual cement is noted on the X-ray taken after implant crown delivery. But can't detect thin residual cement on buccal or lingual aspect of the abutment.

used custom abutment and imagine when stock abutment is used, mesial margin is placed further subgingival and it will not be easy to remove residual cement.

Case with residual cement

This is a case that shows not only that the cement removal is difficult but also hard to find. This is a case that I treated 5 years ago in 2016. The father of a famous actor said he didn't want any metal showing, so the PFM crown was fabricated with porcelain on the occlusal. However, it is just a matter of time for porcelain to break off when restored with porcelain occlusion on the rearmost molars of a strong men. Because the porcelain continued to chip off, the crown was removed to be replaced by a zirconia crown and I was startled by what I saw. There was a white particle around the gingiva where the crown had been removed. I looked closer thinking it must be a bone graft material but it was residual cement. So I looked at the crown I just removed and of course it clearly had cement around

Case where residual cement was found 5 years after abutment-crown delivery

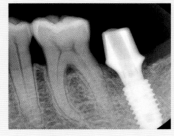

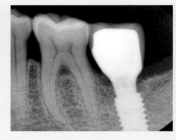

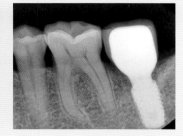

📷 2.5 Standard X-ray after abutment delivery

📷 2.6 Standard X-ray immediately after crown delivery

📷 2.7 Standard X-ray 3 years after crown delivery

Cement is nowhere to be found during the delivery process.

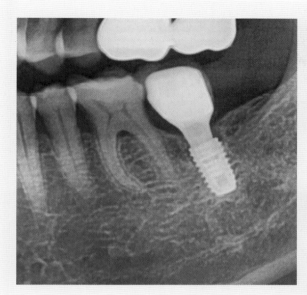

2.8 Panoramic X-ray taken right before implant abutment-crown removal

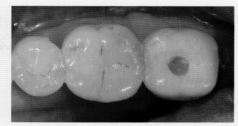

2.9 Clinical photo right before implant crown removal

▼

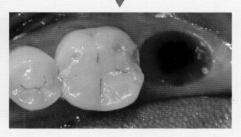

2.10 Clinical photo taken right after implant abutment-crown removal. Residual cement noted on the gingival tissue. It was removed thinking that it was a bone particle but it was cement.

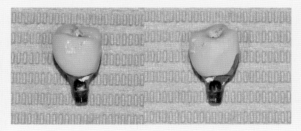

2.11 Residual cement noted on the removed implant abutment-crown.

it. Although the cement had been there for more than 5 years, the color was so vivid and looked fresh. It's very fortunate that there was no inflammation around the implant.

In addition to this case, it is very common to see cement on an old implant abutment that has been removed. Surprisingly, there are many cases where there was no inflammation around the implant, and there was no discoloration. There was nothing that looked like cement on any of the radiographs previously taken. Although I am not a prosthetist, I often emphasize to the prosthetic department that the radiographs should be taken as often as possible with minimum exposure with radiation beam perpendicular to implant and abutment junction.

As seen so far, with periodic exams with recall X-rays, I never questioned having residual cement. Most of the cements do not appear on the radiograph.

Ideal Protocol for Screwmentable Abutment-Crown Delivery

Below is a patient I purposely seated implant restoration myself to take clinical photos. The patient is the father of a current dentist who came in to have his implant crown permanently re-cemented after using it with temporary cement for a longtime.

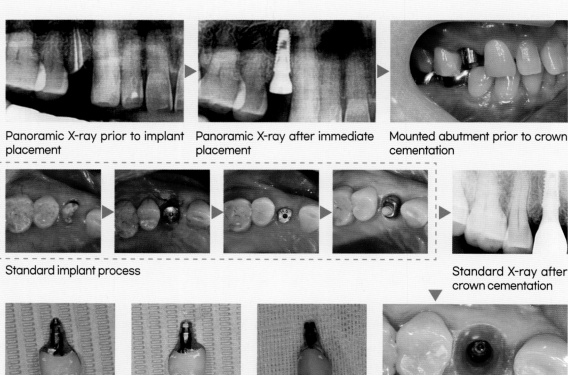

Panoramic X-ray prior to implant placement

Panoramic X-ray after immediate placement

Mounted abutment prior to crown cementation

Standard implant process

Standard X-ray after crown cementation

Screwmentable abutment-crown removed after crown cementation Although the cement was not completely removed yet you can still note residual cement at the abutment level.

Gingiva after removal of cemented abutment and crown
Cement noted on the gingival tissue

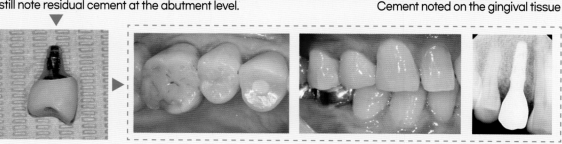

Screwmentable abutment-crown after removal of all the cement

Seated abutment-crown using screw after removing remaining cement on the peri-implant soft tissue
Screw hole was restored using Ketac molar.

📷 2.12

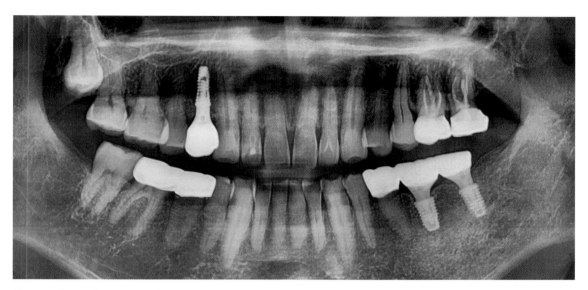

📷 2.13 18 months after seating crown on implant abutment

Abutment-crown was removed while it was still temporarily cemented and then it was re-cemented with permanent cement. Afterwards, the abutment and the crown were removed by loosening the screw, and the peri-implant soft tissue and cemented abutment-crown was photographed right away. It can be seen that the cement remains on the abutment-crown and gingival tissue.

The excess cement on the gingival tissue and implant restoration was removed, polished, and then seated back on the implant using a screw and a photo was taken. It has been 2 years since delivery and still well maintained. In principle, screwmentable abutment-crown are designed to be delivered like this, but as the fee for implants decreases over time, this protocol appears to be complicated and became more like normal cement type prosthesis.

Messages received from the US and Australia simultaneously just before publication

I get a lot of emails and messages from all over the world from my lecturers and foreign dentists I don't know. Some of the days I end up spending all of my free time replying to their messages. It can be annoying, but I think of it as a fan letter and I'm happy to answer most of them. From two dentists who had attended my lecture in the USA and Australia sent me similar messages on the last day of reviewing this book, and I decided to post them here.

Surprisingly, this is a common question asked. These problems mainly occurs after the Ti-base zirconia abutment is fabricated and delivered as a screw type prosthesis. Those of you who have already read this book will know the answer. First of all, the characteristic of Ti-base zirconia abutment is that the abutment is very thick to begin with to prevent fracture at the connection. I only use it as needed for the anterior cases, but I rarely use it in the posterior region. Not only that it is more expensive, but for me, if I design it as I prefer with thin and straight abutment, it has a high chance of fracture. So, if I have to use it, I would recommend using it on the anterior region as screwmentable or cement type only.

If you look at the inquired cases, you can see that they are all designed very thick 1 mm above the fixture. I do not know what healing abutment was used, but it is not easy to passively fit this kind of this final prosthesis to the fixture. Moreover, if it is a screw type, it becomes even more difficult. With this design, even if you invest a lot of money, time, and energy, you may not get a good result. If you want to make a zirconia crown, I would like to recommend the scrwmentable type of abutment, which is made by making a general custom titanium abutment in a thin and straight shape, allowing passive insertion, and cementing the crown on it afterwards. That is why I wrote this chapter.

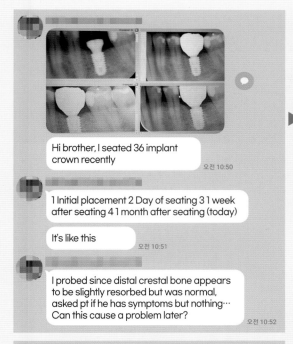

Hi brother, I seated 36 implant crown recently

오전 10:50

1 Initial placement 2 Day of seating 3 1 week after seating 4 1 month after seating (today)

It's like this

오전 10:51

I probed since distal crestal bone appears to be slightly resorbed but was normal, asked pt if he has symptoms but nothing··· Can this cause a problem later?

오전 10:52

Hello~ There is something I want to ask~

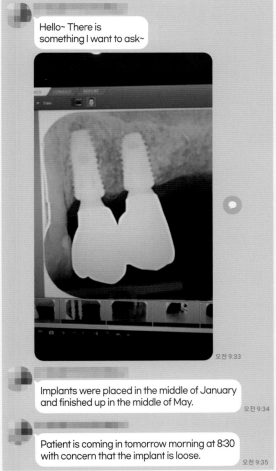

오전 9:33

Implants were placed in the middle of January and finished up in the middle of May.

오전 9:34

Patient is coming in tomorrow morning at 8:30 with concern that the implant is loose.

오전 9:35

📷 2.14 So, in the end, I recommend a thin abutment and screwmentable type crown that extend straight up in the posterior area.

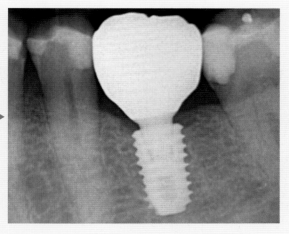

This x-ray was taken right after sitting abutment-crown, but the gap is visible between the abutment and the fixture.

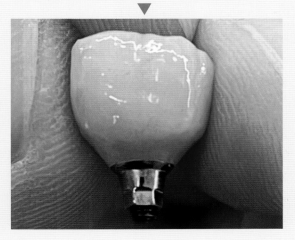

Eventually he sent me a picture of the crown removed.

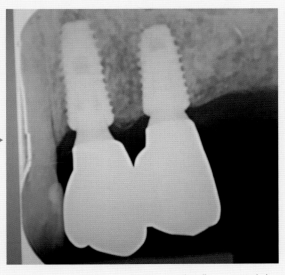

This also shows a gap between the fixture and the abutment. On the day of delivery, even if it seems to have been delivered properly, after a certain period time, pressured gingiva resorbs and mobility is noted and causes problems.

EASY SIMPLE SAFE EFFICIENT

MASTERING DENTAL IMPLANTS

The Essential Elements for Success in Dental Implants

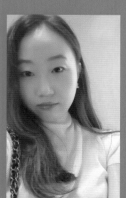

Dr. Shinyoung Park

Honors BSc, University of Toronto
DDS, University of Toronto Faculty of Dentistry

It is such an honor to have participated again in Dr. Kim's 2nd English book. Having taken several of his courses including his live surgery seminar in Mexico, I believe that this book will help many clinicians step up their implant dentistry by providing numerous surgical tips and a better understanding of the implant mechanics.

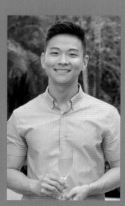

Dr. Byung Jun (Chris) Song

DDS, University of Toronto Faculty of Dentistry

It was an honor to have been asked to help translate Dr. Kim's first implant textbook. Before meeting Dr. Kim, I felt implant dentistry was a scary and unknown field that was reserved only for specialists or the very brave. Dr. Kim's approach to implant dentistry is very accessible to general dentists like me and I hope that other clinicians will be inspired by his passion.

Implant Failures

Implant failure is not the mother of success

8-1 Peri-implantitis

8-2 Fracture of Fixtures and Abutments

8-1

Peri-implantitis

Peri-implantitis

So far this book has emphasized the importance of the right position and depth of the implant fixture and the passive fit of the abutment without micro-gaps and movements. In fact, you will see that most of the peri-implantitis treatment cases you can come across involve either **incorrectly placed fixtures and/or incorrectly made abutments.** Looking at such cases, I think myself, 'Why would one even attempt to treat such cases? The implants weren't placed right to begin with.', 'The abutment and the crown were made wrong.'

As mentioned earlier, when it comes to peri-implantitis, "prevention" is the key. The implant should be placed such a way that it will not be prone to peri-implantitis in the first place. Nonetheless, the majority of the commonly practiced peri-implantitis treatments involve, as the first step, raising a flap to clean the exposed implant surface as much as possible. If GBR is planned in an attempt to regain the lost bone, laser or other tools are used to further clean the contaminated surface prior to the GBR.

Personally, **I do not think that the implant surface, once contaminated, can be reproduced and reconditioned well enough chair-side by a clinician to be osseointegrated again** because as we all know, the implant surface treatment process is quite complex and requires highly advanced technology. If the implant surface has become contaminated with accompanying bone loss, it is more predictable to remove the implant and start from scratch in my opinion. If it is clear that the problem stems from incorrectly made abutment and crown without severe bone loss, those prostheses should first be replaced.

Several implant companies have commercialized instruments to smoothen the exposed implant surface. The most representative are the instruments developed by the president of Neobiotech, Youngku Heo, aka Thomas Edison in the dental world.

As I mentioned earlier in **Chapter 2-1 Dental Implant Materials and Surface Treatments** gingiva

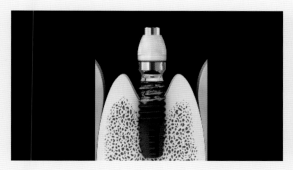
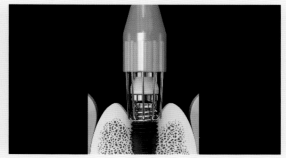

📷 1.1 Cleaning of the exposed implant surface (Ref: Neobiotech)

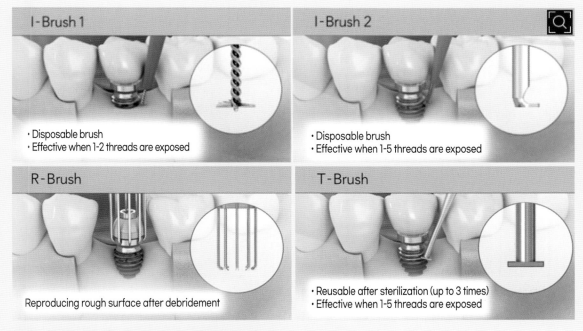

I-Brush 1
· Disposable brush
· Effective when 1-2 threads are exposed

I-Brush 2
· Disposable brush
· Effective when 1-5 threads are exposed

R-Brush
Reproducing rough surface after debridement

T-Brush
· Reusable after sterilization (up to 3 times)
· Effective when 1-5 threads are exposed

📷 1.2 Other Implant Cleaning Tools (Ref: Neobiotech)

do not attach to rough surfaces. Given that bone does not integrate well to contaminated implant surfaces, one may hope for some gingival attachment instead by raising a flap, polishing the exposed implant surface, and closing the flap. I'm not an advocate for such a management, which, I think, is being practiced mostly because the patient is adamant about saving the implant even when advised otherwise. Whenever I see peri-implantitis treatment cases presented in lectures or online I'm often skeptical to consider them successful. Of course, the final treatment decision is up to the patient, but I would try to convince the patient to replace the implant whenever possible.

Then how do I manage peri-implantitis? If there is no clinical symptom, I leave the implant as is and monitor. However, if the bone is lost more than half way down the height of the fixture, I remove the implant and re-implant even if the patient is asymptomatic.

The easiest and most reliable treatment for peri-implantitis in my opinion is to explant and re-implant. Therefore, it is advised not to place implants that are too long for the sake of removal in case things become not so favorable. As being short does not make the implant more prone to failures, short implants are advantageous in many ways.

Take a moment and refer to the products by Neobiotech and the related YouTube videos. It's nice to see their products gradually evolve.

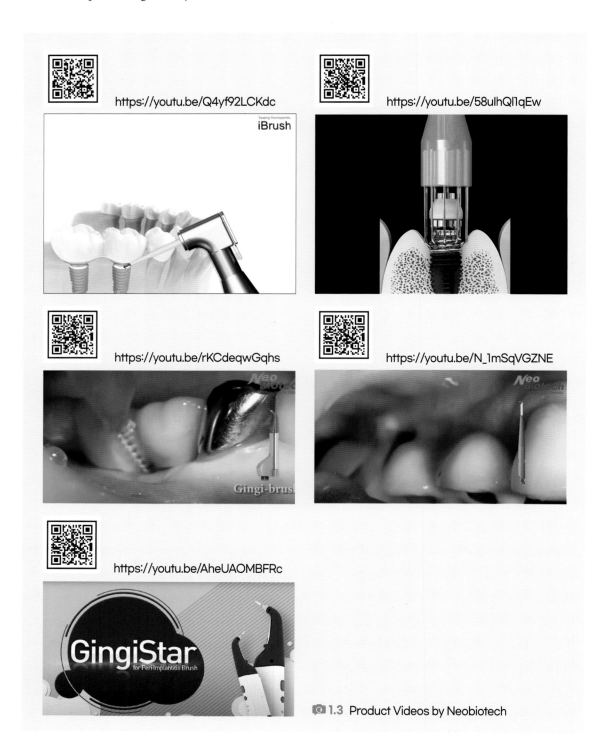

https://youtu.be/Q4yf92LCKdc

https://youtu.be/58ulhQl1qEw

https://youtu.be/rKCdeqwGqhs

https://youtu.be/N_1mSqVGZNE

https://youtu.be/AheUAOMBFRc

📷 1.3 Product Videos by Neobiotech

CASE 1

The first case of peri-implantitis is of Endopore implant, which is famous for its rough surface.

The patient was a male artist in his late 30's, who was referred to me by an acquaintance of mine. He presented on August 19, 2003 to address the pain from tooth 26 and to extract tooth 48. 📷 1.4 is the panoramic radiograph taken during his first visit. I was able to find its digital copy, which I scanned to present at Endopore implant seminar about 10 years ago.

Back in 2003, all his teeth had very poor periodontal prognosis due to severe crowding with malocclusion and poor oral hygiene. His treatment started only after improved oral hygiene had been promised. I often refer to this patient when talking about the importance of good oral hygiene. Being an artist with good dexterity, he has been following my hygiene instructions very well, which is likely how he has been able to maintaine his teeth without further deterioratoin for the last 18 years.

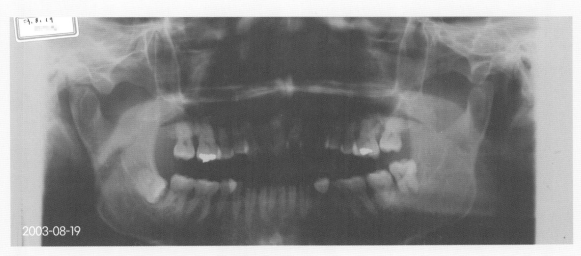

2003-08-19

📷 1.4 Panoramic radiograph taken during his first visit

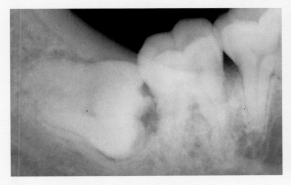

📷 1.5 **PA of tooth 48 taken in 2003**
Digital radiographs are superior. Their resolutions are maintained.

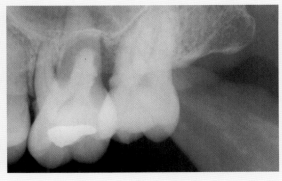

📷 1.6 Tooth 26 which was planned to be extracted and replaced with an implant

Endopore implant placement and restoration in 2003

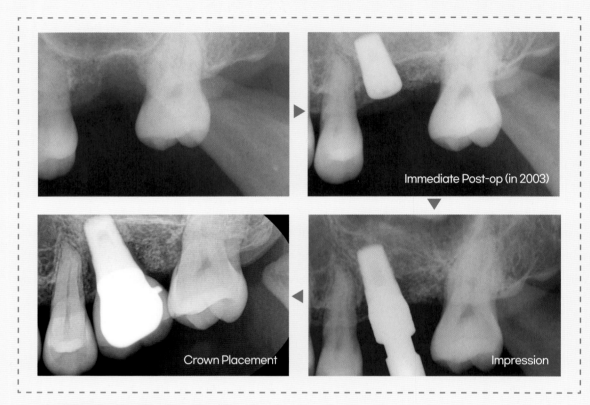

Immediate Post-op (in 2003)

Impression

Crown Placement

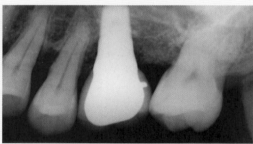

2012-10-20
Other teeth were treated later, but no radiograph was taken for tooth 26 after this. The periodontal improvement at tooth 27 mesial is quite impressive to see even now.

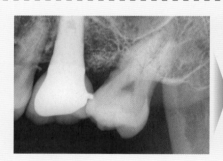

2017-03-09
The patient came in with painful gums around the implant. Peri-implantitis was diagnosed, but since there was no mobility, conventional periodontal treatment was planned.

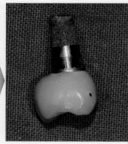

The patient returned with the implant in hand after 23 days.

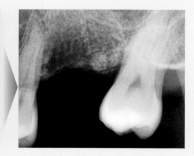

2017-06-05
PA taken after the implant fell out spontaneously. Re-implant surgery was scheduled after a month.

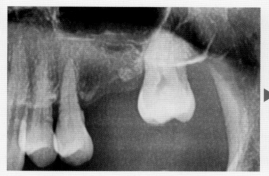

2017-7-3
Panoramic radiograph on the day of reimplantation

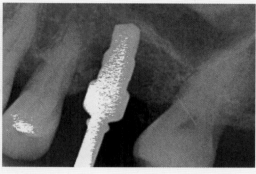

Inadequate bone formation was noted even 3 months after the spontaneous implant loss. Only one drilling was done prior to fixture placement.

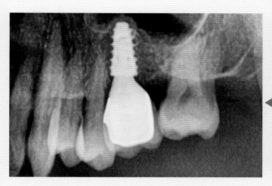

Crown placement 5 months after surgery

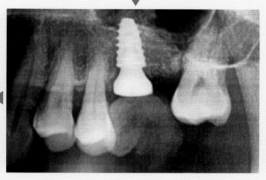

Immediate post-op panoramic radiograph. Hiossen TS4 with deep threads, 5.0 x 8.5 mm fixture was placed following an under-sized drilling as the bone quality was poor.

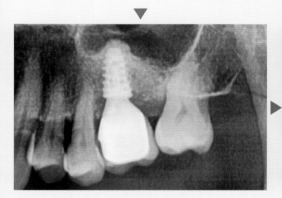

20 months after crown placement

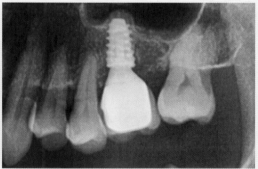

34 months after crown placement

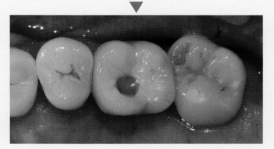

Clinical photo 34 months after crown placement

📷 1.7 **Endopore Implant Placement and Restoration**

Peri-implantitis around Endopore implants progresses very quickly because of the rough surface that Endopore is known for, and once it starts, nothing much can be done other than monitoring since it is impossible to clean between the small particles embedded in the implant surface. In this case as well, the peri-implantitis progressed so fast that the implant came out on its own in less than a month. This also means that there was severe inflammation around the implant, and the bone recovery in the area was therefore slow. Even though the site was re-entered 3 months later, the bone quality was still poor, and it was difficult to correct the implant position properly. In addition, the occlusion had to be taken into consideration as the opposing tooth was lingually tiled due to severe crowding. The patient has been seen on a regular basis every 6 months.

CASE 2

This is a case of a female patient, 32-year-old back in 2009, and the implants were placed by a highly skilled associate surgeon who worked in my office then (📷 1.8). This particular implant line had an atypical shape and was new to us at that time, so we were not yet quite comfortable placing it. The associate left my office soon after, and I took over the case for the remaining treatment course.

If you look at the panoramic radiograph taken immediately after the surgery, you can see that 37 implant was stuck in the middle of the osteotomy that was overdrilled apically. This is a common mistake that unexperienced clinicians make when placing coronally wide implants into D1 bone. Now that I think about it, the surgeon should have used what I call "Ankylos method". It would have been better if the coronal portion of the osteotomy had been done more generously with a full size drill, while the primary stability was obtained mostly from the apical portion. As the implant was stuck coronally, there must have been significant stress exerted on the cortical bone. In addition, the abutments and the crowns were not properly shaped - the abutments being too short and the crowns being too bulbous. Even though one cannot be certain about the exact cause of the bone loss in this case, it is not totally surprising or unexpected to see that it happened.

The bone loss continued persistently thereafter, so the implants were removed 4 years after their placement. Re-implantation was completed in the usual way, followed by the crown placement. So far, the implants have been functional for over 5 years without any issues. You can see that they were placed deeper, but shorter fixtures were used with longer abutments, ensuring adequate gingival thickness. As you can see in the most recent panoramic radiograph, the implants have been well-maintained including 46 implant which was placed at the same time.

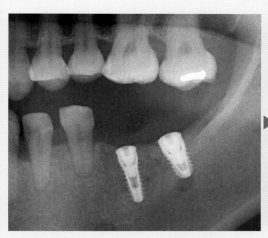 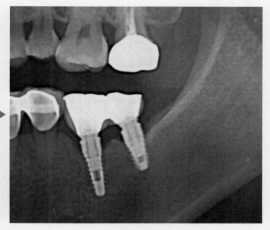

Immediate post-op panoramic radiograph
(Implant manufacturer: DIO Implant)

Panoramic radiograph 3 years after crown placement

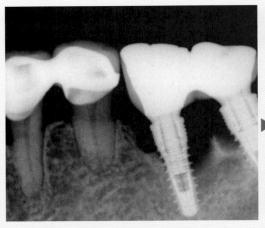

PA taken 4 years after crown placement
It was decided to remove the fixtures due to further bone loss.

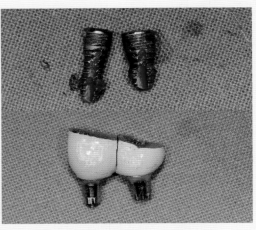

Removed implant fixtures and crowns

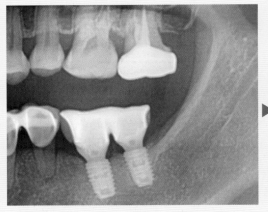

Panoramic radiograph taken immediately after 37 reimplant completion
36 implant was placed 2 years earilier as a single implant.

Panoramic radiograph taken 3 years after re-implantation
(Implant manufacturer: Hiossen)

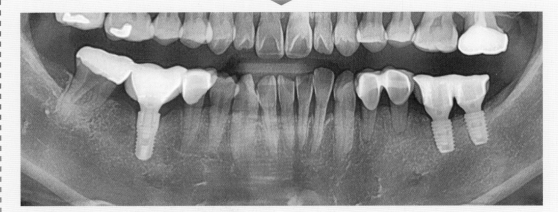

April 2021, 5 years after re-implantation
36, 37 implants - 12 years after initial implantation, 46 implant - placed in 2010 (manufacturer: DIO implant)

1.8

CASE 3

Let's look at the case of a patient whose periodontal condition was very poor to begin with. This was a case of a male patient in his early 40s at that time, and I placed a Hiossen GS3 implant about 10 years ago (📷 1.9). The patient's overall periodontal condition was not good, and the patient himself was quite concerned about it. Looking at it now, the position and angulation of the implant were not ideal, and the abutment was too thick and too short. 5.5 years into function, the implant and the tooth in front of it developed severe periodontitis, so both were extracted and replaced with implants after healing. The implants have been well maintained since the crowns were placed 4 years ago.

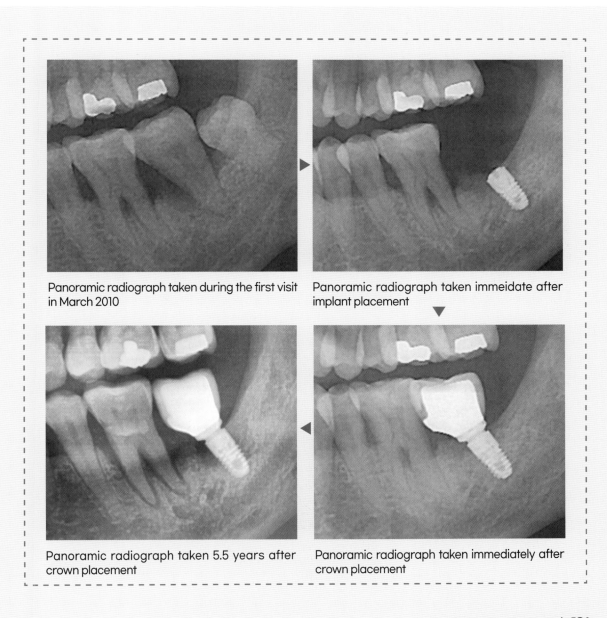

Panoramic radiograph taken during the first visit in March 2010

Panoramic radiograph taken immeidate after implant placement

Panoramic radiograph taken 5.5 years after crown placement

Panoramic radiograph taken immediately after crown placement

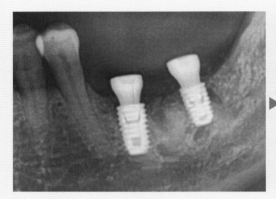

Immediately after re-implantation

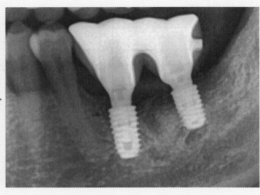

Panoramic radiograph taken after crown placement

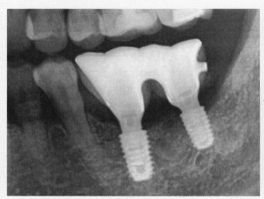

41 months after crown placement

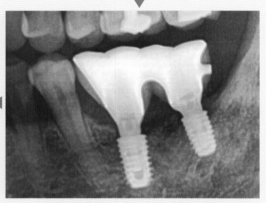

Panoramic radiograph taken 29 months after crown placement

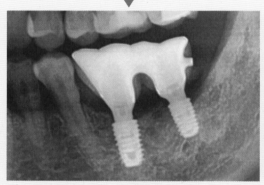

52 months after crown placement

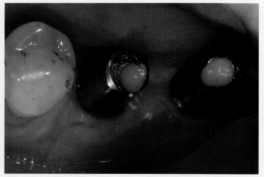

Gingiva prior to crown placement Keratinized gingiva can be seen buccal to the implants.

A. Gingiva 41 months after crown placement
Keratinized gingiva can still be seen.

B. Crowns 41 months after crown placement
PFM with metal occlusal crowns were placed since zirconia crowns were not widely used at that time.

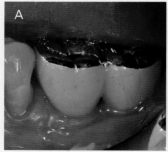

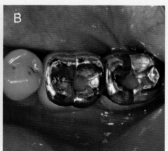

📷 1.9

CASE 4

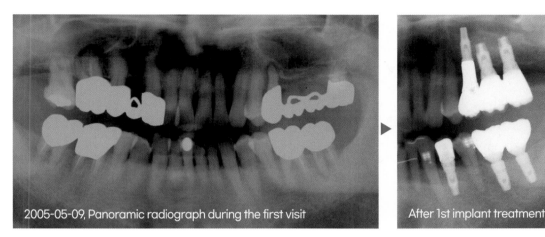

2005-05-09, Panoramic radiograph during the first visit

After 1st implant treatment

📷 1.10

This case has taught me several lessons, so I decided to include it. In 2005, the patient visited for the first time with pain from the molars on the left side, and he has been coming for regular checkups ever since (📷 1.10). Clinicians at that time in general had limited surgical skills and theoretical knowledge of implant dentistry, and their main goal was to make bone to place long and thick implants. You can notice the excessive sinus graft and the 25 implant placed too deep with its significantly long abutment. What we should focus on in this patient's case is the left side, but I'm sharing the entire treatment course including the right side for reference (📷 1.11). It can be seen from the panoramic radiographs that the surgical method used then is rarely performed now.

On May 8, 2015, exactly 10 years after I started to place implants, the patient presented with pain

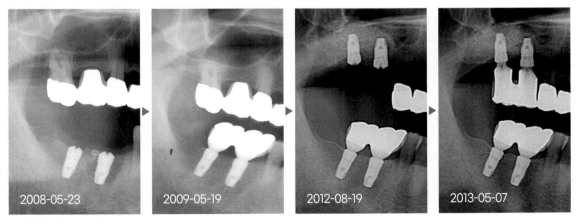

2008-05-23

2009-05-19

2012-08-19

2013-05-07

📷 1.11 Treatment course of the right side implants

from the gums around tooth 24 and the 25 implant (📷 1.12). The gingiva were also edematous with suppuration. After the implant crowns were removed, the 25 implant was buried, and a cantilever bridge was placed instead.

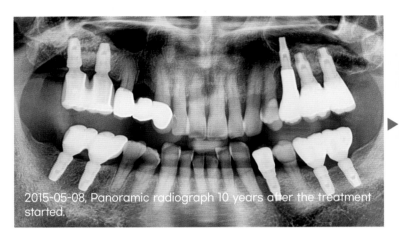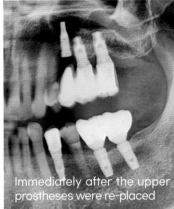

2015-05-08, Panoramic radiograph 10 years after the treatment started.

Immediately after the upper prostheses were re-placed

📷 1.12

After 2 years, some bone loss was noticed around the 36 implant, and it was decided to address it even though the patient was asymptomatic. I was skeptical about treating peri-implantitis even back then, but my associate showed some interest in this case and was confident about his treatment prognosis, so I let him take over. After about a month of healing abutment stage following the GBR, a temporary crown over a stock abutment was placed to monitor the progress. The associate seemed to be quite happy about the outcome, but I was still concerned about its long-term prognosis. The associate eventually left my office, and I ended up removing the implant, 18 months after the GBR, even though the patient still had no discomfort until then (📷 1.13).

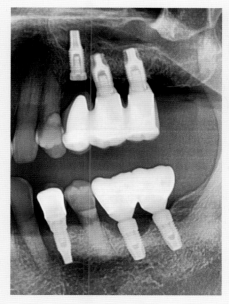

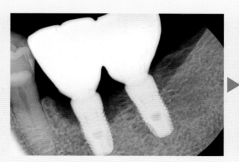

PA taken 2 years after the upper prostheses were replaced. Bone resorption can be seen around the 36 implant.

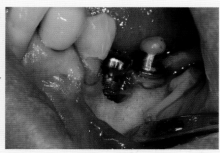

Conventional peri-implantitis treatment followed by GBR

Panoramic radiograph taken 2 years after the upper prostheses were replaced

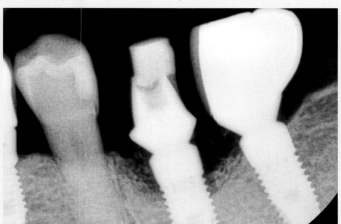

2 months after GBR

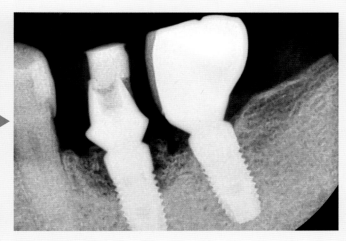

8 months after GBR

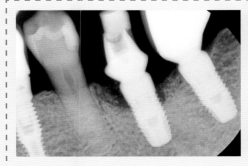

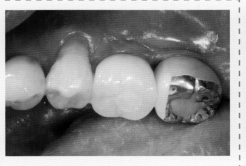

PA and clinical photo taken 18 months after GBR (with temporary crown)

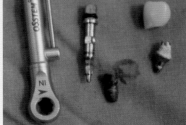

After implant removal

📷 1.13

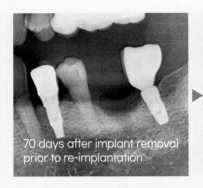

70 days after implant removal prior to re-implantation

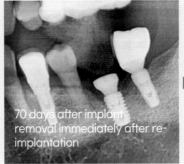

70 days after implant removal immediately after re-implantation

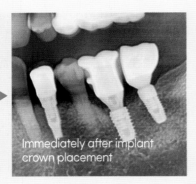

Immediately after implant crown placement

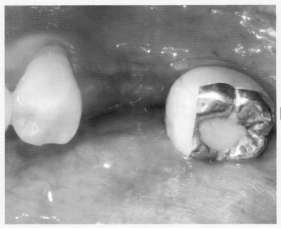

70 days after implant removal prior to re-implantation

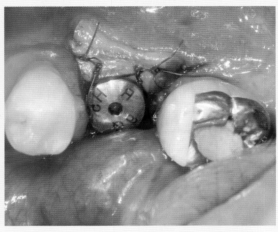

70 days after implant removal immediately after re-implantation

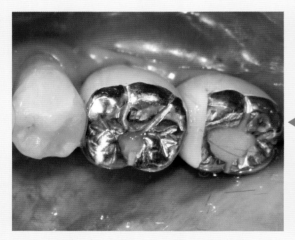

7 months after implant crown placement (following a long-term temporization)

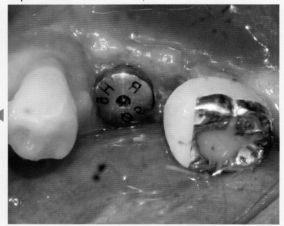

2-week post-op after suture removal

📷 1.14

Re-implantation surgery was performed in my usual way. It can be seen that the vestibule and the keratinized gingiva were maintained with Youngsam flap. The 37 implant still has the crown that was modified from the original joined crowns made 15 years ago. Both the 36 and the 37 implants have

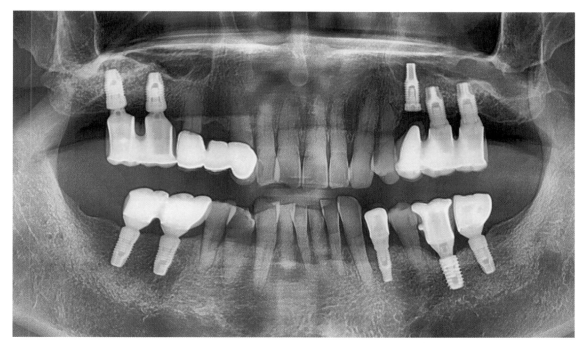

March 2021, 2 years after crown placement, 16 years after initial implant treatment

📷 1.15

long been closely monitored since then.

In this recent panoramic radiograph, it can be seen that all implants remain stable (📷 1.15). Significant bone gain is noticeable between tooth 24 and the 25 implant, and the gingiva have been maintained well. As I mentioned earlier, I wish the implant next to the existing implant had been placed a bit deeper. My implants have always been slightly deeper than others, but they have become 1 mm deeper on average in the past 1-2 years.

From this radiograph, it appears that there is some bone loss around the maxillary implants, but it is likely due to artifacts as the panoramic radiograph taken right before this one showed normal bone levels. Continuous maintenance is required in the future.

How do we remove implants?

In fact, the implant in the previous case could not be removed with a wrench. No matter how much force was applied with the implant tool, it would not budge. Explantation was attempted with a mandibular premolar forcep, to no avail. I even tried a molar forcep, but it still didn't move at all. Considering that I am quite proficient in wisdom teeth extractions using forceps, you can probably imagine how sturdy the implant was in the bone (you have to be very careful not to touch the adjacent teeth when removing implants with forceps).

In such a case, instead of using a Trephine bur, I reduce the bone on one side of the implant (usually the mesial or the distal side further away from the adjacent teeth) using a thin bur or #4 surgical round bur, and luxate the implant from the opposite side with an elevator much as in wisdom teeth extractions.

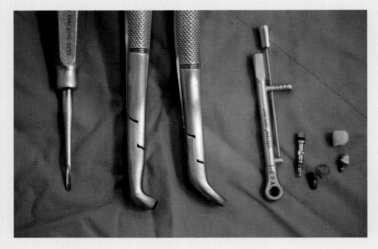

📷 **1.16 Instruments used to remove the implant.** I have the habit of taking photos of the instruments and the explanted implant if unusual instruments were used.

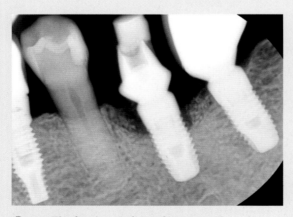

📷 **1.17 The implant prior to its removal**

Once the implant starts to move a little, it becomes easier to remove it from then on.

This is the PA of the implant prior to its removal (📷 **1.17**). Despite the bone loss about half way down the implant height and the poor crown-to-root ratio, it had been functioning as a single unit for a long time without any discomfort, and its removal was very difficult. Implants with even more severe bone loss can be extremely difficult to remove. This is why we should not insist on placing long implants. As mentioned earlier, the length of the implant is important only until the osseointegration is complete, not so much after that. In my experience, it is very difficult to remove implants that are integrated about 4-5 mm, and those integrated less than 3 mm seems to be removed much more easily. Therefore, I believe that 4-5 mm height is enough even for a single-unit implant, and there is no need to stress about placing longer implants when the bone height is limited.

CASE 5

This case was already mentioned earlier in this book, which is about an implant with only apical integration(📷 1.19). The entire family is VIP and has been my patients for a long time. The patient was the father of the family in his 60s, and he presented with the 36 implant, 6 years after its placement.

There were no reported symptoms as the bone loss had occurred chronically without any active inflammation, and at that time, the patient was visiting South Korea for a short period from Bolivia, so he refused to remove the implant. When he returned 15 months later for a longer visit, I convinced him to remove it then even though it was still asymptomatic. We struggled to schedule for the treatments though, as the patient had to travel back and forth between Bolivia and South Korea. Re-implantation was done 1.5 months after the implant removal. Because the patient was unsure when his next visit to Korea would be, the impression was taken 2.5 months after the surgery even though the graft and the soft tissues were still not fully matured. The crown placement was scheduled 2 weeks after the impression.

On the day of the crown placement, however, the worst happened. What I always emphasize to my lab is to extend the abutment straight up to about 3 mm from the fixture before forming the crown, but the crown delivered for this very important case was nowhere close to my expectation as shown in the radiographs. When I called the lab to complain, I was told that it was made by a new technician who had never worked on my cases before. I had no choice other than to place it then because the patient had to fly back to Bolivia very soon. It was decided to replace it later.

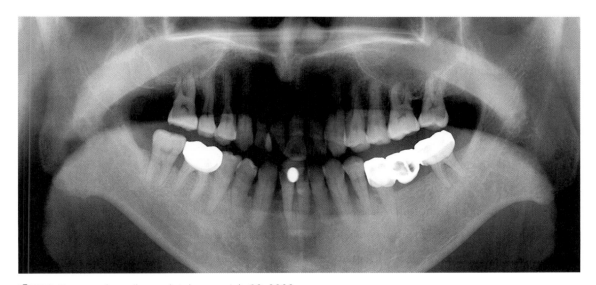

📷 1.18 Panoramic radiograph taken on July 09, 2008

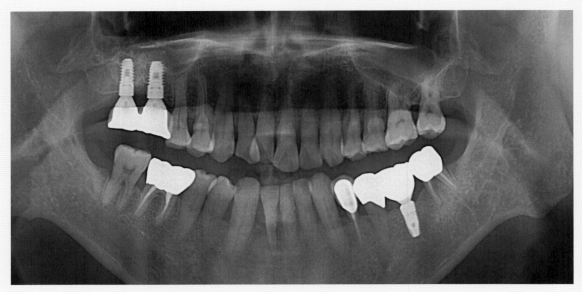

July 2010 (2 years after implant placement)

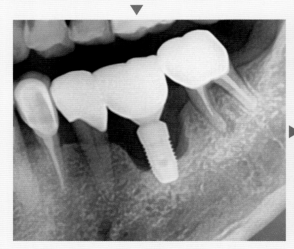

April 2014 (6 years after implant placement)

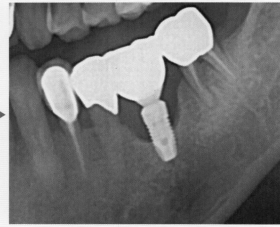

July 2015 (7 years after implant placement)

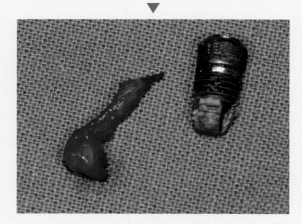

1.19 Immediately after implant removal

1.19

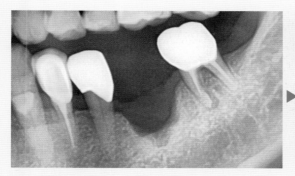

Prior to re-implantation (2015-08-18)

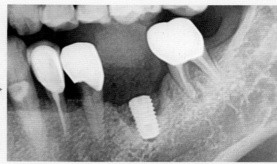

Immeidately after re-implantation

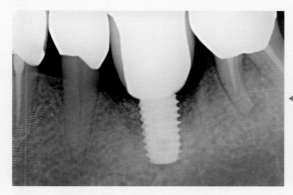

Immediately after crown placement
The incorrectly shaped abutment and crown had to be placed as the patient was taking off soon. In my office, implant abutment should extend straight at least 3 mm from the fixture. Such a shape was probably a result of the immature healing of the gingiva at the time of the impression. It was a mishap by a new lab technician.

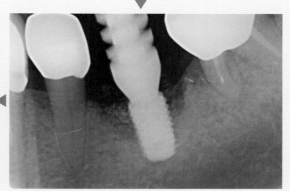

Impression taken Immediately after crown placement 2.5 months later

📷 1.20

When the patient returned to Korea after 4 months, nothing else but a PA could be taken because he was staying for a short time again. When he came back 6 months later, he reported that the tooth behind the implant had been extracted in Bolivia, for which he requested an implant to be placed during that visit. The 36 implant was still of a concern, but I placed the 37 implant as the patient was adamant about it. When he returned after 9 months, again, nothing could be done because he was staying for short. During his next visit after 6 months, it was decided to remove both the 36 and 37 implants, and they were reimplanted 3 months later. The surgery was not straightforward, and I was very nervous throughout. The bone around the 37 implant site was very dense, so it was tricky to adjust the direction and the depth of the implant during the placement. After all, I tried to match the depths of the two implants by placing the 36 implant not as deep and grafting it coronally instead. The final prostheses were placed 5 months later, and the implants have been followed up for 2 years now. Even though the etiology of the peri-implantitis that the patient initially presented with was still unclear, the subsequent failures down the road show us the significance of the contributing factors such as implant position, depth, and crown shape in the success of the implant treatment.

Here are the procedures of the 36 and 37 implant placement.

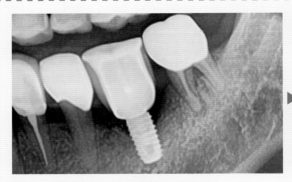

4 monhts after crown placement
As I mentioned earlier, such an abutment/crown shape causes imminent bone loss.

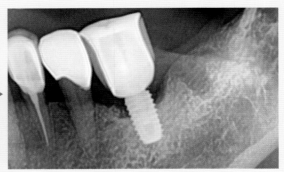

22 monhts after crown placement
Patient presented after having tooth 37 extracted in Bolivia, for which he requested an implant to be placed during his short stay.

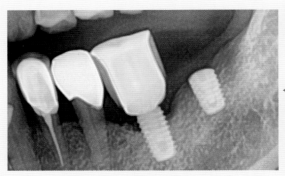

15 months after 37 implant placement
35 months after 36 implant crown placement (Dec 2008)

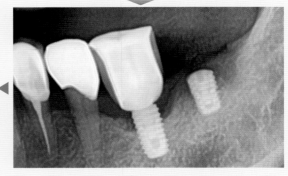

Immediately after 37 implant placement
I couldn't drill deeper as the bone was too dense. The implant should have been placed deeper.

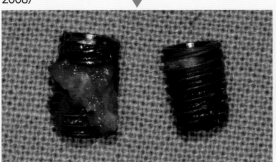

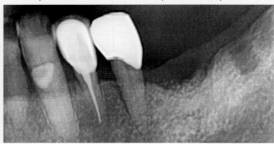

Both implants were removed as it was thought to be impossible to match the implant depths. It was removed easily with an implant mount driver.

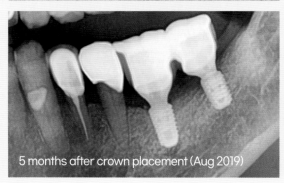

5 months after crown placement (Aug 2019)

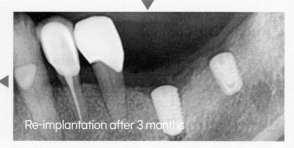

Re-implantation after 3 months

📷 1.21

As seen in the clinical photos, there was limited attached gingiva likely due to the inflammation from the multiple surgeries (📷 1.22). There was also some scar tissue formation, which might have caused the cover screw of the 36 implant to be exposed, and it was immediately replaced with a healing abutment. As mentioned earlier, when cover screws are exposed, I always replace them with healing abutments. Since I could not do Youngsam flap to gain more attached gingiva on the buccal side of the 36 implant, FGG was performed to gain additional attached gingiva and to deepen the vestibule after the second surgery of the 37 implant. I have been following up with these implants closely as I personally believe that scars formed by frequent surgeries can have adverse effects on the long-term prognosis.

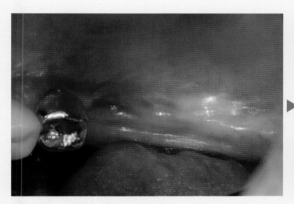

Gingiva prior to re-implantation

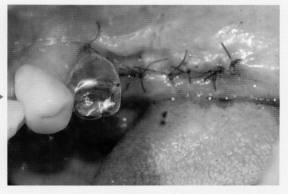

2 weeks after re-implantation prior to suture removal Scar has formed around the 36 implant, which caused impaired circulation and the subsequent necrosis of the gingiva over the implant.

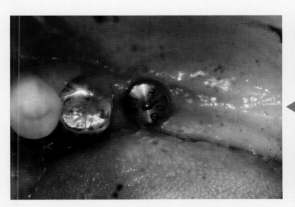

2.5 months after healing abutment was placed Uneventful healing of the gingiva around the 36 implant can be seen.

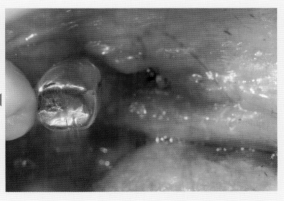

The cover screw of the 36 implant was exposed and replaced with a healing abutment. If cover screw is exposed, I always replace it with a healing abutment.

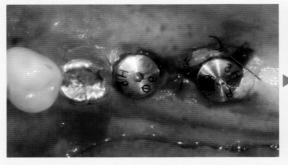

Immediately after the 2nd surgery of the 37 implant
It was done in my usual way with Youngsam flap.

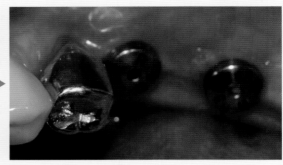

1 month after the 2nd surgery
Even though more than 1 mm of attached gingiva was maintained with Youngsam flap, FCC was decided for better prognosis.

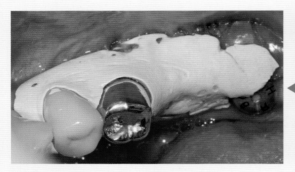

Pack placed to keep the vestibule down

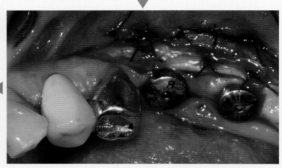

Immediately after vestibuloplasty and FGG

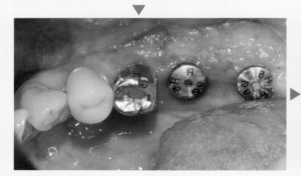

2 weeks after FGG

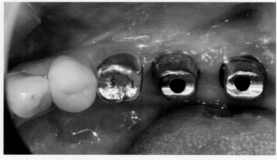

2 months after FGG (5 months after implant placement) prior to crown placement

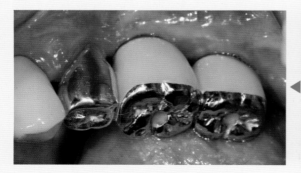

Buccal gingiva after final crown placement

📷 1.22

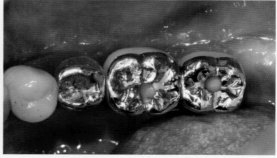

After final crown placement

CASE 6

This case was completed in 2002 (📷 1.23). Thick and long implants were the trend at that time, so presumably 5×13 mm fixtures were placed. There was limited knowledge about keratinized gingiva, vestibule, movable gingiva, etc. back then, and I was not so keen on the soft tissue management as the patient was only 20-year-old.

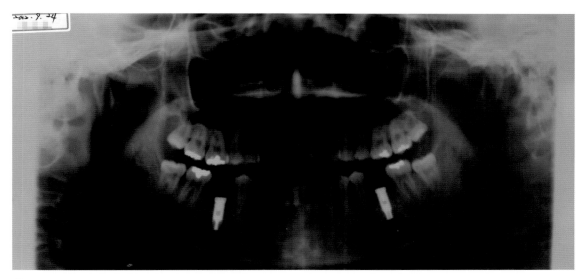

📷 1.23 Panoramic radiograph immediately after implant placement

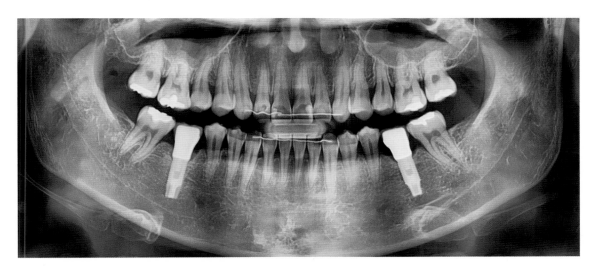

📷 1.24 **Panoramic radiograph during recall exam in 2017. No bone loss is seen even though the implants were external hexa type. I think it is because the gold UCLA abutment and PFG crown were placed.**
Gingival discomfort had been reported from time to time, but this time, the patient requested to remove the 36 implant crown as the gingiva on its buccal side were so painful that she could not even bite on it. I removed the crown, placed a cover screw, and closed gingiva to rule out other issues.

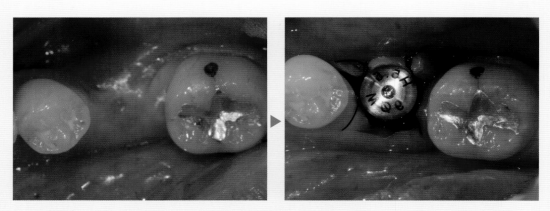

2 months after the 36 implant crown removal Suture closure after the usual Youngsam flap (2017)

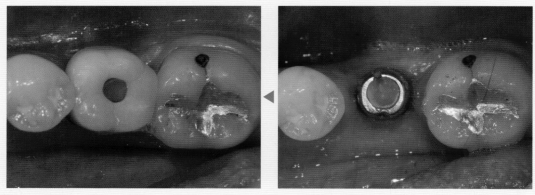

📷 **1.25 Placement of the pre-existing gold abutment and a new crown**
I was not happy with the result to be honest, but at least the gingival pain had been resolved. In hindsight, the buccal gingiva could have been repositioned further apically.

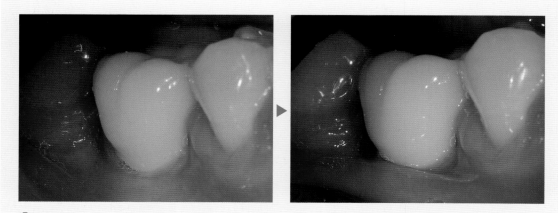

📷 **1.26** The clinical photo I took 10 years after the implant placement in 2012. You can see some marginal fluctuation on the buccal side.

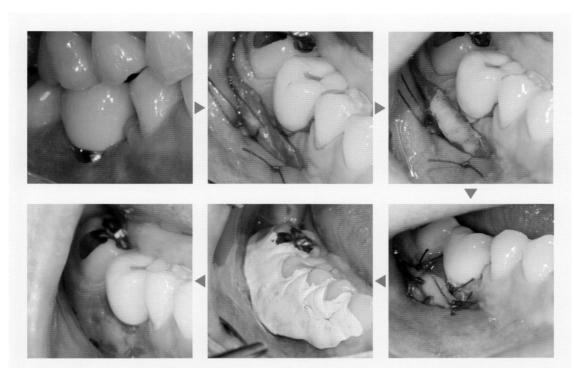

📷 **1.27** Conventional FGG was completed 7 years later to address the abutment exposure and the painful gingiva (2019).

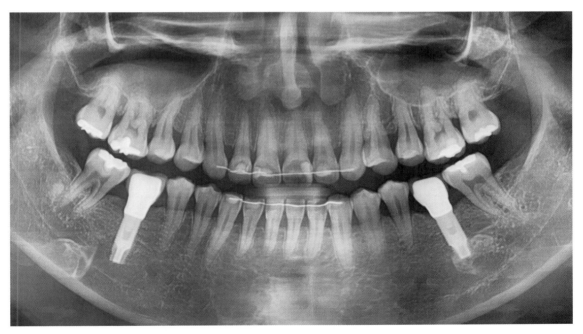

📷 **1.28 May 2021.** The implants and periodontium have been well maintained since their placement 20 years ago.

CASE 7

Last but not least, this case will go down in history a patient for whom I have been placing implants for the last 10 years.

She is the mother of the patient in the previous case (3rd peri-implantitis treatment case). She was 70 years old at the time of her first visit (currently 80 years old), and she has been suffering from diabetes since childhood. She is in poor general health with limited mobility, so every time her children take turns to bring her to my office, which is more than an hour drive away. I suggested dentures instead several times throughout the treatment course, but the patient insisted on implants.

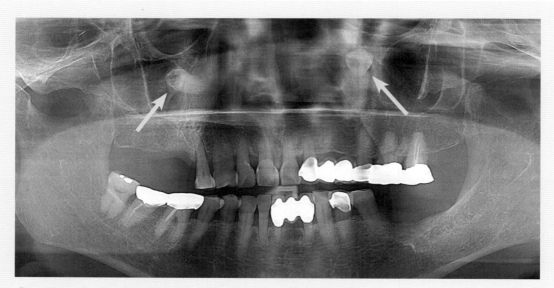

📷 1.29 **Panoramic radiograph taken during the fist visit in 2011**
I know this patient's name by heart because I always show her panoramic radiograph to the patients who ask me to extract their impacted teeth when not indicated. I tell them that it is ok to monitor them as even those canines impacted under the eyes have not been an issue until now.

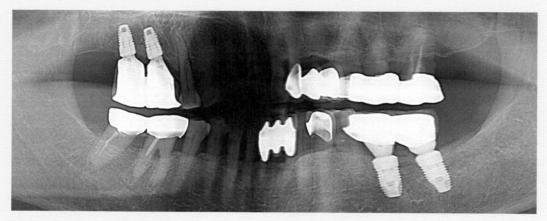

📷 1.30 After 1st implant treatment

When the patient initially presented 10 years ago, the edentulous ridges were first treated with conventional implants (📷 1.30). How the implants were placed is not up to my current standard, but being less skilled at that time, I was quite satisfied with how they turned out back then. The implants in the 1st quadrant are more embarrassing, especially with those prostheses. My prosthetic team must have had some issues with the abutment selection for those Dentium implants. Due to the less than ideal implant positions, stock abutments could not be used, so the custom abutments were made. Still, they are poorly designed according to the current concept.

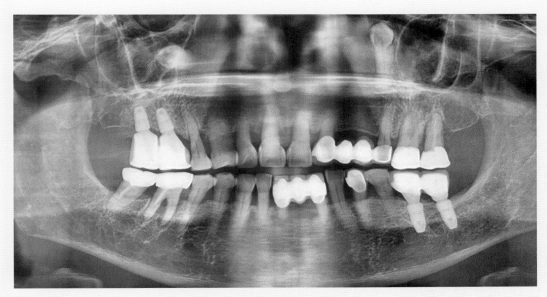

📷 1.31 3 years later, the patient presented with some discomfort from the tooth 46 and the lower anteriors.

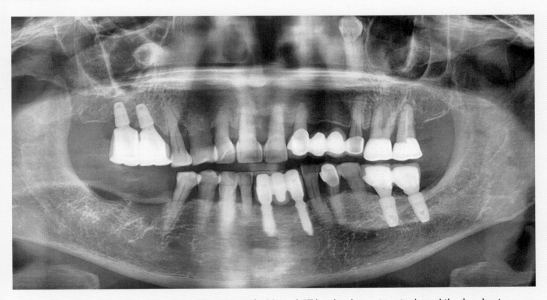

📷 1.32 Despite the periodontal treatment, teeth 46 and 47 had to be extracted, and the implants were placed to replace the mandibular anterioirs.

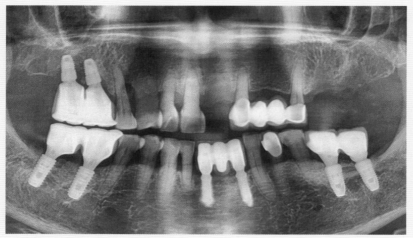

1.33 5 month later, implants were placed to replace teeth 46 and 47. The maxillary left central incisor and the maxillary left molars were also extracted. The mobility of tooth 15 became severe, and some bone loss was noted with the signs of peri-implantitis around the 16 and 17 implants, which reminded me of the significance of abutment shape.

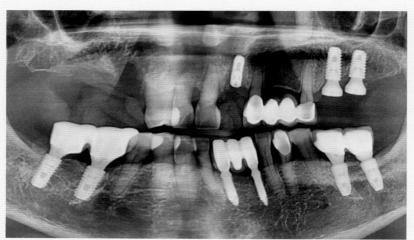

1.34 6 months later the 16 and 17 implants were removed, along with tooth 15. Note that tooth 13 is impacted and unerupted. The 16 and 17 implants were placed thereafter.

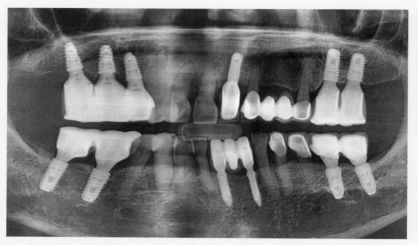

1.35 The implant treatments were completed after 16 months. Because of the long commute, the patient decided to find a dentist close to her home.

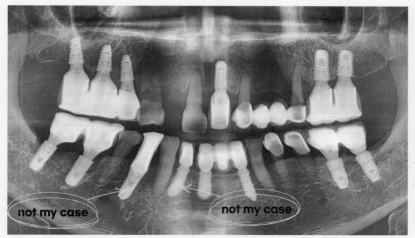

1.36 14 months later, the patient returned with tooth 12 extracted, which she wanted me to replace with an implant. The teeth 42 and 44 were replaced with the implants by her local dentist, but she was not happy with them. Peri-implantitis was noted around the 46 and 47 implants, but there were no reported symptoms. I advised her to postpone further implant treatments for a while.

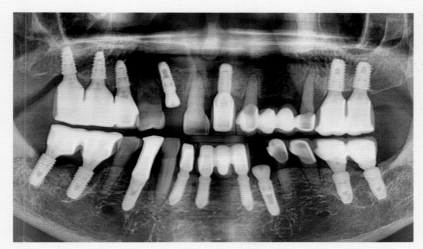

1.37 As the patient was adamant about proceeding with her implant treatments, the 12 implant was placed after 2 months. Tooth 34 also had to be extracted, and it was replaced with an implant 2 months later as in the radiograph. The implants in the 4th quadrant still showed some signs of peri-implantitis with no symptoms.

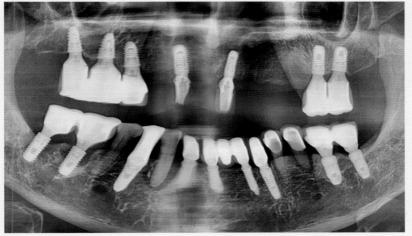

1.38 All the remaining maxillary teeth had to be extracted after 7 months. I was still advising the patient to postpone further implant treatments.

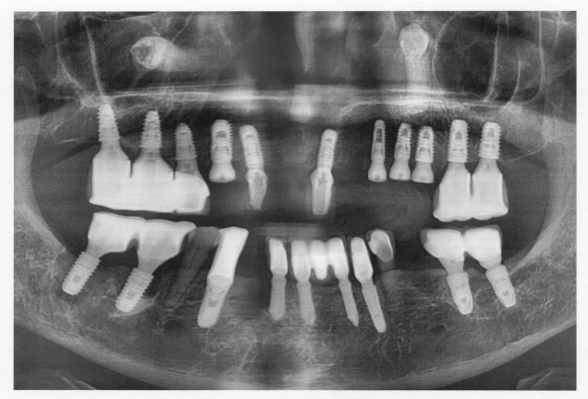

📷 1.39 After 1 month, several implants were placed in the maxilla and two more mandibular teeth had to be extracted. Here, you may be wondering why the three implants on the left side of the maxilla were placed close together. It was inevitable for the prosthetic planning. The 24 and 25 implants had to be joined, and another implant replacing the impacted 23 was needed as an abutment for the anterior implant bridge. In retrospect, those implants could have been spaced out more, but at that time, I was trying to stay away from the 12 socket.

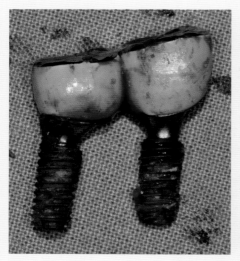

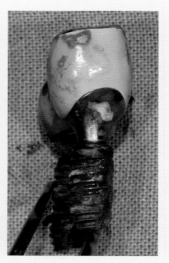

📷 1.40 Excess cement remained on the mesial surface of the implant abutment, which was removed 4 years and 5 months after the crown placement.

In Feb 2020, 2 months after the implants in the 2nd quadrant were placed, the 46 and 47 implants were removed.

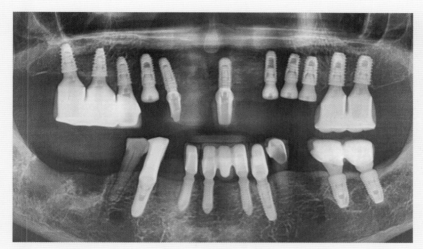

📷 **1.41 Panoramic radiograph taken 2 months after the implant removal (March 2020)**
The patient had no symptoms until the removal surgery.

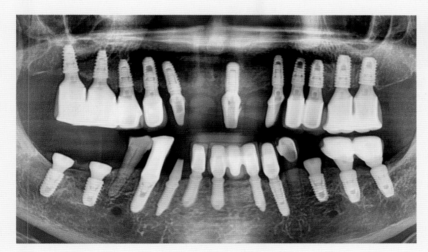

📷 1.42 10 months after the implant removal, the implants were placed to replace all the missing mandibular teeth.

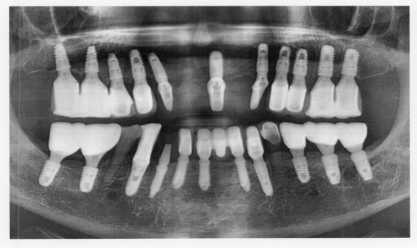

📷 1.43 In March 2021, the crowns were placed for all the implants except for the anteriors, which needed further soft tissue contouring. My prosthetic team asked me why I placed the 23 implant so distally. I explained that the patient's 23 was unerupted due to impaction, so I was trying to place the 24 implant more anterior to make it look like 23.

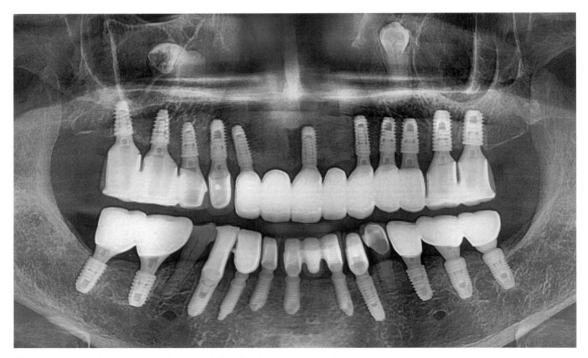

📷 **1.44 May 2021, after the final proethesis placement**
10 years of dental implant treatment has come to an end, but it ain't over until it's over. Implant treatment seems to have no end and is always a process in itself.

For me, this case is like a long movie with endless twists. Who knew that the cements were left on the 46 and 47 implants abutments.

Of course, I do not think that those residual cements were the main cause of the peri-implantitis. The patient was becoming noticeably senile each visit, and her teeth and implants deteriorated suddenly and quickly one after the other, and I did not even try to look for the cause. I was just trying to do my very best as a clinician whenever challenges were encountered. However, those residual cements were indeed humbling, and I will continue to take care of this patient's needs to my best ability.

We tend to associate peri-implantitis with swelling, inflammation, and/or bone loss. However, even without such findings, there are cases where the patient complains about biting pain or pain upon gingival movement around the implant. Of course, such symptoms may eventually lead to the findings of inflammation and/or bone loss. On the other hand, there are many cases where peri-implantitis progresses without any symptoms.

Everyone will agree on the importance of the periodontal maintenance around implants. However, opinions differ as to how. Let's first talk about the proposition that attached gingiva around implants are not critical. Some argue that the lack of attached gingiva does not adversely affect the implant prognosis. However, **it becomes an issue indirectly as brushing around implants with no attached gingiva can be quite uncomfortable, thereby discouraging good oral hygiene.** Therefore, the presence of adequate attached gingiva around implants is very important for continuing periodontal maintenance in my opinion.

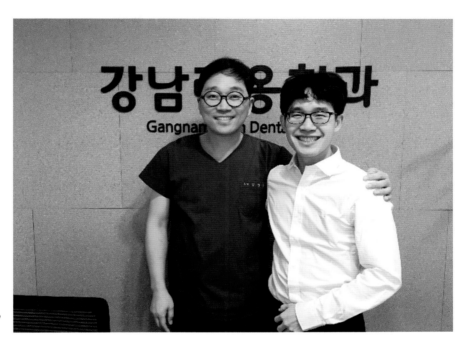

📷 1.45
With my good friend,
Dr. Hyun-Jae Cho

Dr. Hyun-jae Cho, professor of Department of Preventive Dentistry at Seoul National University used to work part-time in my office. Back then, he showed me a case where severe peri-implantitis was treated only with non-surgical periodontal treatments and comprehensive oral hygiene management including interdental toothbrushing (📷 1.46).

As it was such a long time ago, Dr. Cho and I cannot remember the details, but it can be inferred that the bone around the implant was lost due to an acute inflammation, and the bone was regenerated once the inflammation had subsided with improved oral hygiene (likely the bony walls remained intact). In my opinion, it will be difficult to regenerate bone that has been chronically lost over a long period of time only with oral hygiene management. However, in this case, what we need to make a note of is the shape and length of the abutment that extends straight up.

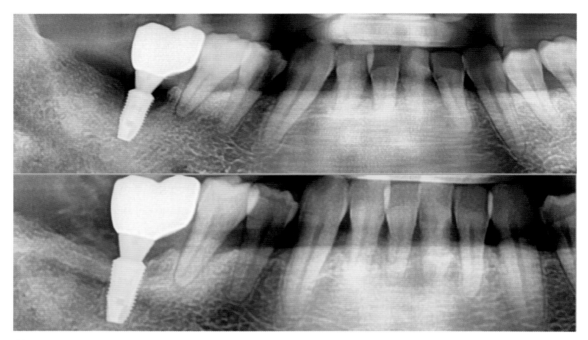

📷 1.46 The case that Dr. Hyun-Jae Cho showed me

It appears that a stock abutment was used, but it extends straight up to more than 4-5 mm before forming the crown, which likely allowed the periodontium to recover and regenerate. Having no micro-gaps and movements between the abutment and the crown might have also contributed. You can again appreciate here what I have been emphasizing repeatedly in this book, the importance of "abutments that extend straight up".

8-2

Fracture of Fixtures and Abutments

Mastering dental implants

Horizontal Fracture of Implant Fixture

Twenty years ago, when I first learned about implants, horizontal fracture of these implants was a common occurrence. However, this seems to have occurred primarily because implants were made mainly of titanium grades 2 and 3, whereas today they are made mostly of grade 4 or above.

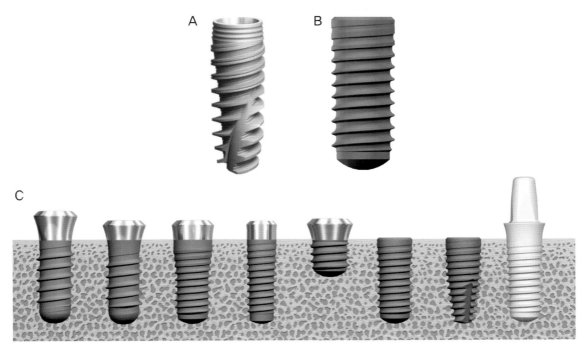

📷 2.1 **A**: Nobel Active Implant, **B**: Straumann BL Implant, **C**: Straumann Product Lineup

A relatively common reported failure is the case of Nobel Biocare's Nobel Active Implant. Horizontal fracture of Straumann implants are rarely reported because most of the threads of the Straumann implants are small (making the basic core of the implant large) and the implant itself is made from strong material known as Roxolid, as described in earlier chapters. Conversely, the primary failure mode for Nobel Active implants is due to a reduction in core size with a corresponding increase in thread size toward the apical end of the implant. In cases where the implant does fail, it is often found that the implant placement direction and height or the shape of the abutment implant crown may be incorrect. Consequently, the implant's crestal bone is absorbed and the apex is subject to frequent horizontal loading and ultimately fractures. When examining the radiographs of a Nobel Active implant, the core often appears thin and brittle. I think Straumann's BLX, which was recently released, also mimics the Nobel Active style and I would like to try it as well, however Nobel is said to be withdrawing from the Korean market. In summary, the most important factor for the success of an implant is the correct orientation and height, as well as proper length and shape of the abutment.

Vertical Fracture of Implant Fixture (Tearing)

The tearing phenomenon (vertical fracture) of the implant fixture is well represented in all implants. As a Korean dentist, I often encounter Osstem TS implant tearing cases. In my view, most of these cases were thought to be **the fault of the operator, not simply the manufacturer's problem.**

Reasons for tearing in implants (Author's opinions)

1. Choosing the wrong size
Osstem recommends a size of 4.5 or more for single premolars. This section refers to the diameter section of Chapter 3-2 Selection of the diameter of the implant.

2. Bone resorption around implant crestal bone
There are various reasons, but in the end, vertical fracture of implant fixture is inevitible if bone loss occurs at the crestal bone of the implant since the implant fixture is not held tightly from the crestal side.

3. Incorrect implant placement
Implant tearing is seen in implants placed in an incorrect direction such that the occlusal force is not distributed and a continuous force is concentrated in a non-concentric direction. This can cause bone loss progression prior to implant tearing, however tearing may also occur prior to bone loss.

4. Wrong implant height

I often observe that a cantilever-type force acts on the margin of the abutment and the fixture even with normal occlusal force because the implant is placed too high. Similarly, it is assumed that this structural error causes bone loss around the implant, resulting in tearing.

5. Improper length and shape of implant abutment

As previously mentioned, bone loss in the cervical region of the implant due to improper length and shape of the implant abutment is thought to be the cause of tearing.

6. If the abutment is not precisely set to the fixture

As emphasized earlier, the abutment must be passively fitted to the fixture. If not, movement of the abutment and fixture caused by a micro-gap will occur, resulting in crestal bone loss. This will weaken the damaged fixture and cause tearing as the surrounding bone disappears.

7. If the implant is placed too hard (strong placement torque)

If the implant is planted with excessively strong torque, the hexa is damaged (residual stress), which causes the damaged hexa to act in combination with the above-mentioned factors, causing vertical fracture.

Looking at these causes, the most important thing is the correct position, direction, and height of the implant, the appropriate length and shape of the abutment, and a passive fit of the abutment on the fixture.

Implant tearing appears in a variety of other companies' products besides Osstem TS. Even in BioHorizon or Zimmer products that make fixtures with alloy, it is clear that the operator is at least 90% at fault, but a manufacturer's defect in the invisible portion cannot be completely ruled out. Such defects may include residual stress or minute cracks in the implant during the manufacturing process.

When it comes to the manufacturer's faults, we cannot leave out Nobel Biocare. In the case of Nobel's trilobe internal fit abutment discussed earlier, many fractures are reported on the thin side of the lobe and thus I suspect that it is rarely used now. In the case of Nobel's flagship product, Nobel Active, even if the implant body is wide, the diameter of the cervical portion is reduced by giving it a back taper rather than making it thicker, such that the collar on the implant crestal side is very thin. In this case, if this product also suffers from the same issues as Osstem, I believe that this product may be subject to more tearing failures than any other product. Even if the manufacturer cannot take into account all the incorrect placement of the clinicians, I think the manufacturers should try to give these issues more consideration.

CASE 1

Let's take a look at one example here.

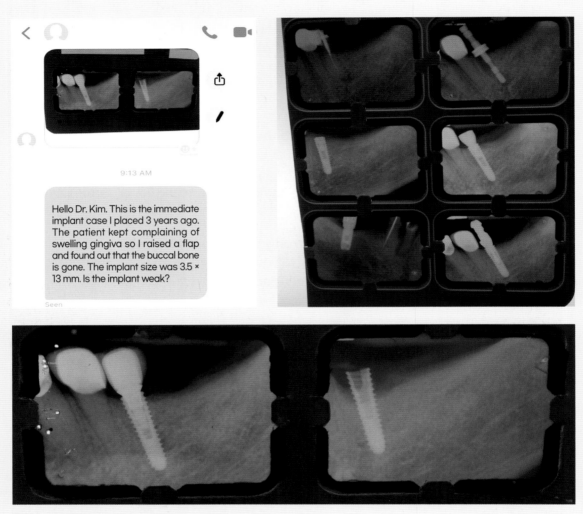

💬 **2.2** Vertical fracture case sent by Dr. Shin in Chicago

Dr. Shin sent me this case (📷 **2.2**) where a 13 mm implant with a diameter of 3.5 in the premolar position of the mandible was placed, but had a tear after 3 years. Just by looking at the size, you can immediately see why it was torn. The implant was also placed too high which resulted in the short length of the abutment. In the end, crestal bone loss and fracturing of fixture were inevitable. There are numerous cases of implant fracture where clinicians blame the manufacturers but their implant placement was not optimal.

CASE 2

My implant tearing case

Here is one of my personal cases of vertical implant fracture. There had not been a fixture tearing case in my office for quite some time, however and it seems that God recently sent me two cases on purpose in order to include in this book. One of these cases belonged to Dr. Pyun Younghoon, a co-author of this book (📷 2.3) and a very talented oral surgeon from whom I have learned a lot. In this case, the 24 implant fractured after just one year. Considering that the abutment shape and the shape of the crown appeared normal, we needed to consider numerous other factors such as whether

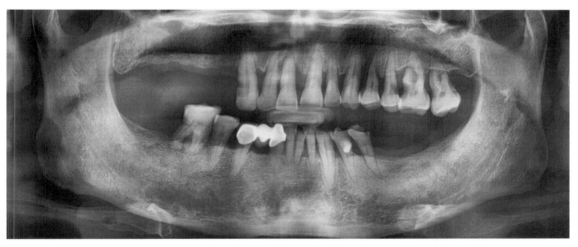

Pre-treatment panoramic radiograph

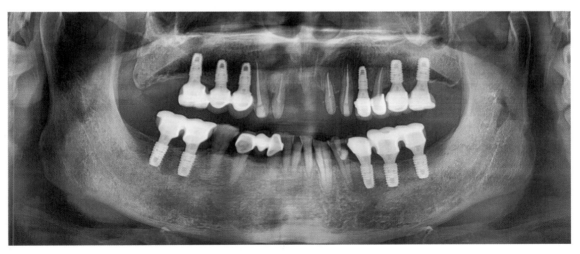

After completion of molar treatment, only anterior treatment is in progress
(2 months after crown placement on implant 24. Crown was delivered 5 months after implant placement)

📷 2.3

the abutment was placed passively and precisely, and whether the failure was caused by impact or excessive occlusal force.

Although just a single premolar, we considered that the primary cause of fracture may be due to the use of a 4.0 diameter implant (although manufacturer's flaws and potential procedural errors by the clinician can not be fully ruled out).

Upon closer examination, it was difficult to pinpoint the exact cause of the implant fracture. Use of excessive torque was also considered but ruled out since initial stability was not achieved based on the doctor's documentation. This case is currently undergoing re-treatment and demonstrates that implant fracturing may occur at any time due to various causes.

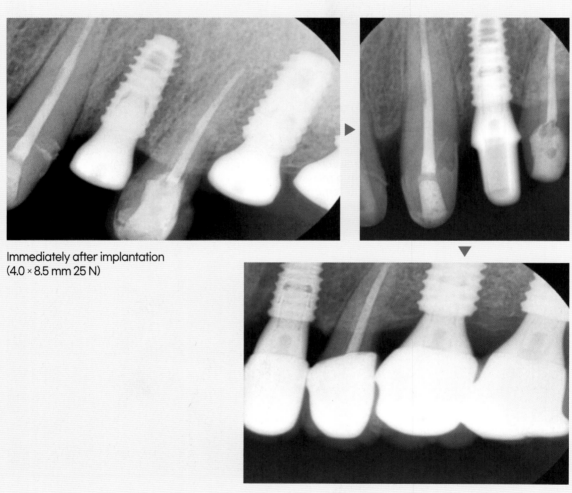

Immediately after implantation
(4.0 × 8.5 mm 25 N)

After 5 months, immediately after setting the abutment and crown

📷 2.4

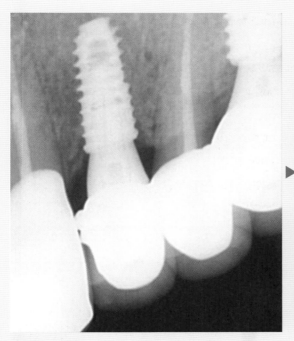

The implant crown became mobile after 12 months

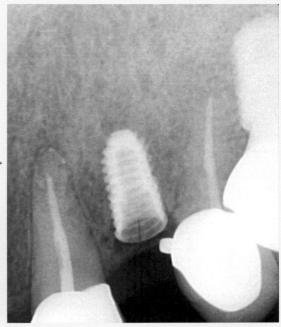

X-ray without the crown
A vertical fracture is evident

Appearance of the removed fixture

Fixture was removed using a removal kit. In the case of the maxilla, the implant can be easily removed with a mount wrench or a fixture removal kit. In the case of the mandible, most cases of fixture removal require adjacent bone removal with a surgical bur or trephine bur.

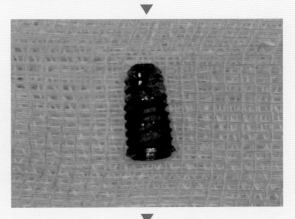

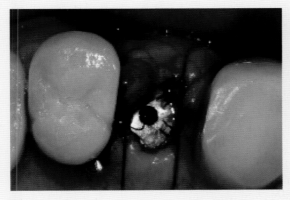

Re-implantation immediately after removal
There was no evidence of bone loss or inflammation, so a new fixture was immediately re-implanted, and treatment is currently ongoing.

📷 2.5 **Conventional treatment course of implant 24**

Now, let's look at another case.

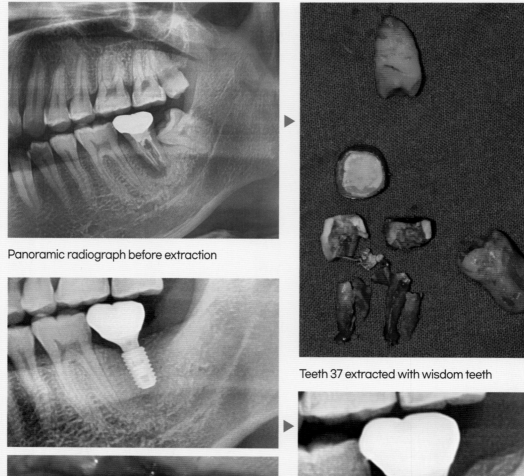

Panoramic radiograph before extraction

Teeth 37 extracted with wisdom teeth

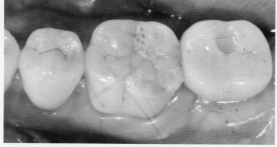

Immediately after setting

📷 2.6

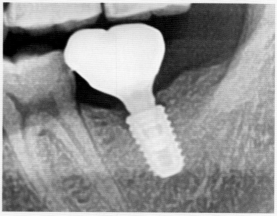

14 months after setting, acute periodontitis around implant is evident. This was not initially diagnosed as a vertical fracture, but rather screw loosening.

Although rare, this is my own case of implant fracture. The wisdom tooth and the second molar were extracted, and implant surgery was performed as usual. Although it seemed as if the implant was placed slightly lingually, it was not considered to be outside the scope of accepted range. Eventually, however, tearing occurred 4 months after implantation (📷 **2.6**).

Since the author delegates the restoration of the implant to the prosthetics department, it is difficult to ascertain if the abutment was set passively (📷 2.7). However, in the photo taken while applying pressure to the crown, it was difficult to see that it was a completely passive fit. However, a tear appeared 4 months later and the patient opted not to see me anymore because he lost trust in my clinical competence. There are a number of considerations as to why the implant may have failed, however it is hypothesized that excessive occlusal force was one of the causes, given that it was incorrectly implanted on the lingual side. This patient was a young man in his 30s whose teeth were severely worn down and his existing anterior prostheses were frequently cracked and fractured. What is clear in this case is that vertical fractures preceded bone loss.

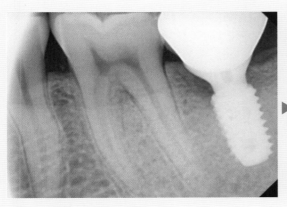

2 weeks after reattachment
There are no special observations.

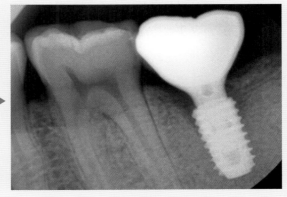

3 months after reattachment. Bone loss is observed.

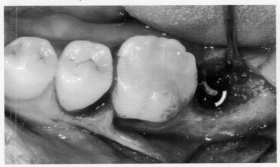

A flap was raised to visualize the fractured fixture.

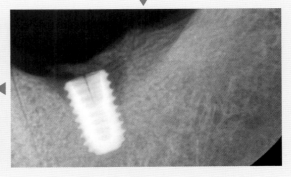

8 months after reattachment. A vertical fracture line and bone loss are clearly visible.

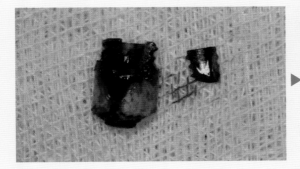

Fractured implant removal

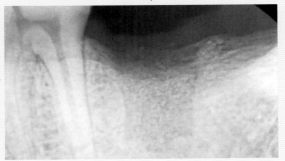

X-ray taken after implant removal and bone graft

📷 2.7

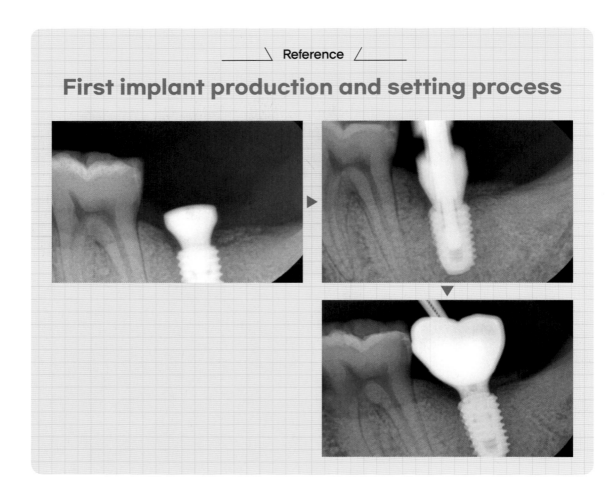

Reference

First implant production and setting process

According to one implant manufacturer, **the fixture does not break even if the fixture is continuously and repeatedly tested for vertical fracture in the laboratory.** It seems that vertical fracture of the fixture by occlusal force is impossible, but some argue that the number of samples for this study was too small. If the number of samples were increased, fracture cases would likely have appeared, and the manufacturer would also be blamed for defective products.

In my opinion, the absence of a passive fit may also be an important cause of implant failure. Since the connection between the abutment and the fixture would have been ideal (solid and passive) in a laboratory setting where this study was conducted, there was no case of fracture. However, in patients, if bone loss occurs at an early stage, vertical fracture is accelerated and inevitable.

As I was about to finish this implant book, three cases of vertical fracture of the implant suddenly occurred in my office, which I will describe below.

CASE 3

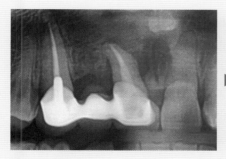

Panoramic photo before extraction & grafting

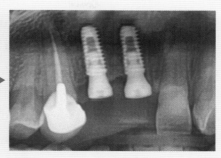

2 months after extraction, new implants were placed.

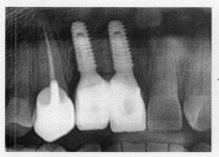

Acute periodontitis 14 months after crowns

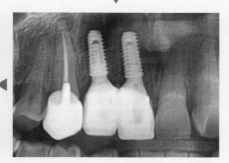

Crowned 3 and a half months after implantation

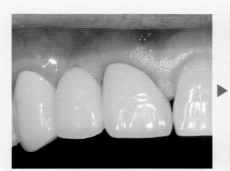

Clinical picture before tooth extraction

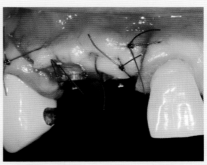

Implant placement 2 months after extraction

Regretfully, I did not pay enough attention to the condition of the gums after implantation. I was living in the US at the time, making it difficult to follow-up. There were many failures: the shape of the teeth, and vertical fracture.

📷 2.8

Clinical picture of gum inflammation 14 months after setting

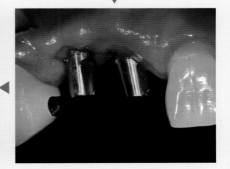

Temporary teeth 3 months after implantation

This is a case in which, while staying in the United Sates, the author returned to Korea for a short while and placed two implants. After implantation, a GP in my office took over from provisional teeth to final setting (📷 2.8). Accurate data for this case are lacking with no detailed medical records or photographic records and the cause of implant fracture is difficult to identify since that GP has left the office. Although I initially thought that the implant was placed deeply enough, considering that the gums are very thin, I now realize that the implants should have been placed 1 mm deeper. When this occurs, I think of implant clinicians who advocate placing implants deeply. Also, I regret that I do not know the details of the prosthetic process. It appeared that the temporary teeth were applying too much pressure on the gingiva between the two implants for too long. The case would have been better managed if gingival remodeling was performed with a temporary crown on a temporary abutment without rushing to the final prosthesis. If the contact was more than 4 mm from the adjacent bone, the papilla would have risen up. As for the factors contributing to the implant failure, firstly, the implant placement was incorrect. Secondly, a bulky crown impinging on the gingiva was also a contributing factor. Thirdly, this 3.5 mm diameter mini implant should not be placed too hard (i.e. with high torque), especially since the abutment wall of the fixture is thin. However, in my opinion, the gingiva-impinging prosthesis seems to be the biggest cause.

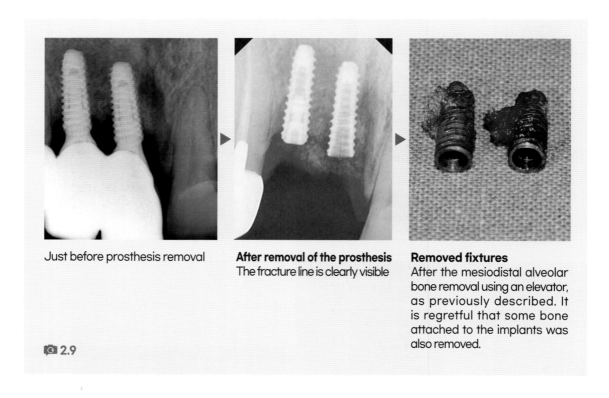

Just before prosthesis removal

After removal of the prosthesis
The fracture line is clearly visible

Removed fixtures
After the mesiodistal alveolar bone removal using an elevator, as previously described. It is regretful that some bone attached to the implants was also removed.

📷 2.9

CASE 4

This is a case where an associate in my office completed treatment 2 years ago. The patient was a 50 year old male patient, and a 4.5×8.5 mm implant fixture was placed at in the 47 site (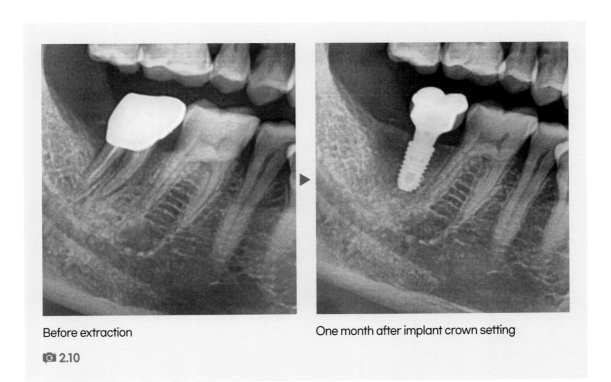 **2.10**). The cause of the vertical fracture of the fixture is only speculated, but in this case, I suspect the fixture size to be the cause. I'm unsure as to why an implant of a 4.5 mm diameter (instead of 5.0 mm) was placed at the rearmost molar location of an adult male.

When this doctor first started placing implants, he placed a long implant resulting in nerve damage, and the direction of the fixture was suboptimal. I therefore shared a lot of my implant philosophy while we worked together. In this situation, there was sufficient space to place a 5.0 mm fixture, thus it is regretful that he used a 4.5 mm diameter implant (although, of course, the exact cause of this fracture cannot be determined conclusively).

Before extraction

One month after implant crown setting

📷 2.10

The implant crown became mobile 2 years later. Even after re-tightening to 35 N, the implant crown became loose again and the diagnosis of a vertical fracture was made. An attempt was made to remove it using a fixture removal kit but was unsuccessful. The implant was then removed using a 5.2 mm trephine drill. A 6.0 mm fixture was immediately re-implanted in place after removal.

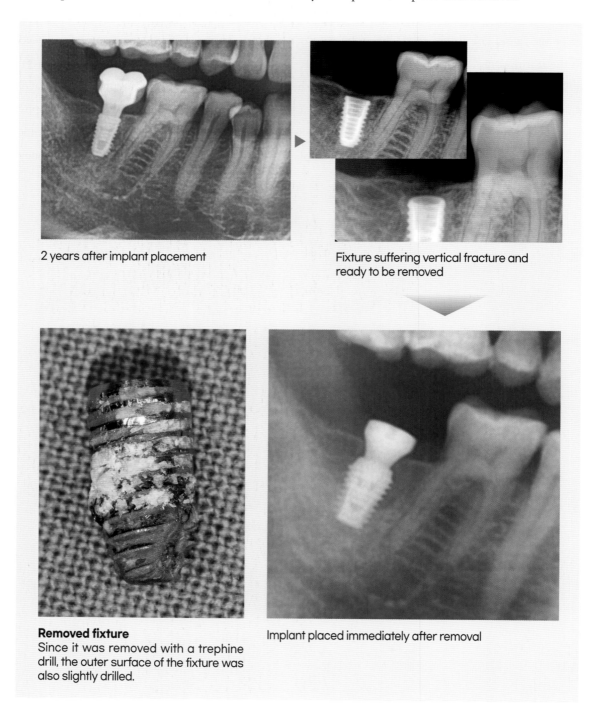

2 years after implant placement

Fixture suffering vertical fracture and ready to be removed

Removed fixture
Since it was removed with a trephine drill, the outer surface of the fixture was also slightly drilled.

Implant placed immediately after removal

📷 2.11

CASE 5

Also in this case, the vertically-fractured implant was not placed by the author. A 57 year old female patient came to the office in 2015 and completed her first implant treatment in 2017. While I was in the United States, the patient returned to the clinic at the end of 2018 and was treated by another colleague in the clinic (📷 2.12). An implant 3.5×10 mm was placed in the canine 13 position. Two years later in April 2021, after the crown was set, the implant was diagnosed with a vertical fracture and was subsequently removed. The patient was very upset with the outcome. In order to avoid a repeat implant fracture, a strong Roxolid Straumann BLT implant was placed instead.

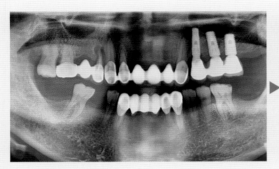 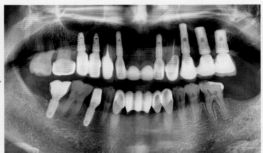

Pre-op panoramic X-ray

Panoramic X-ray after completion of my phase one treatment in 2017.

📷 2.12

There may have been numerous reasons for implant fracture but the biggest cause is most likely the placement of a 3.5 mini implant in the maxillary canine site. Although I placed mini implants in the 12 to 22 region, the patient was not having any problem. This patient is now under the care of my colleague in the same office and we are paying close attention to follow-up care including occlusion adjustment.

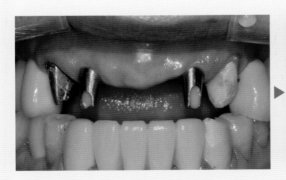 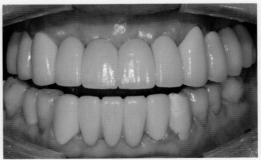

A clinical picture before the implant placement in the maxillary anterior teeth by the author

📷 2.13

Clinical picture immediately after maxillary anterior setting. The maxillary anterior teeth were restored without any gingival remodeling. An unfortunate reality of implants in Korea.

The vertical fracture of implant 13

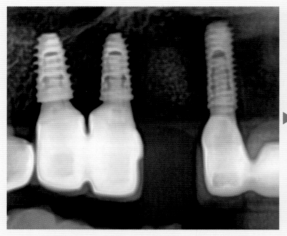

After removal of the maxillary canine (13) by the director of oral surgery department, tooth extraction and preservation were performed.

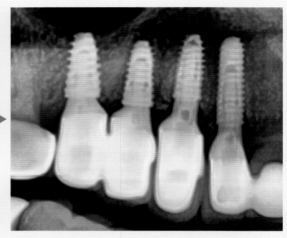

14 weeks after extraction and preservation, the implant was placed and the crown was set in 11 weeks.

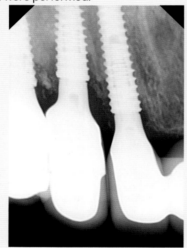

2 years after crown setting

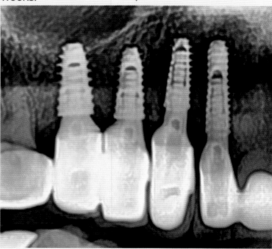

Two years later, the patient returned to the clinic complaining that the implant 13 was mobile

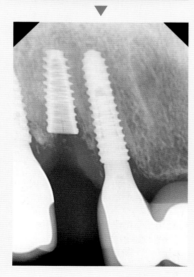

A vertically-fractured fixture can be seen once the abutment was removed

📷 2.14

Disappointing emergency profile of 14 and 15 implant abutments

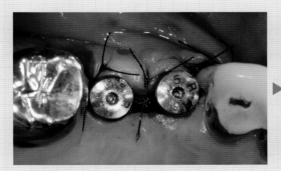 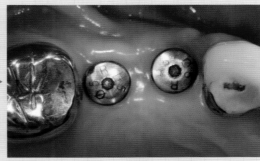

Right after the second surgery

3 weeks after the second surgery

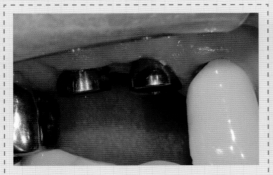

Before setting the crowns for implants 14 and 15
The expected height of the interproximal gingiva between the two implants is about 5 mm. In this photo, only about 2 mm of gingiva was formed. Had we waited longer, more gingival growth would have occurred. Unfortunately with a bulky abutment pressing down on the gingiva, bone loss had occurred between the two implants.

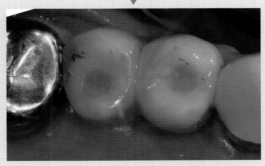

14 and 15 implant secondary surgeries to the final setting Two weeks after the second surgery, the sutures were removed, an impression was taken and the final crowns were seated.

Two weeks after the second surgery, the sutures were removed, an impression was taken and the final crowns were seated. When evaluating the gingiva between the 14 and 15 implants in the clinical photos, one might consider if these implants should have been placed slightly deeper.

However, one should also consider the fact that it takes at least 2.5 months for the thickness of the gingiva to recover between implants with the youngsam flap method. Even if waiting for the complete gingival remodelling is not viable, one should account for the eventual thickness of the gingival fill when creating the emergency profile of final prostheses.

In the more recent photos, bone loss is evident around the 14 and 15 implants. This demonstrates the importance of avoiding excessive pressure on the gingiva (especially between the implants). In **Chapter 7-1**, the topic of abutment length and shape in conjunction with changes in the thickness and shape of the gingiva between the fixture level and the contact point. In order to prevent such fracturing, the author has been placing implants 1 mm deeper.

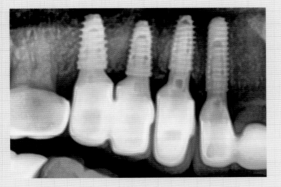

14 weeks after extraction and preservation, the implant was placed and the crowns were set in 11 weeks.

Fracture of the Abutment

Fracture of the abutment is the fracture inside the fixture. Fracture at the crown connection portion outside of the fixture is very rare, although zirconia abutments with titanium bases tend to be an exception. My philosophy is such that I do not recommend the titanium-base (ti-base) and zirconia connection structure not only because of its tendency to fracture but also because the abutment needs to be made thicker. In other words, instead of a thin and straight abutment, there is no choice but to create a fat abutment protruding from the top of the fixture.

Abutment fractures are found in all implant company's products but are most prevalent in the Ankylos implants. Excluding excessive occlusal force, the most likely cause in my opinion is that the abutment is not set precisely. In addition, all issues discussed earlier regarding tearing of the fixture will also affect the fracture of the abutment. It is unlikely that the abutment suddenly snaps and breaks, rather it is more likely that the micro-gap and movement were continuously contributing to the fracture due to fatigue.

CASE 1

This is my second case of abutment fracture (📷 2.15). According to the patient, the author performed the procedure 10 years ago. The shape of the crown was unusual and the implant and abutments were both Dentium products. Since the hexa structure of the internal friction type dentium abutment was introduced to Korea around that time, I had heard that it was structurally a little weak. Therefore, implant hex fractures are very common with this system. I suspect the reason I hadn't had an abutment fracture prior to this case may be attributed to the fact that the implants were placed in the correct position and the prostheses were fabricated by skilled lab technicians. Or maybe, I may simply have been lucky.

The cause of this abutment fracture might have been attributed to the strange shape of the bulky abutment that might have been caught on the mesial bone or gingiva. In addition, the abutment fracture might have been due to the failure to achieve a passive fit within the fixture.

Considering that this patient was a man in his 40s and had been using this implant for well over 10 years and only started to notice the mobility recently, it may be interpreted as a fatigue fracture due to a structural problem of the implant. The crown and the abutment hexa portions were both removed. Since such a case is common with Dentium implants, there is a dedicated removal kit which made removal easy. I followed the instructions of the removal kit but it did not come out because I was being overly careful. Being impatient while watching me struggle, my restorative doctor colleague just pulled it out by force.

If I had to choose between an abutment or fixture fracture, I would always choose an abutment fracture because it is much easier to replace than the fixture itself.

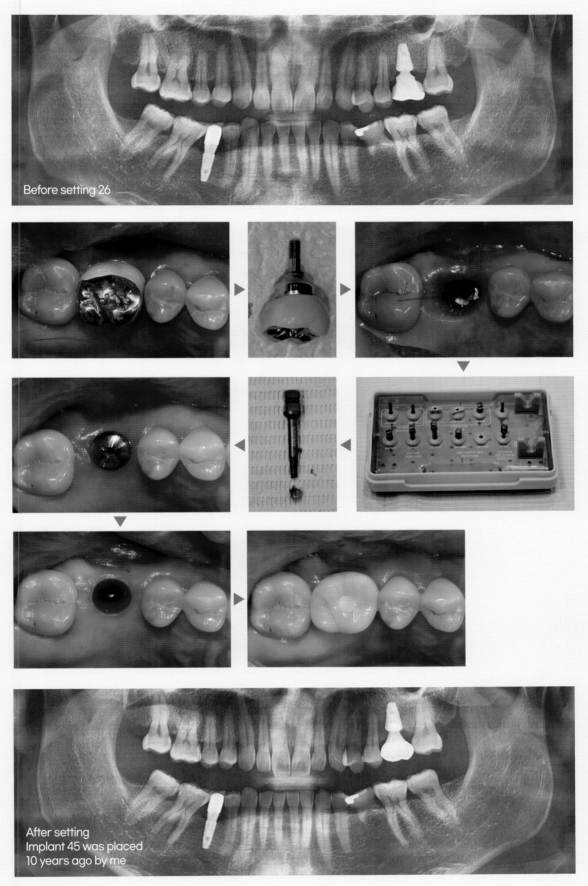

Before setting 26

After setting
Implant 45 was placed
10 years ago by me

📷 2.15

CASE 2

A male patient in his 50s with a large build who completed implant treatment of 26 and 27 in 2011, was admitted to the clinic in 2017 with the chief complaint of mobile implants. Luckily, only the hexa part of the abutment was broken and not the screw. I tried to remove the remaining hexa part, but the 26 abutment fracture fragment could not be removed. Since this was my first broken abutment case, I was unaware that there was a kit dedicated to removing a broken abutment. The fragment inside implant 27 abutment was removed using an ultrasonic scaler and high-speed handpiece. Unfortunately, the fragment inside the implant 26 abutment could not be removed. Eventually, implant 26 was removed and placed again. I wanted to place the implant 26 more mesially but the osteotomy was pushed into the place where the previous implant was removed, and inevitably, the direction of the new implant became similar to the previous one.

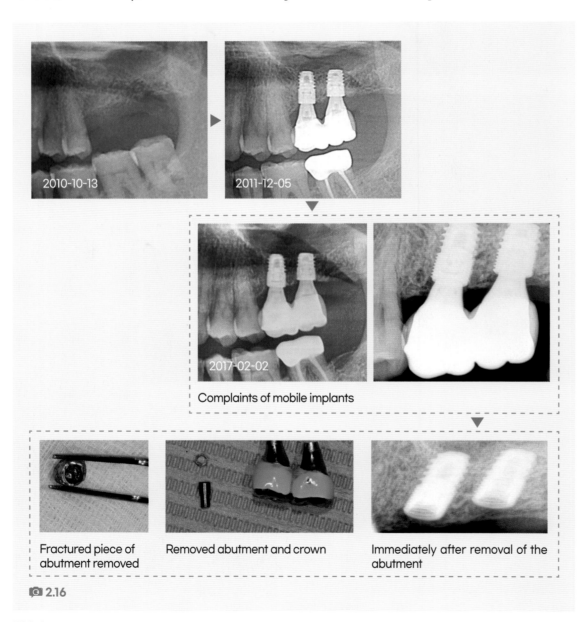

2010-10-13

2011-12-05

2017-02-02

Complaints of mobile implants

Fractured piece of abutment removed

Removed abutment and crown

Immediately after removal of the abutment

📷 2.16

I was puzzled by the cause of the abutment fracture in this patient. It was my first abutment fracture case. Even though the patient had a large build, it was surprising that he managed to fracture two implant crowns that were connected. I was not involved in the prosthetic part of these implants, but I presumed that the abutment was not placed in a passive, precise setting (📷 2.16), so perhaps the patient could not initially feel the movement because the two crowns were connected. In cases where implant crowns are joined, rotation of the abutment is prevented so the patient does not experience any symptoms. In my opinion, it is difficult for two abutments to be fractured at the same time. Most likely, one implant may have fractured early on, but the mobility was not felt until the other one was also fractured. There are numerous possibilities, but in the end, it is author's opinion that precise setting of the crown may have been the likely cause.

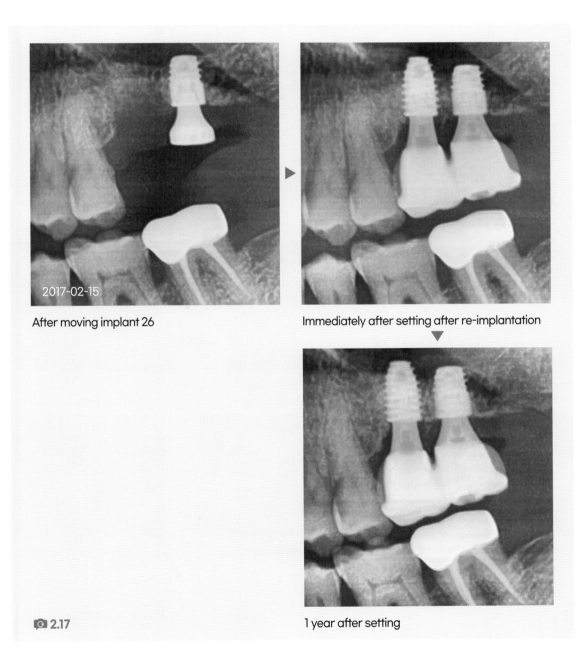

After moving implant 26

Immediately after setting after re-implantation

1 year after setting

📷 2.17

CASE 3

This patient was a male in his mid-40s with a large build. In this case, the abutment of the 36 implant, which I had placed 12 years ago, was fractured and removed. The 37 implant was placed and finished by a student at my live surgery two years ago. If the conditions had allowed, considering that he was a man with a big build, we would have opted to instead re-fabricate two joined crowns for additional support. In this case, I was a little disappointed with the angulation of both implants 36 and 37.

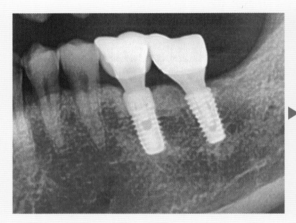

Complaint of mobile implant 36

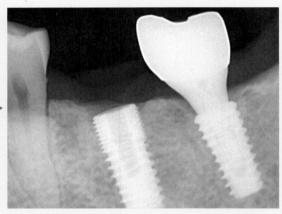

The broken abutment is visible after the implant is removed by loosening the screw.

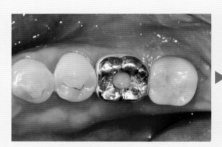

Easy crown removal through SCRP crown screw hole

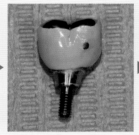

Abutment and crown removed by unscrewing

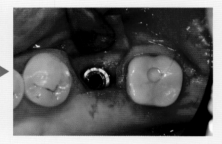

After removal of the crown, a flap was to check the fractured abutment ▼

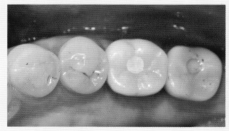

Clinical picture and panoramic radiograph of newly fabricated crown

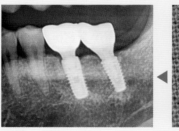

Abutment which fractured at the top level of the fixture was removed. The fragments of the fractured abutment were not easily removable, so the undercut was created inside of the abutment hexa using the high-speed handpiece with a 330 bur to prevent the removal tool from slipping.

📷 2.18

Osstem's KS system

This is the new KS system from Osstem. Although the abutment angle has been increased to 15°, which is clinically convenient for multiple prostheses. However, this is not a big advantage for me since I prefer removing and replanting two implants that are placed with a deviation of more than 30°. Since the abutment angle is increased to 15°, the abutment sync-down (i.e. retightening after it becomes mobile) will occur less frequently, however since I have not had any such cases of sync-down, this is also not a big advantage for me. The reason I'm in favor of this product is due to its strength, as recently, I have also experienced some vertical fractures of the implant fixture. This product is advertised as having a fatigue fracture strength that is 2.4 times stronger than that of the existing TS system, in addition to having increased strength by deepening of the abutment connection.

Further, there are some cases where I hesitate to place 4.0 mm implants (even in the anterior region) due to the thin wall thickness of the fixture, and sometimes there is not adequate bone width to place a diameter of 4.5 mm in the premolar region, so in such cases, I would like to try to use this KS system. Personally, I do not use new implant products that have not been in the market for at least 2 years, and this system has recently reached that threshold.

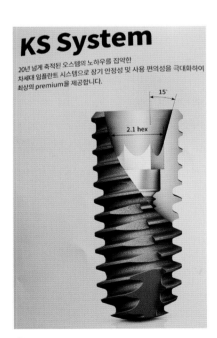

📷 2.19 KS system advertisement that the abutment inner angle is 15°

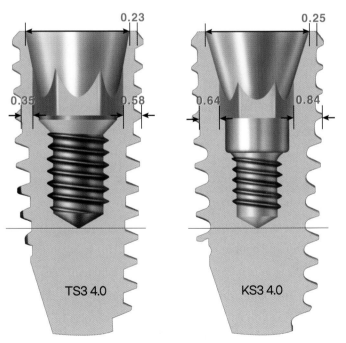

📷 2.20 The comparison of the inner surface of a regular size fixture with a 4.0 mm diameter of TS3 and KS3. It can be seen that the inner wall of the fixture has almost doubled in KS3.

Dentis's SQ New 4.0 regular fixture

The fixture I use most frequently after Osstem is a product called Dentis Implant's OneQ. Although the size is marked as 4.0 mm, the actual size was 4.2 mm. On the other hand, the newly released SQ system is also marked as 4.0 mm, but the diameter is made smaller than the actual size as described above. As a result, the risk of fracture is higher.

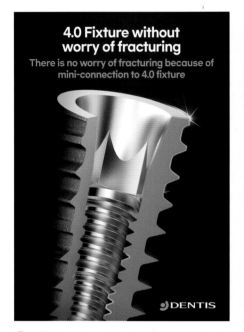 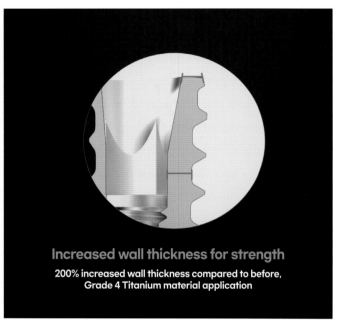

📷 2.21 Dentis Implant's new SQ 4.0 implant advertisement

As a result, Dentis selected a 3.5 mm mini size abutment on a 4.0 mm regular size implant. In an actual 4.0 mm implant, fixture fracture is much more common than abutment fracture. To prevent this, the abutment thickness was reduced and the fixture wall was thickened. Although the company initially expected this implant to be used with existing mini abutment products, a separate product lineup is manufactured dedicated to this 4.0 mm product and that is expected to perform well in the maxillary anterior region due to these advantages.

The primary reason that I want to try this product is that the internal abutment connection angle is 15° (the same as Osstem's KS) and also has the advantage of being compatible with Straumann BL & BLT, the only imported implant I use. At the very least, since even the healing abutment of the Straumann implant is expensive, this product will be cost effective by comparison. Also, I think it will be useful in places where spaces are narrow such as in the maxillary anterior teeth or premolars because it shares several of the same advantages as the Straumann BLT.

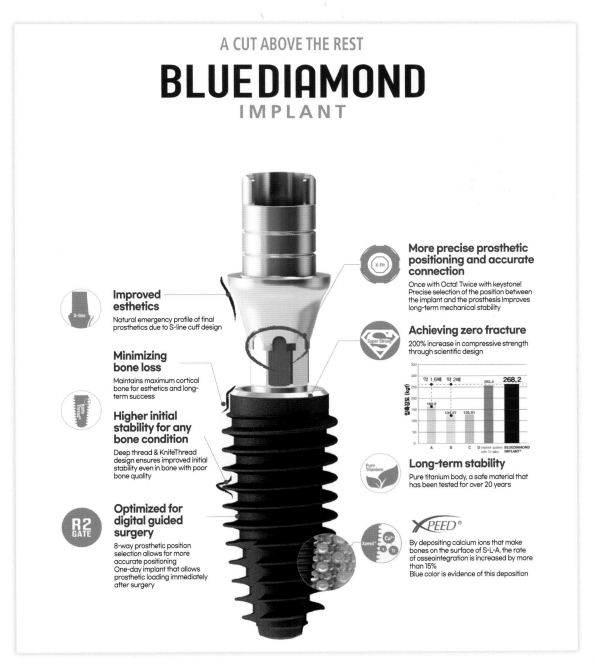

📷 2.22 MegaGen Blue Diamond Implant

Fixture Thread Option for better initial stability

By applying the same core diameter and different thread depth, it ensures better initial stability and facilitates implant placement in any bone density.

Regular thread for hard bones
Bluediamond Implant's KnifeThread Design makes implantation much easier than conventional implants.

Deep Thread for weak bones and poor bone quality
Longer KnifeThread length ensures good initial clamping force

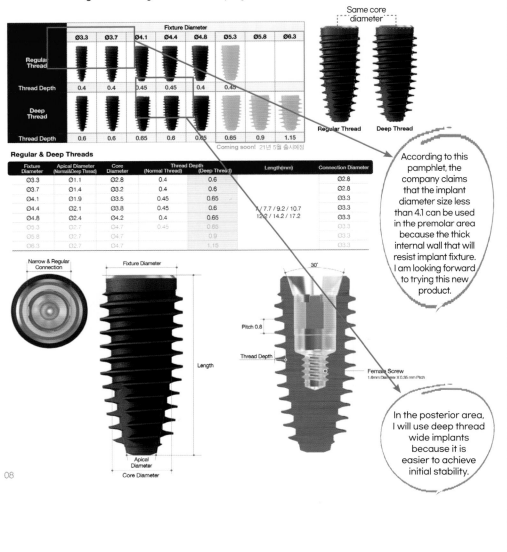

	Fixture Diameter							
	Ø3.3	Ø3.7	Ø4.1	Ø4.4	Ø4.8	Ø5.3	Ø5.8	Ø6.3
Regular Thread								
Thread Depth	0.4	0.4	0.45	0.45	0.4	0.45		
Deep Thread								
Thread Depth	0.6	0.6	0.65	0.6	0.65	0.65	0.9	1.15

Coming soon! 21년 5월 출시예정

Same core diameter

Regular Thread   Deep Thread

Regular & Deep Threads

Fixture Diameter	Apical Diameter (Normal&Deep Thread)	Core Diameter	Thread Depth (Normal Thread)	Thread Depth (Deep Thread)	Length(mm)	Connection Diameter
Ø3.3	Ø1.1	Ø2.8	0.4	0.6		Ø2.8
Ø3.7	Ø1.4	Ø3.2	0.4	0.6		Ø2.8
Ø4.1	Ø1.9	Ø3.5	0.45	0.65		Ø3.3
Ø4.4	Ø2.1	Ø3.8	0.45	0.6	7 / 7.7 / 9.2 / 10.7	Ø3.3
Ø4.8	Ø2.4	Ø4.2	0.4	0.65	12.2 / 14.2 / 17.2	Ø3.3
Ø5.3	Ø2.7	Ø4.7	0.45	0.65		Ø3.3
Ø5.8	Ø2.7	Ø4.7		0.9		Ø3.3
Ø6.3	Ø2.7	Ø4.7		1.15		Ø3.3

Narrow & Regular Connection

Fixture Diameter

30°

According to this pamphlet, the company claims that the implant diameter size less than 4.1 can be used in the premolar area because the thick internal wall that will resist implant fixture. I am looking forward to trying this new product.

Pitch 0.8

Thread Depth

Length

Female Screw
1.6mm Diameter X 0.35 mm Pitch

Apical Diameter

Core Diameter

In the posterior area, I will use deep thread wide implants because it is easier to achieve initial stability.

08

📷 **2.23** MegaGen Blue Diamond Implant

The MegaGen Blue Diamond pamphlet also showcases their EZ Crown which was known to be invented by Professor Heo Joong-bo, a rising star in the field of teaching and research, as well as clinical practice. Although I do not restore my own implants, I have heard a lot of great things about it. Therefore, I would love to try this product after having discussed it with my clinical colleagues.

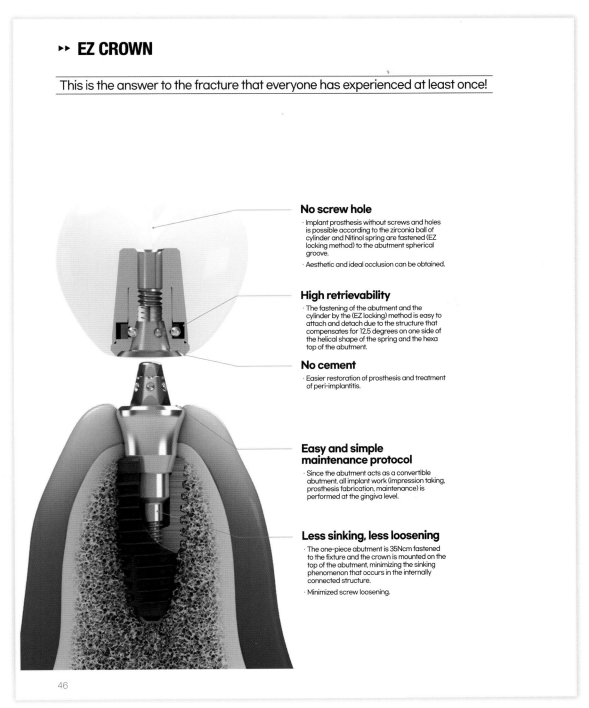

▸▸ EZ CROWN

This is the answer to the fracture that everyone has experienced at least once!

No screw hole
· Implant prosthesis without screws and holes is possible according to the zirconia ball of cylinder and Nitinol spring are fastened (EZ locking method) to the abutment spherical groove.
· Aesthetic and ideal occlusion can be obtained.

High retrievability
· The fastening of the abutment and the cylinder by the (EZ locking) method is easy to attach and detach due to the structure that compensates for 12.5 degrees on one side of the helical shape of the spring and the hexa top of the abutment.

No cement
· Easier restoration of prosthesis and treatment of peri-implantitis.

Easy and simple maintenance protocol
· Since the abutment acts as a convertible abutment, all implant work (impression taking, prosthesis fabrication, maintenance) is performed at the gingiva level.

Less sinking, less loosening
· The one-piece abutment is 35Ncm fastened to the fixture and the crown is mounted on the top of the abutment, minimizing the sinking phenomenon that occurs in the internally connected structure.
· Minimized screw loosening.

46

📷 **2.24** EZ CROWN

Epilogue

The more I do implant treatments, the more inspired I am to continue learning. As I wrote this book, I was able to reflect on my implant work so far, and became excited about my future implant work.

Since I do not restore my own implants, the topics of prosthetics and occlusal issues were not discussed in this book. I feel that if clinicians place implants according to my treatment philosophies, it can become a stress-free and enjoyable treatment experience.

Although not covered here, in the future I would like to continue writing about how to properly place implants in different regions of the mouth, focusing on clinical cases.

Finally, I end this book by saying thank you very much for reading to the end, and I hope that it has been helpful to my readers.

Thank you very much.

With love.